Rationing Is Not a Four-Letter Word

Basic Bioethics

Arthur Caplan, editor

A complete list of the books in the Basic Bioethics series appears at the back of this book.

Rationing Is Not a Four-Letter Word

Setting Limits on Healthcare

Philip M. Rosoff

The MIT Press
Cambridge, Massachusetts
London, England

MIT Press books may be purchased at special quantity discounts for business or sales promotional use. For information, please email special_sales@mitpress.mit.edu.

This book was set in Sabon by the MIT Press. Printed and bound in the United States of America.

Library of Congress Cataloging-in-Publication Data
Rosoff, Philip M.
Rationing is not a four-letter word : setting limits on health care / Philip M. Rosoff.
    pages cm — (Basic bioethics)
Includes bibliographical references and index.
ISBN 978-0-262-02749-6 (hardcover : alk. paper)   1. Health care rationing.   2. Medical economics.   I. Title.
RA410.5.R67 2014
338.4'73621—dc23
2013047166
10 9 8 7 6 5 4 3 2 1

For those whom we serve

Contents

Series Foreword

I am pleased to present the forty-fourth book in the Basic Bioethics series. The series makes innovative works in bioethics available to a broad audience and introduces seminal scholarly manuscripts, state-of-the-art reference works, and textbooks. Topics engaged include the philosophy of medicine, advancing genetics and biotechnology, end-of-life care, health and social policy, and the empirical study of biomedical life. Interdisciplinary work is encouraged.

Arthur Caplan

Basic Bioethics Series Editorial Board
Joseph J. Fins
Rosamond Rhodes
Nadia N. Sawicki
Jan Helge Solbakk

Preface

In late 2006 I began to think seriously about the potential clinical and administrative challenges for my hospital should the predictions about an impending influenza pandemic turn out to be accurate. This brought me front and center up against the many problems associated with scarce-resource rationing. I was then fortunate to be asked to serve on a multi disciplinary statewide task force on pandemic flu convened by the North Carolina Institute of Medicine, an organization created and funded by the state legislature to investigate and issue reports on a wide assortment of health-related topics of concern to the people of the state. These reports could contain a range of policy, regulatory, and statutory recommendations to the legislature and governor. This group brought me into contact with a large number of professionals (and only a couple of ethicists) from a wide variety of professions and areas of expertise, and truly expanded my intellectual and social horizons. Ensconced in both the academy and clinic as I am, I had never before had the opportunity to meet and interact with representatives of professions as diverse as the nuclear energy and power industry, emergency services (including state and local law enforcement), banking, and county public health officials, to name but a few. It was a significant eye-opener and demonstrated the broad array of stakeholders with their parochial interests that wanted to have a seat at the table in any discussion and debate on what should happen. All had their unique viewpoints about how rationing could affect their constituencies. We were fortunate that reasonable discussion and compromise were made the order of the day and we were able to agree on almost all topics, even the especially difficult ones that could potentially involve significant sacrifices for some. Everyone knew the stakes involved and that "grown-up" behavior was expected, that decisions and concrete recommendations were called for, and that all could not get everything they may have wanted.

The report was issued in the spring of 2007 and was comprehensive but contained significant gaps, especially in the area of clinical decision making. The latter task was remanded to the ethics committee of the North Carolina Medical Society by the state health director under the aegis of the governor's office. Our mandate was to develop a detailed algorithm for the rationing of intensive-care resources that could be coordinated throughout the state. In essence, we were asked to create a standard of care in which rationing would be explicit as the norm for medical decision making and the allocation of critical resources. Not surprisingly, this was a major clinical and ethical challenge, but after much discussion and gnashing of teeth a document describing our recommendations was crafted and sent to the governor. There it sat unpublicized and even unopened as far as I know. Perhaps this was not unexpected considering the contents, which included very specific flowcharts on how to allocate scarce beds and ventilators. The document also provided other guidelines on removing patients from life support if they did not improve in a specified amount of time, so as to free machines and supplies for what was anticipated to be an overwhelming number of desperately ill patients. This last part, along with the list of preexisting conditions that would preclude access to ICU care (like advanced cancer, severe dementia, New York Heart Association Class 4 heart disease, etc.), was the most controversial and potentially inflammatory. But the predicted severe pandemic never occurred and so our need to use this plan was unmet. But my interest in rationing was piqued.

This experience made me acutely aware of what could happen with necessary draconian rationing with finite supplies of a given resource, something that occurs every day with organ transplants and potentially with shortages of drugs. But what is most fascinating about these real-life examples, and what could have been the case with pandemic influenza (hopefully we will never know, although pandemics do occur every thirty to forty years or so), is that the fractious, libertarian-inclining, fiercely independent American public accepts what has to be done as a matter of course, even when the consequences of not receiving a medical resource can be death. And, as the North Carolina Institute of Medicine Task Force showed, a group of forty or so individuals with widely disparate backgrounds, interests, constituencies, and goals could come together to discuss what needed to be done and reach a consensus without rancor. Why should the rationing of dollars and the healthcare they can buy be all that different?

Few would disagree with the conclusion that the healthcare system in the United States is a mess. Even with the phasing in of the provisions and benefits of the Affordable Care Act, many millions will still lack health insurance (although the number should be significantly decreased from the unconscionable level it is today), and chances are slim that it will contribute substantively to stabilizing or even lowering the incredible amount per capita that we spend on healthcare. With the looming retirement and aging of the baby boomers leading to a massive influx of Medicare recipients, all demanding what they feel is their rightful benefit, it is probable that unless something drastic is done to rein in healthcare costs, these costs will continue to spiral out of control. Of course that means that this part of our GDP will drain resources from other needs that are also demanding to be met such as education, infrastructure, and the like. The only recourse is rationing in some form. We must limit what is available or what can be had.

But the very word *rationing* evokes fear and engenders visions of "death panels," or the dreaded socialized medicine with big-government bureaucrats rather than doctors and their patients making medical decisions. Or people think about long lines and waiting months to get a hip replaced or a coronary bypass operation as they envision to be the case in Canada and England (it is closer to the truth in the latter country). But that is wrong. It is certainly correct to state that under some conditions of rationing—which I describe in detail in chapter 2 of this book—there is no question that the decisions about the allocation of finitely scarce medical resources are the consensus outcome of committees consisting of both healthcare professionals and laypeople, and that people can wait a long time for a kidney or a heart transplant and most never receive one. But that is only one side of the rationing coin. I argue that in a liberal, wealthy, and culturally diverse democracy like the United States, rationing can only be done in a manner that is both generous and fair so that virtually no one would have to do without what they need and that the availability of healthcare interventions would be both abundant and more easily accessible than it can ever be today. Hence, rationing does not have to be a four-letter word; indeed, rationing is what people would sensibly and rationally choose.

This book would not have been possible but for the help and generosity of a number of people. I would first like to thank Tony Hope of Oxford University, who, during many fruitful discussions while were both resident fellows at the Brocher Foundation in Hermance, Switzerland, encouraged me to embark on a book-writing venture; Alex Rosenberg of Duke's Philosophy Department, for his constant encouragement; Kevin Sowers, who, first as the chief executive officer and now as president of Duke University Hospital, has supported my career both financially and with enthusiasm for what I have tried to do; Peter Ubel and Gopal Sreenivasan, for extremely useful critiques of my ideas; Elizabeth Delong from Duke's Department of Biostatics and Bioinformatics, for her suggestions about continuous variables; Mark Leary of Duke's Department of Psychology and Brain Sciences, for directing me to the studies on "scarcity effects"; and my many colleagues on the Duke University Hospital Ethics Committee, who have been exceedingly gracious and understanding as I have tried out some of my arguments in this book. I also owe a large debt of gratitude to the anonymous reviewers for the MIT Press, whose criticisms and suggestions have improved and honed my thinking about these issues and led to a significantly improved final product. I had the good fortune to have Elizabeth Judd assigned to me as my copy editor. There is no question that the book has benefited immeasurably by her relentless (but always thoughtful, magnanimous, and helpful) cuts and suggestions. My acknowledgments would not be complete without recognizing the contribution of my dog, Sara, whose many long walks with me gave me numerous quiet hours during which most of the ideas discussed in this book were both born and nurtured. Finally, I would like to thank my wife, Dona Chikaraishi, whose patience and encouragement have enabled me to finish this work.

1

The "Evil" of Healthcare Rationing

Some Introductory Examples

Healthcare in the United States accounts for an enormous percentage of gross domestic product (GDP), more so than any other industrialized nation and hence, any other country on earth. Although the United States spends far more per capita on healthcare than anyplace else, its indicators of population health do not reflect this investment (Stabile et al. 2013). This expenditure has been steadily growing for decades, even though the rate of increase has slowed, probably due in part to economic problems (Hartman et al. 2013). As a 2011 report by the Congressional Budget Office predicted, "Total spending on health care would rise from 16 percent of gross domestic product in 2007 to 25 percent in 2025, 37 percent in 2050, and 49 percent in 2082."[1] Moreover, with the expected ballooning of the Medicare-eligible population owing to the retirement of the baby boomers, many are forecasting that healthcare spending could crowd out funding for almost any other kind of federal and state spending and most certainly contribute to the deficit. Assuming we do not wish to continue to spend ever-increasing amounts of our national income on healthcare with so little to show for the investment (on average), something must be done to not only control the rate of growth, but also to possibly reduce the level to a more reasonable amount. At the same time, most Americans (not all, to be sure) believe that quality healthcare should be available to all (or at least citizens and permanent residents) in some basic fashion (Grande, Gollust, and Asch 2011). How can the dual goals of universalizing access to good medical care and keeping it affordable by both individuals and the country be accomplished? Is it a sisyphean task or merely a herculean one?

In late June 2013 there were 75,945 people actively listed for solid-organ transplants in the United States. Many thousands more were deemed ineligible for a variety of reasons, both medical and "psychosocial." The latter encompasses an assortment of reasons, but the lack of sufficient funds to pay for the transplant and its aftermath, including the extremely expensive lifelong antirejection medications, is a major factor (Dew et al. 2007; Dobbels et al. 2009; Flamme, Terry, and Helft 2008; Giacomini, Cook, Streiner, and Anand 2001; Kemmer, Alsina, and Neff 2011; Levenson and Olbrisch 1993; Masterton 2000). Through the first three months of 2013, there were 6,891 transplants (the most recent updated information available).[2] The numbers are clear: most people who could be saved by a transplant won't be, and a significant number, perhaps the majority, will die waiting. It seems as if the decision about who will receive one and who won't—who will live and who will die—is almost a matter of chance, of pure luck. A number of these patients are cared for at my institution. Astonishingly, with so much tragic death and suffering happening as a matter of course, no one seems to be complaining (other than the transplant doctors and nurses bemoaning the fact that there is an insufficient supply of organs). There are no irate letters to the newspapers berating doctors and UNOS (the United Network for Organ Sharing, the organization responsible for creating and setting the nationwide rules for organ donation and allocation) about why their father/mother/sister/son/daughter died waiting for a liver, while the father/mother/sister/son/daughter down the hall received one and could celebrate the holidays at home, *alive*.[3] There are no bloviating, blustering congressmen on Fox TV shouting about "death panels" and how un-American it all is, even though the allocation of solid organs for transplant is an example of unadulterated healthcare-resource rationing that is centrally controlled. Moreover, the people who don't receive an organ—perhaps with the exception of those on dialysis awaiting a kidney—die. Why isn't there a fuss? That is one of the questions this book addresses.

Perhaps the story of a patient might help illustrate this better, using the words of a daughter whose father died without receiving a transplant:

My dad wanted to be an advocate for organ and tissue donation after he received his heart transplant. His unfulfilled wish is what compels me to share our story—he died waiting for a second chance at life. I remember my dad, Denny Hile, as a warm, loving man who was the foundation of our family. He was one of the most positive people I knew, and was dedicated to our family. He listened, really listened when I needed him, gave great advice and was a source of strength for me. He taught me "Never say you can't until you try" and I live by this each and every day of my life. . . . When he was just 52, my dad was diagnosed with congestive heart failure/arrhythmia. I was only a teenager when doctors told us that he was "a walking time bomb" and required an immediate bypass surgery in

November 1986. Fortunately, the surgery was a success and he lived a relatively normal life for just under seven years. In 1994 my father's heart started failing again and another triple bypass wasn't enough to fix it. By August 1995 he was listed for a heart transplant as his health continued to decline. He had numerous hospital visits, was drained of energy, forced to retire and got to the point where daily activities became too much for him and he was confined to his recliner. My dad remained optimistic, in spite of growing weaker. He made plans for "when" he got his heart transplant, never "if," and looked forward to enjoying his retirement years with my mom, Margaret, and advocating for donation by sharing his story and encouraging others to register as donors. He was the model patient, doing everything doctors asked of him, and had no ailments beyond heart failure. We all remained hopeful that after a heart transplant his health would be restored and he could live his life again. After 16 months waiting for a heart, my father got "the call" on December 31, 1996 ... [but the] ... doctors learned the heart was not viable for transplant. We remained hopeful that another heart would come along but a few months later, my father's health caught up with him. He collapsed and never returned home from the hospital. My dad was only 62 when he died on May 1, 1997, and he had a lot to live for. He missed weddings, graduations and spending time with his growing family. He has seven grandchildren and four great-grandchildren, many of whom he never knew—including my youngest son.[4]

Mr. Hile died waiting for a transplant, like so many thousands of other patients each year. But other than advocating for more donations, his grieving daughter was not angry at the system that relegated organs to others and not to her father. One problem was that there are far too few organs for those who could benefit from transplantation, but it was also the allocation system—the rationing method—that let him die and another live. Why was this not a death panel, or a threat to the American way of life? Why was Mr. Hile's family not permitted to raise money and "buy" an organ on the open marketplace? Why is this system viewed as fair—tragic, perhaps, but fair—when the very mention of general healthcare rationing seems anathema?

Consider another case. At any given time more than 100 drugs are in critically short supply in the United States. This is an ongoing crisis that does not seem amenable to a quick or simple solution in a complex market where production and demand are susceptible to government regulation and the freedom of manufacturers to respond to profit and loss irrespective of the effect of these considerations on vitally important goods is relatively unimpeded. Some of these medications are so arcane I suspect most readers will never have heard of them (unless you were prescribed one and it wasn't available), but many others are commonly used and have been available for years—medications such as diazepam (also sold as Valium®), doxorubicin (a chemotherapy drug used in a wide variety of cancers from Hodgkin's disease to breast cancer), and azithromycin, an antibiotic.[5] Most drugs that are scarce are administered intravenously (also known as sterile injectables; pills are rarely affected). Many patients needing these drugs can be switched to an adequate alternative, but sometimes there are none, and they may suffer the consequences of not receiving an effective—possibly life-saving—treatment. This is especially true for anticancer drugs. Just as with organ transplantation, where the supply does not equal the demand, doctors must make decisions about which patients receive a scarce drug and which do not. This is rationing, pure and simple. There is a lot of anger about the failure of the prescription drug market and other economic concerns, but no one seems to be screaming about the tragedy of rationing and the threat this poses to our freedom.

Other kinds of rationing or scarce-resource allocation decisions by the government abound. For instance, each year Congress debates how much money should be allotted to the Department of Defense. A budget is approved by Congress and signed into law by the president. It is broken down into money for hardware, salaries for uniformed military personnel and civilian contractors, general support needs, and other items. But there is a cap, and if the armed forces want or need more money sometime during the fiscal year (say, for events like an unanticipated war such as the NATO-led air war in Libya in 2011), generally they have to request an additional allocation and Congress has to approve it. Otherwise, the Pentagon has to shift money around from one internal budget to another in order to supply the funds to pay for their new needs without exceeding the limits set by the overall budget. And aside from the usual arguments about how much to spend on defense versus other budgetary priorities, everyone agrees that there has to be a ceiling on how much is voted for this part of the overall federal budget.[6] There is also an "internal" budget in that the generals and admirals and their civilian masters decide how to divide the total amount and determine which items should take precedence over others. Both the portion of the federal budget devoted to defense and the prioritization within the department as to various needs are examples of rationing, rather lavish rationing to be sure, but rationing nonetheless. But, except for the usual fights about *how much to spend*, there is little squabbling about the fact that there is a maximum amount. This is not to say that the Defense Department might not wish for more money each budget year, but they get what they get.

It is often argued that healthcare budgets and expenditures must expand to meet the needs of an aging population, and the efficacy (and hence expense) of medicine is mostly fueled by the ever-increasing ability of expensive technologies to extend life (Callahan 2009). But the same is true of military technologies. The Pentagon brass and their friends and supporters in the defense industries are constantly demanding the latest gizmo and device that will expand high-tech warfare. Despite the ever-present cost overruns, military hardware inflation and the oft-cited $1,000 toilet seat or $500 hammer, there is an absolute amount that we spend each year on this part of the total budget. Even though there is intense lobbying for one thing over another, at some point choices are made, priorities are set, and a budget is passed. Decision making within financial limits is the essence of rationing. But somehow healthcare seems different and operates as if there is no upper limit, even in the federally supported programs such as Medicare. There is no preset cap on Medicare costs; it is whatever gets spent.[7]

But why do we accept restrictions in the military budget, often the part of the federal budget that generates the most intense public and private argument, but can't even seem to discuss the topic for healthcare? One could argue that the value of effective healthcare to people is considerably greater than the things the defense budget pays for. On the other hand, one could also make a reasonable case that possessing the means to defend one's home (country) in a dangerous world filled with people and organizations that dislike us and have made efforts to harm us, is also essential, and one would not want to scrimp on funding. But we also set limits on funding for education, scientific research (much of which has contributed to the expensive technologies that constitute a major portion of the increasingly large healthcare budget), and many other areas of what we consider important—even vital—domains of federal and state spending. Many people would argue that devoting more money to National Institutes of Health (NIH)–sponsored research would be a good thing; we could fund more research proposals from investigators, knowledge would be produced, and new discoveries and treatments might be the result. But we consciously say no to an ever-escalating NIH budget and tell scientists, "This is what you get, do the best you can with it; good luck and don't ask us for any more."

Why is healthcare so special? Many would suggest that it isn't, at least in comparison to other important areas of societal life that can be supported by government funding. However, I am not alone in suggesting that highly effective healthcare—which is what we have available in wealthy and technologically sophisticated countries—can contribute in a major way to improving people's lives. This occurs both in a primary way by relieving suffering, but also from what good or better health can enable people to accomplish (the opportunities it offers people to attempt and achieve). Daniels has argued that there is a unique moral dimension to sickness and health due to the way they can reduce our well-being and our ability to formulate and achieve our life goals (Daniels 2000, 2008; Daniels and Sabin 2008). The increasingly effective medical interventions thus offer a unique potential to interrupt what might be called the natural history or trajectory of disease. This is true, but healthcare is only one of many significant sectors that compete for the public dollar, all of which can lay claim to substantive priorities for our attention. And while healthcare can be substantively important to human welfare, so can good education, which often goes wanting in vying for a piece of the budgetary pie. Indeed, Daniels and others suggest that one of the best arguments against unbridled or limitless healthcare spending (and thus the need for rationing) is the funding competition for more or less equally valid and essential components of our social lives. So these are the facts: an ever-increasing and somewhat open-ended healthcare budget, highly variable distribution of healthcare resources and access in the population, and other budgetary needs claiming our attention and money, all contributing to the necessity of admitting that we can't buy everything for everybody that modern medicine might conceivably offer. The solution is rationing or setting limits on what and when healthcare should be available.

The "Problem" with Rationing

In a 1995 paper titled "Straight Talk about Rationing," Arthur Caplan asked, "Can Americans talk publicly and reasonably about how to ration?" (Caplan 1995). It is the lack of reasonable public discourse on this subject that has led to our present situation, where healthcare rationing has been demonized to the point that even raising the word *rationing* in polite conversation is worse than cursing in public. The term turns people off. It raises their hackles. It makes them angry. And what follows is anything but a sensible and level-headed discussion.[8] Many of my colleagues have suggested that I should go to great lengths to avoid using the "R word" in this book. Some have proposed that it would be wise to change the title to avoid turning potential readers off right from the start. They have recommended that I instead employ euphemisms such as "scarce resource allocation" or "supply prioritization," anything to avoid using the odious *rationing*. But throwing caution to the wind, I will stick with rationing. And that is because I don't think it is necessarily so bad; it all depends on what it means. My goal in this book is to rid rationing of its demons.

What exactly do we mean when we speak of rationing? The *Oxford English Dictionary* gives several definitions, including "allocation of a fixed allowance of a specified type of food, clothing, fuel, etc., to each civilian during time . . . of shortage," and "restriction of the supply of any commodity or service as an economic policy."[9] In essence rationing implies that there is a limited supply of some good that people value (which could be almost anything), that there is a demand for that good exceeding the amount available, and that decisions must be made about how to distribute the good among those who want to possess it. To a certain extent, the operation of normal markets is a relatively unregulated form of rationing, in which the price of something is the rationing point and the amount and to whom a specific commodity (for example) is distributed is governed by supply and demand. In the kind of rationing I refer to in the healthcare arena, it can take the form of poorly regulated, uncoordinated rationing (which is what we have now), where millions of small and sometimes large allocation and prioritization decisions are constantly being made on how to allot existing resources. Alternatively, there could be centralized, controlled, or managed forms of rationing in which the rules of distribution are fair, equitable, and open to scrutiny and debate, and I provide examples of these later. It also doesn't necessarily matter what is in limited supply, be it food after a drought or a flood, or money to buy things that actually could be plentiful (or seemingly inexhaustible).

What are people scared of when they think about rationing? No doubt some believe (or remember) stories they have heard about America in World War II and the scarcities of meat and eggs, along with the allotment of ration coupon books that limited the amount of these items one could purchase. It is thus possible that they are concerned that they won't get enough of what they want (irrespective of whether they could obtain it without rationing) and that someone else will make the decisions about what they can have and how much of it. While it is doubtful that anyone starved or even went hungry because of this forced privation, they did go completely without some things (i.e., new cars) and had less of what they might have wanted of others (Bentley 1998). But it wasn't that bad and it was for a good cause (winning the war). People got used to it (Wansink 2002), and it certainly wasn't nearly as draconian as rationing in England, where many people lost significant weight due to a drastically reduced caloric intake (Zweiniger-Bargielowska 2000, chap. 1, 31–44). So rationing can be unpleasant—at least until one gets used to it—but it doesn't have to kill anyone who wasn't going to die anyway. Indeed, even during the depths of the war, Americans did not go hungry and many actually thrived. Moreover, most people embraced it as their patriotic duty to help win the war. So what is the problem, especially for a very rich country like the United States? Well, our fears may be far worse than reality.

The goal of this book is to examine and, I hope, dispel the commonly accepted public trope of healthcare rationing as evil, corrosive, and erosive to individual and collective liberty, not to mention dangerous (think of the label "death panels"). I base my argument on the following premises. First, healthcare costs in the United States are spiraling out of control, with annual percentage increases often well above inflation (even though the rate of growth has slowed in the past few years). These costs are unsustainable for the country and some mechanism must be found to rein them in. Moreover, it has been amply demonstrated that we don't get much value for our money: we spend more per person than any other developed nation, but our overall health outcomes are near the bottom for many indicators of population well-being. This is what might be termed the "economic premise" of this book.

Second, we have an unconscionable number of people who are either uninsured or underinsured and whose access to healthcare is tenuous at best. Even when the Affordable Care Act is fully implemented, many millions with no health insurance will remain—to be sure, some by choice, but mostly because they fall through the cracks or loopholes in the law.[10] Many millions more elderly poor will also remain whose only income is Social Security, and whose only healthcare coverage is via Medicare. It is indefensible for a wealthy country like the United States to have such callous disregard for the welfare of its people. I will call this the "moral premise."

While the first premise is a given with which few disagree, I suspect there are many people who would question the second premise, contending that in a free society, there is no "right" to healthcare or to the means to obtain it. I will not argue this point, except to state that it is not unreasonable to propose that in a country that grants its senior citizens the "right" not to live in abject poverty or completely without medical care, or extends a social safety net (however filled with holes or meager it may be) to its poorest and most vulnerable citizens, similar societal concerns can be broadened to include all who may fall sick (which is everyone). So I will go out on a limb to suggest that, at least theoretically, a significant number of Americans would not object to the proposition that decent healthcare is, if not a "right," something that it is not crazy to think should be available to us all. If this is plausible, then ethical rationing is the only option available to both control costs and give everyone access to healthcare. And to do it well, it must be centralized and unified and must be carried out fairly, equitably, and in a manner consistent with our values. In this book I show that we already do this in acceptable ways for resources much more scarce than money, and in so doing, I try to dispel some of the animosity that the thought of healthcare rationing inspires.

Bioethicists, health policy analysts, politicians, economists, and many others have been talking about healthcare rationing for years. Indeed, ever since it became apparent that a byproduct of effective medical care was an ever-burgeoning budget for more and more expensive technologies, it became "obvious" to most astute observers that healthcare expenditure inflation had the potential to be limitless, fueled by new research discoveries, patient demands for curative therapies, and the enormous profits to be had from exploiting a marketplace with customers who seemed to have a bottomless pocketbook.[11]

A continuing source of frustration to policymakers, bioethicists, pundits, and others who think, write, talk, and often bloviate about healthcare rationing is the seeming inability of "the public" to understand their clear-headed, logical, and (they think) simple and straightforward arguments for setting reasonable limits on what we spend on healthcare, and hence rationing. "Why don't they get it?" they bemoan with annoyance. Well, aside from the fact that many people have difficulty comprehending arguments about many different topics, especially ones as complex as healthcare, this one also is laced with emotional overlay. After all, we are talking about human pain and suffering from illness and restricting what we will make available to relieve it. Naturally, people get passionate and scared about this, and this clouds their ability to reason, especially when academics or thinktank pundits try to convince them that saying no really won't be so bad (except sometimes when it will), and that they will still be able to get what they need (except when they won't), and that they should be able to get what they want (except when they won't). Moreover, this subject is immensely complicated and we will need lots of time to discuss it, so it's best left to the experts. This doesn't sound like an easy sell, it hasn't been and it won't be.

Moreover, we Americans have a pervasive dedication to individualistic self-determination and a corresponding apparent loathing of government intrusion and control of many, if not all, aspects of our lives. This makes policy discussions of a communitarian society-wide healthcare system that limits some types of personally specified medical desires and needs off limits. Almost two centuries ago de Tocqueville noted this "go it alone and control my own destiny streak" as characteristic of Americans, and it is still with us (de Tocqueville 2004). Of course, people in the United States have a dualistic and contradictory relationship with government intrusion in their lives: while loudly lambasting any notion of increased state or federal sway over them, at the same time they protest any attempt to decrease government programs from which they personally benefit (e.g., "Don't touch my Medicare").[12] But within this oxymoronic and Manichaean approach to government, may lie the seeds to a strategy to think about rationing healthcare: maybe it just needs a better sales job. One way to think about this might be to consider already-existing healthcare delivery systems *in this country* that openly employ rationing techniques and are in general accepted by almost everyone, especially those most directly affected by them.

To repeat, there seems to be general agreement or convergence on at least two truisms describing the discussion/debate on healthcare rationing:

• We must ration or financial chaos will ensue.

• The American people will never accept rationing for a variety of intrinsic (e.g., rugged American libertarian individualism) and/or extrinsic reasons (e.g., Americans are easily swayed by entrenched interests who have too much to lose with any reasonable rationing scheme: doctors, hospitals, insurance companies, and so on: think of the "Harry and Louise" commercials that helped scuttle the ill-fated Clinton healthcare reform proposal).[13]

These narratives have come to simplistically represent and dominate the debate about how (or whether) we will move to formal rationing. But they ignore an important fact: we already engage in rationing and it is accepted, even praised, by many. I am not speaking of the informal rationing that goes on around us, little noticed by the public (except perhaps by its victims), which is accomplished by insurance companies, including government ones like Medicare.

Perhaps a different approach to discussing this sensitive topic may have a better chance of convincing at least a few more people. One of the things I examine in this book is how we already do open and honest and publicly acceptable medical rationing in actual life-threatening situations, and the results have been accepted by most as fair and reasonable. The best example may be the organ transplant system. Even though patients who don't get these resources frequently (if not always) go on to die, they are not left lonely and bereft of everything, because they still receive compassion and palliative care. If we can figure out a system to allocate such important, but severely limited, items like livers, hearts, and kidneys in a way that is both just and accepted as such, surely we can apply similar approaches to healthcare limitations in a wider arena, where virtually everyone should be able to get what they need.

Of course, some might say I am engaging in exactly the same sort of unsuccessful (and therefore pointless) kind of argument I just analyzed as having been tried and failed. And, to a certain extent, that is true. Except that here I am simply pointing out what we already do, how we do it, how we decided how to do it, and most significantly, the details of why it has been tolerated and even accepted as honest and legitimate. I am not partaking in a facile "bait-and-switch" approach, but taking one that is both simple and straightforward. My hope is that the realization that planned rationing systems already exist among us that work well will lead to a gradual understanding that the next step is not too scary to take. Many reasoned arguments have been raised to support why we should ration healthcare. I will not add to those, almost all of which have been met with implacable—often vociferous—opposition from a variety of groups. No, I will argue from a position that we already do planned rationing and it is not only accepted but admired. I will join this claim with another in which I will suggest that any consensus position to ration equitably (i.e., fairly) will have to coalesce around a decision that a resulting healthcare system would necessarily have to be generous and comprehensive to beget acceptance by a broad-based and skeptical public.

What Is Healthcare Rationing?

It is very curious that so many people regard the concept of healthcare rationing with such disdain and even fear. In other domains we have viewed it much differently. Soldiers eat their MRE rations, and the World War II "Greatest Generation" tell tales of butter, sugar, and gasoline rationing in which the entire country shared the pain together, enhancing citizen solidarity in the face of the enemy. Of course there was grumbling and complaining, and regret that circumstances compelled such shortages, but on the whole, the state of affairs was accepted. And there are many other examples in which decisions have been made to limit either access or amounts (or both) of resources or commodities, some of which we find inconvenient and irksome, but all of which we tolerate. When it comes to healthcare rationing, on the other hand, illogical, even irrational, apprehensiveness, worries, and fears take over. It is only then that the alarm and dread of "death panels" grip us.[14]

What is rationing? What do we really mean when we use this word, especially in healthcare? While the term is conceptually vague, it generally refers to states of affairs in which decisions are made to limit access of a specific patient or group of patients to a healthcare intervention—be it diagnostic or therapeutic—that has the potential to benefit that patient or patients.[15] This could include substitution of one form of treatment for another, or the wholesale removal of some treatments or diagnostic tests after a determination that the one eliminated is on average just as effective as the other, except that it is more expensive. Other types of treatments could be done away with altogether if the benefit they bestow is only marginally greater than that with which they compete. It is also possible that it may not better at all. In addition, some types of treatment or testing may have secondary effects (not necessarily toxic side effects) that diminish their overall effectiveness and evaluation as worthwhile. For instance, if a diagnostic test detects some false positives as well as "real" positives,[16] leading to further testing (such as biopsies and the risks of surgery and anesthesia, or more x-rays and hence radiation exposure, both of which lead to more expense and patient anxiety), it may not be judged worthwhile for the few actual diagnoses it leads to in a given population of patients.[17]

There are obviously some major challenges associated with this approach. The big one is how decisions about benefit are to be made. One might view this in a number of ways by asking certain probing questions, such as "How small a benefit for a person or group of people is too small to support?," and "Will a gross, population-based scheme be able to distinguish the subtle, potentially important differences between individual members of a given population that could make the difference of receiving benefit or not?," or "How many people will be affected?" These are important questions and any decent rationing plan that aims for both inclusiveness and fairness must consider them and provide some acceptable answers.

A popular way of calculating benefit (especially among healthcare economists) is cost-effectiveness analysis (Levin and McEwan 2001; Ubel 2001). But this approach has its attendant issues, not the least of which is the way it puts a definitive price tag on medical interventions and judges their worthiness on how much "bang for the buck" can be demonstrated. Many people find this distasteful, especially the part of the system that uses the much maligned "QALY," or "quality-adjusted life year," which aims to calculate what effect a given treatment has on an individual's quality of life and for how long. If you think that defining "benefit" is difficult, trying to figure out the quality of a life is even more so. One person's acceptable quality of life is another person's worst nightmare. Should both views count equally? Or should only one, based on some arbitrary scale of majority rules or norms, especially if one view is much more expensive than the other? It really boils down to a clash of values: different people placing greater or lesser importance on different things. As with many disputes about values that individuals hold dear, people tend to be resolute and immune to logical argument from the other side. You can see how complicated and morally and socially challenging this can get. But I will describe situations in which these types of disagreements seem to matter not so much, where rankings of what's important are open to scrutiny and comment by all, and the people directly affected by life-or-death decisions abide by them as fair and honest. And amazingly, this state of affairs exists in the United States for cases of explicit healthcare rationing.

Any kind of rationing system, short of one in which everyone can have whatever they want, means having to say no to someone or some group of people, even if they continue to want it by insisting that it will help them. This fact implies that some claims of entitlement to certain treatments (even assuming they might be effective for some small number of persons) must be declared illegitimate because they cannot be justified by any appeal to medical efficacy, cost efficiency, and so on.[18] For instance, by deciding to offer kidney dialysis to virtually everyone who could possibly benefit from it (defining benefit as a minimal physiological term, meaning someone who has complete kidney failure and whose blood chemistry values improve after the procedure) and having the Federal government pay for it, we are now blessed (or burdened) with a program that is ballooning in total cost to an estimated $23 billion per year.[19] If we limited the availability of dialysis to those who could more reasonably benefit from it, such as those who do not have metastatic cancer, progressive dementia, irreversible heart failure, or other conditions that rule them out as kidney transplant candidates,[20] what would that look like? Would those denied dialysis be truly worse off than they would be with it? Of course, they would be dead, but sometimes that may not be worse than a miserable life filled with unremitting suffering, considering that a leading cause of death for people on chronic hemodialysis is *voluntary cessation* of the treatment because they can't bear that kind of life anymore (Murray et al. 2009).

We could also look at this differently. Let us say we had 50 percent fewer dialysis machines (by choice or for some other reason) and we had to think very carefully about who among the population of patients with end-stage kidney failure should be permitted to use these now much more valuable and scarce machines. What information would we use to inform our decisions? How would we allocate (i.e., ration) these life-saving devices? Would we be saying to those denied access that their demands were not valid or important enough to be met, given the severe constraints on resources, hence implying that someone else's claims were more significant? I suspect we would be able to come to a consensus decision that some people could benefit more than others from this life-saving, and very expensive, technology. How different would this scenario be from one in which we said that dialysis would only be available to people with some reasonably good cognitive function and without other fatal diseases—that is, patients who might otherwise be eligible for a kidney transplant?[21]

Another example might be observed with certain chemotherapy drugs that are extremely expensive, that do not cure cancer, but that do extend life for some months on average. Others may not extend life at all, but do slow the growth of cancer for a few months, except that it then returns explosively, leading to death very rapidly.[22] Either way, is this "benefit" cost-effective (you could also ask the same question independent of whether we were trying to slow down the growth of healthcare costs)? At least some patients who get the drug might agree that it's worth the cost, but others might not. And the latter number might increase if we could assure people that the money being saved by not using this drug was going to be spent on another, perhaps more worthwhile cause. But some patients might still insist that they receive a benefit and that their insurance company or Medicare should pay for the treatment. The point is that what we call beneficial is complex and may be difficult to agree on when we think that resources (including money) are unlimited. We have a totally different mindset when we know that the resources are limited.[23]

We Already Ration

I am not going to be making a case for the need to formally and coherently and ethically ration *general* healthcare in this country. Others have done so in books almost too numerous to count.[24] Most of the arguments point to the fact that the ever-increasing costs of relatively unregulated and seemingly limitless, profit- and market-oriented healthcare in the United States are spiraling out of control, with no end in sight. Without some effort to put a stop to the escalation in the amount of our GDP that is devoted to healthcare, we may go bankrupt, or at least shortchange many of the other things we think are important and worth spending money on. The last point—to me—is the most persuasive argument for rationing. As most eloquently stated by Norman Daniels, effective healthcare is but one of many important things available among the universe of things we can buy with our economic output, either personally or governmentally, but most particularly as a society (Daniels 2008; Daniels and Sabin 2008). No doubt healthcare is one of the most important priorities, especially in the last fifty years as medicine has become ever more powerful in making people healthier. However, there are still other things we want or need to pay for. These include national security, roads and bridges, national parks, education, research, and so forth. All of these compete with each other for their share of the budget dollar. Without being too simplistic, how much we have to spend and where we spend it is a complex formula that plays out each year at the state and federal level in legislatures and Congress. If there weren't all these other important "goods" that we value in our society, we could potentially spend all we have on healthcare. But obviously, we do value other things, and that's where the problem lies: we have to put a cap on how much we spend on health and determine what percentage of our national budget should be devoted to this sector of the economy. Unless it is to be virtually infinite, the only plausible response is rationing, or placing limits on what we can offer people within the budget we have set. At least some of the objections to rationing are based on the idea that it would lead to a radical change in the way we get medical care in this country. While it's undoubtedly true that ethically justifiable rationing would lead to thoroughgoing changes to U.S. healthcare, a substantial part of the opposition is based on the misapprehension that rationing is something new, something vaguely foreign and un-American. And many people think we don't ration now. Nothing could be further from the truth.

Currently, we ration mostly by happenstance, not by design, although there are well-known examples of overt rationing that are accepted, even embraced, by most patients, healthcare administrators, and doctors (well, maybe not so much by doctors: see below). It would be reasonable to say that two main forms of rationing exist today in the United States: informal and formal. The first is pervasive and quotidian, but most people (and I suspect their healthcare providers) are unaware of it by the name *rationing*. Access to both basic and advanced healthcare is limited in a variety of different settings. For many people the rules of the marketplace (in a somewhat distorted and skewed manner) govern what they can get: we see this in the variety of differently priced health insurance plans with an enormous diversity of available options for a range of prices. For those who obtain their health insurance via their job, the choices are restricted in innumerable ways, from the few (or no) options of available plans from which to choose, to the list of medicines they can buy (via their inclusion or exclusion on the plan's drug formulary), to the restrictions on specialist referrals and even which primary-care doctors or hospitals they can use. While this is not often called rationing, it most certainly is.

In addition, enormous numbers of people are completely excluded from the insured healthcare system by not having any insurance at all, either because they are unemployed, underemployed, self-employed, or work for a business that does not offer insurance. Some minority of these people could potentially afford to purchase policies for themselves and their families but have chosen to play a sort of sickness "lottery," opting to spend what money they have elsewhere. However, most of the uninsured simply fall in the gap between the very poor, many of whom have access to Medicaid, and those at the other end of the spectrum, who have some form of employer-provided health insurance. Thus, almost everyone, except perhaps the wealthiest segment of the population, is constrained in their choices at least at the basic, entry level, and therefore faces rationing.

One can label this "system" by any name one wants (I have called it "informal"), but make no mistake: it is a form of de facto rationing in which what kind and how much healthcare one can get are determined by how much money one has. Even many of those who are insured are limited in some way in their choices. As I have suggested, insurance companies or collective formularies restrict what drugs are available, or policies may control which doctors one can see, or what kind of hoops one has to go through to get a specialty referral or expensive radiology studies (such as magnetic resonance imaging or MRI). All of this "fine print" limits choices from the universe of what could be available and potentially beneficial and hence constitutes rationing, although most people don't call it that.

Unfortunately, the many books and policy white papers declaring the necessity of healthcare rationing have been unsuccessful in convincing those who need to be convinced. They argue not only about the impending financial doom we face if we fail to rein in healthcare costs, but also that we waste enormous amounts of money on healthcare administration and overhead and on paying for treatments only marginally beneficial if at all. They also point out that we already engage in the informal rationing I have just described (Ubcl 2001). All to no avail. Those that need to be convinced are still scared or obstinately opposed. It seems as if we may have to wait for change until the entire system collapses or goes bankrupt.

One should not get the impression that this country does not have any experience with planned or "formal" rationing of healthcare in general.

Indeed, a noble experiment was undertaken by the state of Oregon in the 1980s. In an attempt to control its burgeoning Medicaid budget, the state elected to see if public health goals could be achieved by limiting the kinds and amounts of healthcare it offered, in essence delivering as much health benefit as possible for the money it believed it could devote to this effort.[25] There were a number of high-level and community discussions held to decide what services would be included. An initial effort to employ strict cost-effectiveness analysis was a notable failure when surgery for acute appendicitis (a potentially life-saving operation) somehow came out lower on the scale than treatment for temporomandibular joint (TMJ) pain (Ubel 2001, chap. 1). In addition, there was an interesting experience when certain types of extremely expensive procedures were not included on the list due to their limited efficacy and their very high cost, such as bone marrow transplantation for leukemia. When the mother of a young boy with relapsed acute leukemia was denied payment for this treatment, she and her son went on television and appealed to the public for help. Not surprisingly, there was an immediate outcry and bone marrow transplantation (and other types of transplants) were then included (Hadorn 1991; Lindsay 2009; Oberlander, Marmor, and Jacobs 2001). While this could be viewed as caving to public pressure, there were other issues at stake, as I will discuss further in chapters 2–4. It should also be noted that the Oregon plan applied exclusively to poor people who received Medicaid, and most, if not all, of the ultimate decision makers of what would and would not be covered were not affected by the decisions made, except by virtue of being taxpayers. (Of course, one could also imagine that this would expose them to a potential conflict of interest since a significant portion of Medicaid funding is supplied by the individual states and thus by the taxpayers. One aspect of fairness I will examine in chapter 2 is the principle that rule makers should be bound by the rules they make.) Nevertheless, Oregonians, especially Medicaid recipients directly affected by the rationing plan, generally felt that it was fair and accepted it without too much complaint. One could argue that these people had little choice, but it is also true that many of them were much better off with the rationing plan than they had been before, because the plan actually enhanced the availability of healthcare both in the number of people it covered and the breadth of services offered. It is unlikely that this would hold if analogous rationing were implemented for people who already had good insurance, since they would undoubtedly experience a contraction of choices rather than an expansion, and they might be less than pleased with the change. However, if the funding were reasonably generous, this outcome could be avoided.

But there is another excellent example of now three decades' worth of national, universal, federally mandated, explicit (i.e., formal) rationing (of course not named as such) that while irksome to hospital administrators and some doctors, was accepted with nary a whimper or declaration of a mysterious plot on behalf of some murky "other" to steal away Americans' hard-earned right to have freedom in their healthcare. Of course I speak of that well-known (at least well-known to people like me and others who spend a lot of time in hospitals) system called "diagnosis-related groups" or "DRGs" (Iglehart 1982). Launched in the early 1980s by none other than Ronald Reagan, this was an attempt by Medicare, based on a feasibility project undertaken earlier in New Jersey, to control what were then quaintly thought to be health costs spiraling wildly out of control (little did they know). It basically dictated from on high what would be paid for a given hospitalization for a given medical problem. If a hospital could do it for less, they got to keep the difference; if not, they ate the cost. Because of the buying power of Medicare, private insurers (and of course Medicaid) quickly embraced the same approach, which was soon universally adopted. Amazingly, it was accepted and (sort of) worked. Indeed, it has proven so popular that the model has moved abroad and been introduced into many European countries in one form or another.

Why has this system, which has the explicit goal of reducing costs by restricting the amount of healthcare to patients *ex ante*, been accepted so readily? Some have argued that it is an example of so-called invisible rationing, meaning that it is hidden from the ordinary view of patients (but certainly not hospitals and doctors). The only effect patients notice is that new mothers get discharged from the hospital within a day or so of giving birth, and if one has an uncomplicated heart attack, one doesn't get to stay in much longer than that.[26] It is difficult to imagine that after thirty years, DRGs are all that much of a secret, but that is beside the point. The important thing is that this system was imposed by fiat and universally, lots and lots of people knew about it and knew what its purpose was, and, most crucially, they knew that it was rationing under the guise of cost containment. But it has been accepted without much fuss. One wonders why. One other significant thing to note about DRGs: they apply to everyone. Unless you can pay your hospital bill yourself and are a patient in a hospital with so many extra beds and nurses that they don't care how long you stay, you obey the rules (barring complications). Rich or poor, whatever your ethnic group, when it's time to go home, you go home; it's a great leveler.

There are several other situations in which unavoidable and formal rationing occurs and with which we have a lot of experience. The two best known are in solid-organ transplantation and battlefield triage. In the first, no matter what we do, we have been unable to increase the supply of livers, hearts, and kidneys to keep up with an inexorable demand, despite the fact that we expend enormous effort to convince the public to "give the gift of life." Even when we know that the "value" of donated organs has increased over the last twenty years as our ability to prevent graft rejection has improved, we cannot keep up with the growing need. Indeed, the truth is that even if everyone who could were willing to be a donor, there still would not be enough organs to meet our requirements (that is why there has been such an intense research interest in developing artificial organs). In response to this situation, we have developed relatively straightforward algorithms to allocate organs, generally following the principle of sickest first, with certain caveats including the ability to "take care" of the organ the best (there are variations on this theme depending on which organ we are talking about). Surprisingly, this system is generally viewed as fair, with relatively little controversy, except for the occasional kerfuffle when a prisoner or undocumented immigrant is being considered for a transplant (I discuss this subject more fully in chapters 3 and 6). Even more remarkable is that there is little objection to the fact that this system is about as stark an example of healthcare rationing as one could possibly find, and one in which the "losers" really lose: they die.

The second system, battlefield or emergency triage, is also an example of rationing in action and under pressure and without choice: too many sick people need care in a short period of time and there are not enough doctors, nurses, or operating rooms to take care of everyone all at once, when they really need care. There are variations on this theme such as sickest first, or those most likely to survive first (who may or may not be the sickest) but, as with organ transplantation, this rationing approach (and it is most certainly rationing, in that it is a decision on how to allocate limited resources) is an accepted (perhaps regrettably, but accepted nonetheless) component of standard medical care.

There are also instances of proposed rationing of projected shortages, such as vaccines and ventilators during the feared influenza pandemic of 2008–2009. Though the pandemic was not nearly as serious as was initially forecast, enormous energy was devoted to preparing for the possibility of a healthcare system overwhelmed by very sick and potentially dying patients. The first issue was how to allocate what was anticipated to be a relative scarcity (at least initially) of influenza vaccine: Who should get the first doses? A variety of plans were advanced.[27] Interestingly, focus groups of the public demonstrated not only an acceptance of the need to ration what could be a life-saving resource, but also provoked suggestions on how we might do it better by altering the distribution priorities to better represent the values of the public (Quinn et al. 2009; Bernier and Marcuse 2005). Thus, like the public's knowledge and acceptance of the necessity for rationing in organ transplantation and emergency triage, they also seemed to understand and accept this need in the case of the flu pandemic. Finally, over the last five to ten years the industrialized, developed world has been plagued with a seemingly never-ending series of sudden and severe shortages of prescription drugs, most often those that are both generic and must be used intravenously. The causes are numerous and complex, but the situation has demanded that the dwindling supply be allocated (i.e., rationed), something that doctors, pharmacists, and hospitals are now doing on an everyday basis, with little outcry from the public (Rosoff 2012a; Rosoff et al. 2012). All of these are examples of publicly known and accepted explicit rationing systems, although perhaps they are not viewed as such.

Why Do People Object to Rationing?

When people talk about why they don't like or why they fear healthcare rationing, they think of stories like that of Coby Howard (whose case I alluded to earlier) (Crawshaw, Garland, and Hines 1989). Coby was a seven-year-old boy in Oregon who was diagnosed with acute lymphoblastic leukemia, the most common form of leukemia in children. While he initially seemed to do well—going into remission and staying there—his disease returned and his only hope for a cure, and hence survival, was an expensive and risky bone marrow transplant. This was in 1987, shortly after the state had instituted its Medicaid rationing plan (see above). Coby and his family did not have private insurance (which may have funded the transplant), and were on the Medicaid rolls that denied his application for the procedure, estimated to cost about $100,000 at the time. Aside from the fact that Coby was not in remission at the time the transplant was being proposed, making its chances of success virtually nil (Klevit et al. 1991), his family tried to raise the money by various philanthropic means, including taking the story public via the news media. If ever a story was made for television, this was it: a nameless and faceless bureaucracy refusing to give a young boy his only chance at life solely because of money. Unlike other types of organ transplants, say for a liver after a life of alcoholism or a heart after many years of smoking or even kidneys after adult-onset diabetes, Coby's illness was purely a result of misfortune and "not his fault." What could be more tragic and cruel than to deny him a transplant? Unfortunately, Coby's family was unable to raise the full amount needed—they were apparently short about $30,000—and he died. This is the kind of story that gives currency to wild accusations of "death panels." These narratives are also useful to buttress passionate claims of unfairness, and they are rarely countered by the far more numerous accounts of people dying from delayed medical care because they didn't have health insurance. The truth of the matter is, while healthcare rationing can seem heartless and unfeeling to a few, it is overwhelmingly balanced by the good it can do for the vast majority.[28]

Unfortunately, people are even scared of the word *rationing*. A recent article called it the "R word," stating that "the R word's power to stop conversation reflects the popular belief that cost should be no object at the bedside" (Bloche 2012, 1951; also see Meltzer and Detsky 2010). Conversely, another author who is intimately involved in rationing (or "allocation") decisions every day in his job as a transplant surgeon suggests that we should call a spade a spade because it lets us know of the dire scarcity of kidneys and other solid organs needed to save lives (Matas 2009). As scary as this term may be, I use it throughout this book, not because I want to frighten people, but to get them accustomed to its sound and real meaning as a referent to a process and not an outcome. It need not entail a situation in which some must unavoidably do without something that could potentially help them a great deal. While I discuss the organ rationing system in some detail, I do so only as an example of a system that we accept as fair and tolerable even when the consequences for those who do not receive organs because of the inherent scarcity are so grim. I contrast it to what should (and could) be available in a wealthy and generous country like the United States were we to rationally ration healthcare, hopefully to show that it's nothing to be afraid of. We have been rationing solid organs for transplantation on a national basis for almost thirty years, and for the most part we have been doing it well. The system is under constant scrutiny for fairness and on the lookout for doctors and patients who try to "game the system." Aberrations exist, and when they are discovered, the transplant regulatory authority (the United Network for Organ Sharing or UNOS) institutes changes to make the system more equitable (I discuss this in greater detail in chapter 3).[29]

What reasons do people give who reject (formal) rationing? Some use balanced, grounded reasoning and logical arguments that can be potentially overcome by effective counterarguments. Others are simply afraid of what the effects of rationing will be: this can potentially be answered by arguments with facts. Many others, however, have an irrational, emotional fear that is most likely immune to any kind of reasoned argument since it can be better classified as an unsupported belief, if not faith. Indeed, one could draw an analogy between people who reject formal and planned (and ethically justifiable) rationing and those who are vaccine refusers and maintain an unshakable belief that vaccines cause autism or other severe and irreversible ills. These individuals ignore the fact that vaccines prevent massive amounts of diseases that are far worse than the terrible side effects they mistakenly attribute to the inoculations (Bearman 2009; Gross 2009). The same can be said of those who advocate for the existence of such entities as chronic Lyme disease despite the lack of any evidence for its existence (Auwaerter et al. 2011).

Why this resistance? Almost everyone agrees that the current spending on healthcare in the United States in unsustainable and that economic catastrophe awaits us without some check on spending. Almost everyone acknowledges that many other countries spend less per patient per year and have aggregate health outcomes that are as good and often significantly better than ours in such signature areas as infant mortality and longevity (Berkman 2009; MacDorman and Mathews 2010). And again, everyone accepts that these foreign "miracles" occur even though most, if not all, of these countries have limited access to some services—that is, rationing. And almost everyone agrees that it is a shame, if not an immoral tragedy, that the United States has so much of its population without any health insurance at all (most not by choice). Those who maintain that we should avoid rationing at almost all costs advance a sophistic argument that has little basis in fact; those who continue to believe that rationing is elective and does not currently exist in this system—the "best healthcare system in the world"—are selectively blind to reality.

Why are the instances of unalloyed formal healthcare rationing tolerated so well—indeed, accepted—by the public when the mere mention of rationing of anything else brings about accusations of "death panels" and the like? Perhaps it is because of a unique feature of organ transplantation, emergency triage, pandemic influenza preparations, and drug shortage allocations: we have no choice in the matter. We either ration by developing as fair a system as we can to allocate an inescapable and immutable shortage of resources, or we do it arbitrarily, capriciously, and unjustly (or maybe we don't do it at all). Now there are many who would maintain we don't have any choice about limiting the amount of money we spend on all of healthcare if we wish to control the ever-increasing costs. Doing so will of course involve rationing of one form or another. But in this case, it *seems* as if we have a choice, because it's elective, even though it really isn't. Perhaps it is because money is fungible, unlike livers or ventilators. The fact that it can buy healthcare or schools or roads and bridges endows it with apparent powers that it doesn't have. And the money we "decide" to devote to healthcare can buy any number of different goods, from universal childhood vaccination to the latest MRI scanners to nose jobs. Cash is almost infinitely malleable and hence makes allocation decisions more difficult (a donor heart can *only* be used for a heart transplant).[30] Moreover, it is what we might call a second-order resource: it is used to obtain what one really wants, such as medicines, surgical operations, and so on, while organs are first-order resources, because they will directly affect one's life. If a patient needs a heart and none are available, all the money in the world won't help. And this may be a crucial psychological difference, especially in a society so accustomed to borrowing to buy what we want.

However, we could also simply say that we will auction off the drug or the ventilator to the highest bidder, letting the rules of the marketplace determine who gets better and who doesn't, or who lives and who dies. This would obviously privilege those who are already privileged by virtue of their superior financial situation in life. This would have the consequence of increasing the disadvantages experienced by those who cannot afford to buy these "commodities" (of course, something like this situation already occurs with the millions who lack health insurance not by choice). Naturally, that doesn't seem right, and there are many other ways that we could allocate the scarce resource(s) that may be preferable, ways that would offer the best chances to use the resource both wisely and well, so that those who did not receive the resource may be disappointed, but they would be unable to say the system was unfair. There are also things we could do to make the loss easier to bear, such as the provision of excellent palliative care or other compensatory forms of compassionate support that would lessen the burden of being denied access to what is believed to be a precious asset.

Of course, it should be pointed out that healthcare rationing is not inherently benign. While we would like to think that whoever manages the allocation system does so in a fair manner in which the most people get access to the most healthcare that is conceivably possible given whatever resource constraints exist, there is no guarantee that this will happen. For instance, there could be a decision that different classes of people will have access to tiered levels of healthcare. So, for example, we could imagine a state of affairs where Medicaid recipients (poor people) would be eligible to receive certain types of interventions, but those who had private insurance could receive another (as envisioned by the original Oregon Health Plan). There is no built-in reason to believe that interventions on the poor peoples' list would be inferior to those appearing on the list for the more financially secure population. Indeed, they probably would not be so; they just would be fewer in number and cheaper. And who is to say that the extra stuff on the longer list would actually be anything more than marginally beneficial for the recipients? But the situation could be more nefarious. Poor people, being poor, tend to have less political clout than those with money and their ability to argue for an expansive range of services may be muted if those in charge of setting funding levels decide to scrimp on the backs of the impoverished, as has happened so often in this country.[31] Or there could be overt forms of discrimination against those who are marginalized for all sorts of reasons (Rosoff and Decamp 2011; also see chapter 6). This point emphasizes what many people erroneously think is self-evident: that any rationing scheme must be equitable and have adequate safeguards for the most vulnerable members of society. Most proposed systems have more of the former and less of the latter; some types of healthcare allocation and prioritization decisions may need to be excluded a priori because of their very nature (see chapter 3). In this regard, it bears mentioning that what many people may fear about rationing is its explicit emphasis on what is *not* available, rather that what is. People naturally apply this to themselves in their own lives and thus worry about what this might mean for them—that is, about what they can't have, even if they don't need it.

There is an interesting story from the hospital where I work that illustrates the illogical, perhaps even incoherent, way we often approach rationing, in which common sense is seemingly absent. Just before the North American influenza season began in the fall of 2004, a very worrisome event occurred: the British government shut down the vaccine production facility of the Chiron Corporation, located in Liverpool (Treanor 2004). The concern was that there might be contamination of some lots of the vaccine currently in production. Unfortunately, Chiron was one of only two manufacturers of the influenza vaccine to supply the entire United States. Thus, the country was looking forward to a flu season with only half of the usual vaccine supply. At the time my institution did not require annual influenza vaccination of personnel with direct patient contact, although it was strongly encouraged and the vaccine was supplied free of charge. In the past, the average overall vaccination rate varied from between 35 and 50 percent, although there were some groups that did better, such as physicians. When vaccine refusers were asked why they did not get the annual flu shot, they often cited their fear of getting the flu (even though the vaccine was composed of either attenuated or killed virus, making this virtually impossible), frequently recalling a past bad experience with vaccination. That season looked to be a repeat of prior years' experience with the usual abysmal immunization rates—that is, until it was announced that there was a vaccine shortage. All of a sudden, it seemed as if everyone, refusers as well as acceptors (but procrastinators), wanted to get the flu vaccine. All it took was for them to learn that they might not get what they had previously not wanted (remember, I said this didn't make sense). Indeed, at the end of the flu season that year, our immunization rate set a record: about 65 percent of eligible personnel got vaccinated. Unfortunately, this effect was short-lived, because it then fell back to the historical low averages the next year when the vaccine was plentiful. In this case, scarcity—the necessary precondition for rationing—stimulated the desire for the vaccine in those who previously didn't want it or care about it.

Psychologists call this phenomenon the "scarcity principle" (Cialdini 2009, chap. 7). I think there is an important lesson here that can be instructive for thinking about healthcare rationing. This phenomenon is also crucial to my analysis in chapter 2 of rationing during drug shortages. There are a number of interesting aspects of this psychological trait that are pertinent to the emotional, and thus less-than-rational, fear of planned (and presumably fair) healthcare rationing. For instance, Cialdini points out that when our options are limited (or we become aware that our options are limited, meaning that they could have been limited before but we never knew about it), we believe we have curbs or boundaries on some conception of absolute freedom. And in the United States, at least, that thought, however unconnected it may be to reality, is anathema. It is psychologically irrelevant what the actual truth of the matter may be or how minimally our freedom may have been curtailed, or for that matter, whether the curtailment had any effect on our freedom whatsoever.

For example, if a restriction on the availability of some resource was announced (say, our ability to have a PET scan whenever our doctor recommended it),[32] we may be quite upset to find out about this, even if we don't have a disease or condition in which such a scan would be potentially useful. Another instance might be changes to the medication formulary used by our health insurance company. Even if we don't take, say, Synthroid® (an expensive brand-name form of thyroxine, the main hormone from the thyroid gland, for which there are quite a few generic substitutes), we would be dismayed to learn that we couldn't obtain it if we might need thyroxine for hypothyroidism in the future. This response is maintained, regardless of the fact that we don't have an immediate need for the item in question. We just want to have the illusion of its potential availability at some unspecified time. To quote Cialdini:

> According to the theory, whenever free choice is limited or threatened, the need to retain our freedoms makes us want them (as well as the goods and services associated with them) significantly more than before. Therefore, when increasing scarcity—or anything else—interferes with our prior access to some item, we will *react against* the interference by wanting and trying to possess the item more than we did before. (Cialdini 2009, 205; his emphasis)

This feature of human psychology, which some think is both universal and evolutionarily adaptive (Haselton and Nettle 2006), can do much to explain the difficulty of implementing any kind of rationing system *unless there is no choice*. For in those situations, there is no illusion of perfect and unlimited freedom; the very nature of the shortage is integral or inherent in the resource itself, like solid organs for transplantation or even unavoidable drug shortages. While it may be impossible to react to such structural scarcity by hoarding organs, due to their very short "shelf life," that may not be true of drugs, as I discuss in chapter 2. Finally, there is also evidence that a relatively new scarcity of resources, especially when knowledge or memory of previous abundance is still current, results in a greater desire for the scarce resource (whatever it may be) compared with conditions in which scarcity is common or when one has become acclimated to such resource constraints (Aggarwal, Jun, and Huh 2011; Worchel, Lee, and Adewole 1975). It is the novelty of this new situation that seems to be the driving factor, which suggests an important lesson about rationing to which we should pay heed.

It has been observed that Americans sometimes cannot distinguish between what they want and what they need (Young 1994). Of course, advertisers thrive on taking advantage of this conflation and indeed spend enormous amounts of money and effort to encourage its continuation. Thinking you need something that is not necessary or even frivolous is the essence of the consumer society, and blurring the line between need and want so the two are merged is essential to stimulating demand for goods that are arguably either unnecessary or at least a matter of choice. Examples from the medical world might include some types of cosmetic surgery such as tummy tucks, nose jobs, and refractive keratotomy (Lasik™), or even access to cash-on-demand whole-body CT scans that frequently park their mobile machines at the local mall. In the universe of medical treatments and diagnostic tests, absolute free and unfettered choice offers the supposed benefit, but also the attendant risk. When the indication for the treatment or test is subject only to caprice or personal whimsy or desire, the harms could easily outweigh any conceivable good.

Did this principle apply in a real-life rationing experiment? It is interesting to note that there was very little negative reaction to the general idea of overall healthcare rationing in Oregon, once the bumps were worked out. There could be a number of reasons for this, including the possibility that Oregonians are a very sensible and balanced-thinking group of people, different from many others in the rest of the country in seeing the wisdom of what was being attempted. Alternatively, Oregonians could be immune to the psychological effects of the scarcity principle, but that seems somehow very unlikely. More credibly, the people affected by the Oregon plan were poor by definition (otherwise they would not have been included in the plan, since it was restricted to Medicaid patients). And poor people tend to have less political clout that those of more significant financial means, resulting in less input in the decision-making process. So, in the Oregon rationing case, the acceptance of the plan by its recipients may be more similar to the rationing of solid organs or scarce drugs in that those covered by the plan had no choice: it was that or nothing.[33] However, the people who insisted on getting the newly scarce vaccine which previously they had refused, most certainly seemed to hew to the scarcity principle.

Unfortunately, the long-term success of the Oregon plan was neither assured nor stable. Oberlander (2007) has illustrated the problem of having people make rules for others when they are not personally bound by those rules. They are not accountable in the same way other approaches might have them be. Indeed, in Oregon, the lawmakers who drew up the plan and, most importantly, voted on how much funding to devote to the plan (and hence how much healthcare could be offered to individuals and how many could be covered), were truly answerable to the taxpayers (i.e., voters), and not necessarily to those people covered by the OHP. The eventual cutback and decreased commitment to the plan demonstrated that it was a political football, susceptible to easy manipulation by the political and financial winds of fortune. And the people who were on the receiving end could do nothing about it. Poverty is generally equivalent to powerlessness.

Nevertheless, we are all susceptible to the effects of the scarcity principle: it respects neither socioeconomic class nor educational level nor individual tastes. A little bit of honest self-examination would reveal the veracity of this statement. True, some of us can resist the pull of this emotion more than others, but the overwhelming majority of us are suckers. Which is why the fear of, and reaction to, the very idea of rationing has the effect it does. It is also important to emphasize the emotional nature of the reaction to this form of scarcity, which may help explain some of the seemingly over-the-top responses to any proposal to ration or restrict access to certain healthcare resources. Indeed, "knowing the causes and workings of scarcity pressures may not be sufficient to protect us from them because knowing is a cognitive act, and cognitive processes are suppressed by our emotional reaction to scarcity pressures" (Cialdini 2009, 222).[34]

Now of course healthcare resources—drugs, various surgical procedures, x-rays and scans, and so on—are not really the same as things sold in stores, even though our behavior may be similar when we become aware of the scarcity of either type of item and even though healthcare resources are often commoditized in our society. So it may be possible that we would take a collective big breath, recognize the illogic of these responses, and think carefully about what we want and, more importantly, what we reasonably *need* from a healthcare system. At least in the United States, people seem to want the freedom to want everything and have it available, even if they don't need it or don't have the means to obtain it. It's just the thought that it is there waiting for them that is significant.

Furthermore, Americans are massively susceptible to what has been called the "moral hazard" of health insurance: once one is shielded from most of the cost of what one wants or thinks one needs (such as healthcare interventions), there is an incentive to use as much of it as one likes (Stone 2011). One area in which this plays out most graphically is in end-of-life care in intensive-care units in the United States. Despite the phenomenal growth of the hospice movement over the last two decades and the recognition of palliative-care medicine as a distinct medical specialty, the majority of Americans still die in hospitals.[35] More important, a large percentage of annual Medicare dollars is spent in the last six months of life, often for only marginal benefit (Riley and Lubitz 2010; Hanchate et al. 2009). Is this right? Should people be allowed to have whatever they or their families want, irrespective of the costs to us all, even if there is little benefit to themselves? Actually, this question implies that all of us have the ability to demand all healthcare services or interventions, but that is somewhat deceptive, because not all of us are equally insured. And even though in the heat of the moment we may get what we or our families think we need, the bill will only come later and it may very well be devastating.

What Is Different in This Book

Calls for the rationing of healthcare—setting limits on what should be available and for what reasons—have been made for years. Innumerable books, essays, newspaper articles, government reports, and noisy and pleonastic statements by countless pundits of various political stripes have stated that the current unregulated and hodgepodge healthcare system in the United States is financially unsustainable and is leading to the bankruptcy of the country. I would not disagree, but I do not wish to add yet one more voice crying out in the wilderness. My hope is that by focusing on a specific and somewhat restricted area of rationing accepted to a remarkable extent by the people directly affected by its decisions as well as—most importantly—by the general public, we might be able to ease into a discussion of more general rationing. This is the discussion required to keep our healthcare system (and country) solvent as well as to stimulate thinking about better utilizing resources that work and discarding those that don't.

In the preface to his book *Taming the Beloved Beast*, Daniel Callahan (2009, x) declares that persuading the public and doctors to accept healthcare reform (and necessarily rationing) will guarantee "that any plausible solution will require pain and sacrifice." But is this true? Would reasonable limits placed on access to certain types and amounts of healthcare in a country as wealthy as the United States actually cause widespread suffering? I suspect not for several reasons, as I argue throughout this book. For any conceivable and publicly acceptable allocation or rationing scheme would mostly restrict the availability of the kinds of medical interventions that people could arguably do without, and not cause increases in both the aggregate and particulate kind of suffering due to illness. Hence, it would be generous, but not necessarily overly or unreasonably so. Of course, if it were too munificent, the ability to both save money and distribute the benefits of decent comprehensive healthcare to most (perhaps all) Americans would be either severely compromised or impossible.

As I discuss in detail later, eliminating waste, including intemperate administrative overhead inherent in a polyglot insurance system and ineffective or marginally effective treatments, could enable us to meet these dual goals without breaking the bank. Furthermore, extending health insurance to those currently uninsured—especially preventive health services—could reduce the overall costs of medical care simply by reducing emergency service needs and excessive costs associated with caring for those who wait until they are very sick to seek help (Bradley et al. 2012). The expansiveness of coverage would be a precondition to "sell" the plan to the public and to minimize activation of the scarcity principle.

The more difficult challenge would be in deciding how to approach rationing: budget first or benefits first. In the former, one would set a ceiling on the amount of funding available, and then figure out what one could buy with the allocated budget; this method intensifies the fungibility problem, as demonstrated in Oregon (see chapter 2). In the latter approach, which I think preferable on a national scale, one decides what a decent benefit package should contain and the budget is then determined based on this list. Of course, there are risks associated with this strategy. Not least of these is what might be called "list inflation" (which of course inevitably results in budgetary inflation) due to the danger of the attraction of new—and often unproven—treatments and devices, which Leff and Finucane label "gizmo idolatry" (Leff and Finucane 2008; also see Callahan 2009).

I will argue that healthcare rationing need not be the bogeyman that its naysayers and fearmongers believe it to be. Indeed, I will elaborate on situations that I have already introduced in which we overtly ration care, because we have to: organ transplantation and treatments during unexpected crises like an influenza pandemic or drug shortages. In both these situations, patients and their families accept—reluctantly perhaps, but accept nonetheless—that they may not get what they want and need, which could lead to death. This is a clearcut case of rationing truly leading to "pain and sacrifice," making it radically different from the rationing most healthcare analysts talk about. But people not only comply with these systems, they do so quietly. Why is this so, and what lessons can we learn about how to ration healthcare in general? While many may argue persuasively (and do) that the DRG system is an exemplar of "invisible" rationing, and hence is in a class by itself when compared with the other arrangements I have introduced here and will discuss in depth later in the book, it does represent a national attempt to rein in costs by limiting access to healthcare, and it does so with little fuss. That may happen because of its invisibility, which may contribute to it being unjust in some sense (which I will also discuss); my point here is only to note that it is a rationing method that people accept.

If people tolerate these forms of rationing without complaint—indeed, the overwhelming majority of Americans embrace them and endorse them as a public good from which all can potentially benefit—then we may be able to discover what it is about this kind of rationing that seems to work.

Maybe it's because we rarely refer to the organ transplant allocation system as "rationing," thereby avoiding the four-letter word that scares so many people. But if I can speak about these "scarce-resource distribution and prioritization schemes" without needing to employ these anodyne euphemisms, and rather use the term *rationing*, I may be able to go a long way toward toning down the argument about rationing as a *method*, and steer the debate toward what we should be talking about: *how* to ration. If people are truly worried about what they won't get or what they might lose in any type of comprehensive rationing system, and if we approach its development and implementation the way I and many others suggest—openly and with true dialog and some form of democratic deliberation—then it is inconceivable that any system that results would not be generous (perhaps to a fault). It is implausible, if not unthinkable, that those who would be charged with coming up with a system that most people would accept would not try to make it as liberal and lavish as economically feasible, especially if it applied to them as well as others. Some might argue that the problems with the rollout of the Affordable Care Act rebut this claim, but it is plausible that these issues have less to do with the generosity of the benefits offered than the contentious political climate, the disastrous problems with the federal government website for the program, and the false promises made by the president about the ability of people to keep their own privately purchased health insurance. Nevertheless, one could easily imagine that if we took the plunge and really embraced healthcare rationing as a way to control costs and bring a more fair and equitable mechanism for delivering medical care to everyone, the (ironic) danger actually might be that we could have a rationing plan that would throw fiscal cares to the wind, if only for both political and self-serving reasons. But of course, we can worry about that once we get over the psychological mountain range that is rationing itself.

It is fascinating how often the discussion of healthcare rationing is framed around the idea of life and death, as if all medical decisions about the allocations of resources involved the distribution of life-saving medicines or technologies, rescuing patients from the rapacious jaws of death, or condemning them to oblivion.[36] The truth of the matter is that a wealthy country like the United States could ration expansively, generously, and fairly and would not have to make this choice. What will go a long way to ease the "pain" of rationing—if there is any to be had—will be the generosity of our funding, so that all but the most ineffective interventions would continue to be available. Few, if any, people would die or indeed suffer solely because they could not have access to some potential curative therapy; undoubtedly, the overwhelming majority of these patients would die anyway. But this is the fear that is stirred up by the very mention of the word *rationing*. I hope to dispel some of this fear.

However, I should also add a comment about what I do not attempt to do in the following pages. Most important is that I do not try to rehash the rationale as well as any disputes over the need to rein in healthcare costs, possibly by some form of rationing, because this has been done by many others in great detail. I will assume that this is a settled matter, since even the most vociferous opponents of any sort of nationalized, government-run healthcare plan agree that healthcare expenditures are out of control and some kind of restraint on growth—which will entail refusing to provide some things to some people—is necessary. Even though they avoid the use of the word *rationing*, rationing is what they mean.

This is the essence of my argument. While most commentators have focused on the hidden or unregulated (what I have termed the informal or hidden) system of rationing, such as DRGs and the ways the less fortunate suffer at the hands of powers beyond their control, I turn my attention elsewhere to formal systems. I have already introduced a discussion about how we ration some sectors of the healthcare system openly and strictly and with grievous consequences for those who fail to receive the resources they want and need. Whether it is too many patients with liver or heart failure and insufficient organs to save their lives, or desperate and grievously injured patients awaiting triage in an emergency department, we go about our business deciding who should receive the absolutely scarce resources that have the possibility of saving lives, knowing full well that those who fail to obtain them may die. We do so because we have no choice. And perhaps it is because we lack options that this practice is so well accepted.

The truth is that we are facing a similar lack of choice about the money we use to fund healthcare in this country. It, too, is becoming increasingly scarce. But unlike livers, which are strictly limited in number, we have much more money and are willing to devote considerably more resources to fund healthcare than we will ever possess for organs, even when we factor in the necessity of controlling costs and saving money. While this means we must ration money and what it can purchase, the ramifications for patients may not be that severe at all; people should not die unnecessarily simply because there are inadequate resources to buy and provide them with what they need. Moreover, a system that is just would ensure not only that we don't bankrupt ourselves but that we deliver what should be our moral imperative as a nation: caring for the health and welfare of the people who live here. In essence, I am making a moral argument: a comprehensive, centralized, and fair rationing system created by the public for the public is truly the only method we can employ to both control costs and bring the undeniable benefits of modern medicine to all Americans. I will attempt to present a convincing argument that rationing, the only plausible way to accomplish this task, is not to be feared; it is not a four-letter word.

I develop my argument as follows. I first make my case that rationing, done in a specific manner and incorporating certain essential features, could be palatable. I leave to the final chapter any detailed discussion of what rationing could actually look like and what might be done to accomplish the twin goals of saving money and offering a decent set of healthcare benefits to the entire population, all the while packaging it in a way that it could be plausibly sold to the American public.

In chapter 2, I describe some existing and clearcut rationing systems that we (mostly) know about, understand, and accept; these include organ transplantation, the Oregon Health Plan, and the allocation of scarce drugs during a shortage. In particular, I note key characteristics of these approaches that may help make them both justifiable and acceptable to the public (albeit not immune to criticism).

I then move to a more detailed discussion in chapter 3 of fairness, the essence of any just distribution system that would enable both buy-in and the endorsement of those it affects.

In chapter 4, I consider the real and potential constraints that must be reckoned with in any comprehensive overhaul of a national healthcare system. These include what I am calling the "cutoff problem": the issue of where to draw the line(s) about which benefits or interventions should be included and which should not. This chapter also includes a detailed analysis of the problem of the fungibility of money and proposes a possible solution.

Next, in chapter 5, I discuss the challenge of how to consider the claims of people who feel they have been treated unfairly by the system and whether or how to judge these assertions as legitimate.

In chapter 6, I examine the very difficult issue of what can practically be accomplished in a democracy or what some have called the "tyranny of the majority." This is especially relevant in a nation like the modern United States, in which speech is almost completely unbridled and free and but is also subject to the ability to purchase a platform from which to broadcast whatever one wishes to say, irrespective of its truth content. Thus, the potential to skew the conversation with innuendo or even outright falsehoods that appeal to people's basest instincts (not to mention their fear of change and susceptibility to the scarcity principle) could easily lead to restrictions on the fairness and inclusiveness of any plan that could win support and be implemented. In chapter 7, I will bring together all of these considerations to argue that rationing of the kind that I am discussing need not be hypothetical or a pipedream.

Deliberate and sensible rationing is the only way to deliver good healthcare to all: deciding what works (and thus should be available), what doesn't work (and shouldn't be offered), and what might be experimental (and hence should be properly investigated). Significant cost savings will almost necessarily follow as a "side effect," if you will. This is the approach we take with organ transplants. But we have a lot more money than we will ever have donor hearts or livers, so the recipients of reasonable and morally justifiable rationing in a wealthy (and presumably generous) country should be notably better off—even those who feel they may not receive what they want—so long as they get what they need.

Lastly, I want to state clearly that I understand perfectly well the substantial practical obstacles to implementation of the proposals that I make in this book. No one should be under any illusions—or delusions—that achieving comprehensive healthcare reform of the kind that forms a recurring theme throughout this book, will be simple. The knockdown and often savage fights over the Clinton-era reform proposal and, more recently, the ongoing vicious battles over the Affordable Care Act should provide more than sufficient evidence of the obstacles that await. Some might maintain that it is a sisyphean fight. However, I believe that the conversation and topic are vitally important, and so I hope that this discussion will initiate debate and argument about the need for rationing. This book represents an attempt to demythologize and wash away the demons that have embraced the whole topic of healthcare rationing. Essentially, I am making a moral argument. It holds that maintaining the status quo delivers a message that we as a people care so little for those among us—citizen or not—that we do not seem to mind that they suffer from ills when we have the means to offer them help. The misguided notion that people who are poor or otherwise marginalized deserve their fate is an anachronistic belief harking back to ill-conceived tenets of social Darwinism. The goal of delivering decent and affordable healthcare to all who live in this country is a meritorious and virtuous one. And, like any virtue worth pursuing, it will take time, dedication, and practice to perfect.

2

Existing Rationing Systems: Organ Transplantation, Scarce Drugs, and Oregon

To begin my argument about the possible acceptability of widespread and tolerable rationing, I will start with a discussion of some existing systems of explicit—what I have called "formal"—rationing arrangements in distinct areas of healthcare. Two of the examples will demonstrate what might be described as the extremes of rationing, in which there is an absolute limit on the available resources, thus forcing the prioritized allocation of the extant supply to recipients whose numbers far exceed the quantity available. The third case (Oregon) is a demonstration of an approach to rationing in which money (not organs or drugs) is the limiting factor and the goals mirror those I have suggested should be the goals of any coherent, morally based, nationwide system. My objective in this chapter is to present real-life models of rationing methods that have proven acceptable to those affected by them, even if they are not ideal and those who fail to gain access to the resources often pay a steep price. I am proposing that these satisfactory arrangements can serve as potential models for more widespread applicability and can demonstrate that rationing can both work and be endorsed by the public. Some features of these systems are notable for contributing to their acceptance by the public and hence can add to our understanding of how they could be incorporated into more comprehensive approaches. But first, a story to starkly illustrate a challenge in rationing.

In late 2006 and early 2007, epidemiologists and infectious disease specialists became concerned about the very real possibility of a worldwide influenza pandemic. They feared that it could be a public health catastrophe of the magnitude of the global disaster of 1918–1919, which killed an estimated 50–100 million people in as little as 18 months (Barry 2004). Most of the people who died in the early twentieth century succumbed to respiratory failure, either primary viral pneumonia or secondary infection with bacteria. Therefore, it was felt that in the modern era most patients could be saved if there were an effective vaccine that could be administered on a massive scale, if there were extensive access to antiviral medications, and if advanced technological intensive care were used judiciously. The challenges were that the entire six billion–plus population of the world was potentially at risk, only wealthy countries could afford to even think about prevention or treatment (Rhorer et al. 2009; Sasaki et al. 2011; Osterholm, Kelley, Sommer, and Belongia 2012),[1] and even those nations had inadequate supplies should the worst predictions be realized. While it is true that we were lucky and dodged the bullet then, another potential pandemic may be looming again with the threat of a possible jump from animal to human transmission of the H7N9 virus, requiring only a few mutations to achieve this status (Uyeki and Cox 2013; Gao et al. 2013; Pavia 2013).[2]

Ironically—in a particularly heartrending way—the predicament in which we found ourselves was a direct result of the scientific and technological advances medicine and society had made since the second decade of the twentieth century during the Great Pandemic. Ninety years ago, little could be offered to victims of the flu beyond pain relief and comfort care. Many patients died at home or in large dormitories set up to house and quarantine the massive numbers of the sick. Today, we would expect (no, demand) that these people be hospitalized in order to receive intravenous fluids and antibiotics, supplemental oxygen, even intensive care if it were clinically indicated. The full panoply of modern medical interventions would be brought to bear to heal the ill. But if the number of patients were large enough, we would anticipate running out of virtually everything we routinely use in these clinical scenarios. And without our contemporary tools, we would be reduced to using treatments not dissimilar to those from 1919. This state of affairs presented a classic rationing situation as well as a profound test of distributive justice. I will discuss these issues in detail later in this chapter, but for now (perhaps to whet the reader's appetite), I will mention a real-life dilemma related to these problems.

On the evening of October 16, 2009, I received an urgent phone call from the chief medical officer of the hospital where I am on the faculty and a member of the medical staff as well as the chair of the ethics committee. There had been a number of cases of H1N1 influenza (the presumptive pandemic strain) diagnosed in the United States, and quite a few in my state. While the total cases by no means met the criteria to be labeled a pandemic, experts were still very concerned that the outbreak could occur at any time. Many patients were getting quite ill, requiring intensive care and mechanical ventilation. For some unknown reason, pregnant women were particularly susceptible to getting very sick. Unfortunately, for some patients the standard types of ventilators were insufficient to provide their blood with enough oxygen and to rid it of carbon dioxide. People were literally suffocating to death, dying in their own respiratory secretions despite maximal care. In some cases of severe respiratory failure similar to what was being observed, a special kind of intervention could be used in a heroic attempt to let the lungs heal on their own. This is ECMO, or extracorporeal membrane oxygenation. ECMO utilizes a variant of a heart-lung machine, comparable to the ones used in the operating room for open-heart surgery (Allen et al. 2011; Almond et al. 2011; Lee et al. 2012).[3] As a center for the use of these devices (mostly in children who have congenital heart disease, but increasingly for adults awaiting lung transplantation), we were already experienced in using this technology. There was some early evidence from New Zealand that suggested that ECMO might be life saving in this disease (Davies et al. 2009). However, even though pandemic conditions did not yet formally exist, we were seeing many more patients with influenza-related respiratory failure than we could accommodate with the number of machines we possessed as well as the highly trained technicians needed to run them.[4] The problem that stimulated the phone call was that all of our ECMO machines were in use (one for a patient with H1N1 and the other three for patients with noninfluenza disease), no patient could be removed without causing their death, and there was a young pregnant woman with influenza in the medical intensive-care unit who was doing worse with conventional ventilation: her only hope was ECMO. Our choices were grim. We could remove a current patient from a machine (he or she would then die quickly) or there was another possibility. We could take one of the heart-lung machines from a cardiac surgery operating room and use it. But that would mean closing that room to operations for up to three weeks (experience had shown that patients could require ECMO for this long to recover). Not only would that make the cardiac surgeons angry, but heart surgery was a very busy service at our hospital, often being performed on extremely sick patients in an urgent or emergency setting. Would we still be able to meet the needs of those patients, or would they be placed at risk in an attempt to save this one patient's life? What would be the right thing to do?

Fortunately, it turned out that this situation was resolved on its own without having to make any difficult choices. The condition of one of the patients already on ECMO suddenly deteriorated and it was decided to terminate life support, so that she subsequently died. That machine was now available; the new patient was placed on it and did well, making a full recovery after a prolonged ICU course. But what happened next was perhaps most interesting. A high-level meeting was called with many of the concerned parties: administrators, Respiratory Therapy, critical-care doctors, an ethicist (me), and members of the lung transplant team. We could have confronted the problem directly and addressed questions such as how to reasonably, equitably, and fairly create a procedure by which we could allocate (ration) these complex and strictly limited machines, who should be eligible for the few machines available, and whether the technology should even be accessible to influenza patients should we be faced with an overwhelming pandemic. But it was decided to take a different approach. This potential crisis was seen as an opportunity. The lung transplanters had wanted to expand their program for some time, and they viewed the small number of ECMO machines as a limitation on their ability to do so. Why not accomplish two goals at once: buy more machines, which we could use immediately for flu patients in respiratory failure, and then "repurpose" them as bridge devices for waiting transplant patients? And that is what we did. To a certain extent we tried to buy ourselves out of having to make difficult decisions.[5] This is very similar to what the U.S. Congress did with hemodialysis machines in 1972 (see below) and what we effectively continue to do with such programs as Medicare. It is also a very curious way to confront the moral and medical challenges imposed by a strict scarcity of resources in the face of increased demand. Most important, it avoided having to think about (formal) rationing.

My goal in this chapter is not to concentrate on the minutiae of different rationing systems or modes of rationing. Rather it is to describe in general several systems that are already in existence and accepted, one of which is "mainstream" enough that no one really thinks about it much as rationing. I want to focus on these three systems because they serve as existing examples of rationing in which there is a finite scarcity of resources that may be critically important to people who receive them (and those that don't). One of the main reasons this discussion is relevant is that people accept these forms of rationing with minimal fuss, resentment, and anger. Why is that so? For instance, while there was a great deal of open discussion about various ways of prioritizing people for vaccines and other forms of therapy for an influenza outbreak (and what their professional roles were and how that should influence their place on the priority list), there was little-to-no controversy over the necessity for doing it. In a similar vein, we have suggested ways to approach the allocation of critically scarce drugs, and again this appears to have been accepted as required by the gravity of the circumstances. Most significant, these rationing schemes concern resources that can be justifiably described as "life saving": when a patient receives them appropriately, he or she is offered the opportunity (not the guarantee) to live, whereas those who do not obtain the ventilator, vaccine, liver, or drug (assuming they meet reasonable medical criteria) very often die (Gatesman and Smith 2011; Hoffman 2012; Link, Hagerty, and Kantarjian 2012).[6] The consequences of such decisions could not be more grave or dramatic, but they are received with reasonable equanimity, albeit with sadness and resignation.

Organ Transplantation

In 1971 the U.S. Congress held hearings about proposed amendments to the Social Security Act. After approval by an overwhelming majority of both Houses in 1972, the End-Stage Renal Disease Program was created.[7] Over the preceding decade, improvements in the technology of hemodialysis had made it increasingly practical to offer this life-preserving therapy to as many patients as could afford the expensive machine time, the highly specialized and skilled personnel necessary to administer the treatment, and the required costly medications needed to combat the side effects of renal failure. If funds were made available to support dialysis, there were no technical barriers to prevent virtually all kidney-failure patients from having access to this intervention. All that was needed was the money to pay for it, hence the newly created ESRDP.

This newly established program would pay for renal dialysis (both at home and at specialized centers) as well as kidney transplantation and its associated costs for all American citizens and holders of permanent residency status irrespective of other comorbidities or considerations, medical or social. All that would be required was a doctor's order and the expenses would be reimbursed for as long as the patient needed the treatment (Blagg 2007).[8] The initial cost projections were on the low side, to say the least: "Estimates of the cost of the kidney provision were wildly off. According to the NKF [National Kidney Foundation], the cost would be $35 to $75 million the first year; the SSA [Social Security Administration] Office of the Actuary, which had had little time to come up with figures, estimated $100 to $500 million the first year, increasing substantially in succeeding years" (Blagg 2007, 492). The annual bill for this program now exceeds $25 billion and is increasing every year.[9] More importantly, the lack of effective controls on who should receive this life-saving therapy means that it is provided not only to people who are waiting for a transplant (so-called bridge therapy), but as an end in itself, to people who are not now or ever could be kidney transplant candidates (this is called "destination" therapy). Furthermore, there are few incentives *not* to provide this treatment, and many reasons for physicians to order it, since it can be a lucrative form of medical practice (Blagg 2007, 488).[10] Indeed, many (if not most) nephrologists earn the bulk of their income supervising and providing dialysis services.

Nevertheless, the significant point for my purposes is that the resources needed for dialysis are never scarce: there are more than enough facilities, dialysis machines, associated drugs and supplies, and personnel to meet the demand. Thus, it does not need to be rationed because of a choice that was made more than forty years ago and that has never been officially questioned, much less reversed or substantively modified. But the costs of the program have ballooned and have led some to inquire whether it is reasonable for this expensive therapy to be used with the sole criterion being renal failure (I discuss this point more fully in chapter 4). Indeed, with the rapid increase in the population of older adults due to the aging of the baby boomers and the burgeoning of those with (mostly obesity-related) diabetes, it is almost certain that the cost of this program will continue to escalate rapidly with almost no end in sight. This is not to say that destination dialysis is not a reasonable treatment for some patients, including older ones, but it is perhaps not appropriate for all. However, the universal availability of kidneys for transplant, or for that matter, any other solid organ cannot be said.

There are at least two substantive questions that I want to address about transplantation. The answers will help us understand how rationing organs works. First, what should the goal or goals of an organ transplantation system be? As a prerequisite, such a system must acknowledge the fact of a continuing shortage of organs that will never keep up with demand. Indeed, the mismatch between available livers, kidneys, hearts, and the like and those patients who could possibly benefit from receiving one continues to increase. Ironically, this state of affairs only exacerbates the acuity of scarcity and entails that more and more patients will die while waiting for transplants. Thus, this is a clear case of necessary healthcare-resource rationing, and one in which the result of not receiving the organ is almost certain death (Melnitchouk et al. 2011; Kirklin et al. 2011).[11] And second, what characteristics of the system as it exists today endow it with the credibility and legitimacy that ensure that it continues to be viewed as by and large fair and thus acceptable, even though the stakes for recipients are so high?

In the United States, the supply of organs is entirely dependent on the generosity of the public. We do not utilize such devices as "opt-in" or "opt-out" to increase the percentage of organs donated by individuals or their grieving families (Johnson and Goldstein 2004; De Wispelaere 2012; Forsythe 2012). We also strictly obey the "dead-donor rule," which states that organ donors must be declared dead prior to retrieving organs for use; this limits potential donors to those who have experienced whole-brain death or met cardiac criteria (Halpern and Truog 2010; Collins 2010; Khushf 2010).[12]

Moreover, we have made the considered moral decision to not com-modify the process by transforming it into a market, where patients with sufficient financial means could purchase a kidney or part of a liver or even a lung from a "willing" seller (as far as I know, this illicit market, where it exists, is almost exclusively restricted to kidneys, perhaps for obvious medical and logistical reasons).[13] We also do not pay the relatives of the deceased as an incentive to donate their loved one's organs if they are wavering in their decision, although there is at least one example of a transplant system that gives transplant priority to patients who them-selves had previously indicated their willingness to serve as donors, as an inducement to increase the availability of organs.[14] The upshot is that the entire system is completely reliant on the generosity and willingness of in-dividuals, and especially of grieving families, to make what is often called (for marketing and promotional purposes) the "gift of life." Other than deriving satisfaction from memorializing their dead relative, these fami-lies are engaging in a completely altruistic act for which there is neither tangible remuneration nor even knowledge of who the recipient(s) might be. (Although there are certain situations in which both parties may be introduced to each other, this is uncommon and requires the consent of all concerned.)

The organization responsible for collecting organs, organizing their dis-tribution, and overseeing quality control in the United States is a private, nonprofit group called the United Network for Organ Sharing, or UNOS. UNOS operates under contract to the Organ Procurement and Transplant Network, which is part of the federal Department of Health and Human Services and its Health Resources and Services Administration (HRSA).[15] Thus, the entire bureaucratic apparatus of organ transplantation in this country is a government—and hence, civic—concern. A national(ized) group that is both in charge of, and accountable for, the total process is a quasi-governmental institution. Since there is only one legal way that a patient can receive an organ transplant in the United States, he or she must cooperate with this system and agree to abide by its rules (as must the healthcare professionals who are also a necessary component). So OPTN, UNOS, the regional OPOs (Organ Procurement Organizations), institutional transplant doctors, nurses, coordinators, social workers, and so on are all part of a countrywide network of cooperating and collaborating professionals whose duty it is to administer the system, perform ongoing audits, reviews of its rules and results and who operate under the auspices and authority of a central government body. In other words, it is a nationalized healthcare delivery system, albeit limited in its scope.

The regulations demonstrate that there are two overriding aims that are frequently in great tension (Childress 1989; Egan et al. 2006; Fox 2003; Frader 2012; Neuberger 2012; Tong et al. 2010). First, organs must be used responsibly. This is often interpreted as transplanting them into people who can live the longest with the best quality of life possible. This duty reflects a public, fiduciary responsibility to utilize this life-saving communal resource in a manner that derives the most public welfare or benefit, normally translated as equivalent to years of functional life with the transplanted organ. This is commonly referred to as the "efficiency" argument (Ladin and Hanto 2011; Segev 2009).[16]

Second, organs must be used to benefit individuals. Unfortunately, what helps one identifiable person may not be the wisest stewardship of a publicly held and controlled resource. For example, if a patient has cirrhosis of the liver and liver failure (from say, chronic hepatitis C infection), but has several comorbidities such as poor lung and heart function from years of cigarette smoking, the chances are much lower of him or her living as well and as long as another patient with similarly grave liver disease but with relatively normal cardiopulmonary function. All things being equal, one would allocate the organ to the latter rather than the former patient, even though it might save the lives of both (i.e., both have an equal personal interest in receiving a transplant). Everyone desiring a transplant presumably values life to the same degree and wants to live, even if it is only to get out of the hospital and attend the wedding of a daughter or son or to play with the grandchildren one more time. And perhaps if we had enough livers for everyone who could possibly benefit—for everyone who could conceivably be saved—the prognostic differences between the two patients could be ignored. Indeed, this is what we often do in practice with hemodialysis because we have decided that, for the most part, even a little benefit may be enough to justify the use of this expensive technology. But we do not have that "luxury" with solid organs, and discriminating (though not discriminatory) decisions—sometime tragic ones—must be made.[17]

That being said, significant efforts have been made to try to level the access playing field in order to counteract some of the existing inequities in healthcare delivery in the United States (especially in advanced, technologically sophisticated care). Not surprisingly, disparities in entry into the system and then eligibility for transplantation mirror those found throughout the medical system (Patzer et al. 2012; Mathur et al. 2011; Amaral, Patzer, Kutner, and McClellan 2012; Kucirka et al. 2012; Thabut et al. 2012; Wells 2009; Joshi et al. 2013; Mathur et al. 2010; Norris and Agodoa 2012; Patzer and Pastan 2013). Indeed, much of the recent discussion about revising the prioritization scheme for cadaveric kidney transplant is centered on making the system more fair (by changing the weighting between social and personal stewardship), especially to those most affected by end-stage renal disease, while at the same time trying to maximize the overall benefit (number of lives and number of years saved) (Segev 2009; Ladin and Hanto 2011; Norris and Agodoa 2012; Poli et al. 2000; Hippen, Thistlethwaite, and Ross 2011; Reese and Caplan 2011). Some deference is paid to what some might describe as the worst off (in a patient population where everyone is of course "worst off" in one sense), which also supports the intuitive opinions of both patients and healthy people obtained from surveys (Ayanian et al. 2004; Kroeker et al. 2008; Secunda et al. 2012; Stahl, Tramontano, Swan, and Cohen 2008; Tong et al. 2013; Ubel and Loewenstein 1996).

On the other hand, the strain between the dual goals of transplant is once again brought to the fore, since one could easily argue that the sickest patients may not be the ones who could best benefit from transplant; there is such a thing as being too sick, where patients with preexisting comorbidities as well as those that are brought about by the state of prolonged organ failure may predispose them to a poor outcome after transplantation. Hence "sickest first" may not be the best use of such a rare resource. And again, the vast array of expensive medications, psychosocial support, frequent clinic visits, and costly transportation required in order to not jeopardize the viability of the organ after surgery, are themselves often a barrier to transplant for those without insurance or those whose other resources are insufficient. In the absence of a comprehensive, universal healthcare system that can help defray some of these costs, very often organ transplantation is unavailable to many patients from lower socioeconomic strata.[18] Short of a total reform of healthcare in the United States, these inequities are likely to remain.[19]

Nevertheless, this balancing of the inevitable tension between the often-competing and frequently incompatible—if not contradictory—goals of a public transplantation system that is applied uniquely to "private" individual patients, is a constant work in progress. Deciding which should have precedence—the needs of a patient versus the demand by society that this communally derived, "owned," and distributed resource be used responsibly to benefit the most people for the longest period of time—is an unceasing medical and moral struggle. Doctors are naturally inclined to be the strongest advocates for advancing and securing the health and well-being of their own patients, an objective that can be at odds with systemwide aims. Indeed, many of the reforms of prioritization that have been introduced over the years have attempted to counteract the individualistic and parochial advocacy (however well intentioned it might be) of physicians who are only trying to fulfill their professional duty to their patients.[20]

All of this is well and good and suggests that most of the people and organizations involved in solid-organ transplant in the United States are trying to do their best to achieve a reasonable balance between equity and efficiency. But how do patients and potential patients (or potential donors) view their efforts? Is the system acceptable only because there is no choice if they want to live? Do people simply tolerate how things work, applying a public veneer of perhaps grudging acquiescence because the circumstances are so grave (an ever-worsening shortage of organs available for transplant and gravely ill, dying patients and their families desperate for a chance to live)? Or are the rules viewed as reasonably fair, with the occasional "gaming" and manipulation of the system by the rich and powerful (see chapter 3) taken to be somewhat anomalous and thus not a threat to the overall impartiality and justice of the methodology?

Significantly, a number of surveys of the public (and of many patients, including those on the waiting list for organs—i.e., those whose lives hang in the balance) report that they view the system by and large as fair, even with the publicity surrounding cheaters, gamers of the system, and others who might threaten the legitimacy of the allocation procedures factored in (although there are exceptions) (Tong et al. 2010; Neuberger 2007, 2012; Neuberger et al. 1998; Volk et al. 2011). This does not translate into overwhelming support for organ *donation*—as measured by the absolute quantity of organs available and the omnipresent challenge to increase donation rates. Many members of minority groups, such as African Americans, are very reluctant to participate in a system that requires the death of a patient in order to function (Boulware et al. 2002; Bratton, Chavin, and Baliga 2011; Davis et al. 2005; Randall 1996; Siminoff, Burant, and Ibrahim 2006; Siminoff, Lawrence, and Arnold 2003). Since the declaration of death is almost always in the hands of a physician, the best donors are those declared dead by whole-brain criteria. And since patients who are brain dead are still physiologically alive (and more important, certainly look alive to the uninitiated and even to experts), it is not surprising that people who may not implicitly trust the medical system would be reluctant to permit the withdrawal of intensive-care support under emotionally trying circumstances from someone who is still warm, breathing and has a beating heart.

In sum, my reading of the relevant literature suggests an interesting dichotomous—even schizophrenic—situation in which similar or identical groups of people seemingly accept the allocation and receipt of organs as fair enough, but the collection of them as deeply suspect. Of course this cannot be taken as a blanket statement, applicable to all ethnic and potential donor groups, but the ability to increase the number of available donor organs has proven stubbornly resistant to attempts to dispel commonly held opinions about the motivations of doctors and organizations charged with harvesting organs, by and large due to recalcitrant populations that appear immune to persuasion. At the same time, the transplant process itself has apparently become more fair (although this should not be taken to imply that all is well and that substantial work does not still need to be done to reduce or eliminate lingering disparities in both access and outcome).

Even with these qualifiers noted, the conditions of organ rationing may offer us a lesson in how to use resources judiciously, even wisely. The system is viewed as just, and while tinkering with it is an ongoing process that continues to yield improvements, the reluctance of certain people to become donors or to permit the donation of organs from their dead relatives is due less to mistrust in the rationing component (the prioritization and allocation part) of transplantation, than it is to a deeply ingrained, culturally determined, and an historically not unreasonable suspicion of the aims of organ harvesting. While the latter remains a problem to be overcome, the former offers strong support for my argument that ethical rationing is not only feasible but can be accomplished without the taint of maleficence believed inherent in all healthcare rationing schemes.

Drug Shortages

In late December 2010, the central pharmacy at my hospital was notified by its main wholesale distributer of drugs that there was an unexpected and severe nationwide shortage of cytarabine, a chemotherapy agent critical in the treatment of childhood acute lymphoblastic leukemia (ALL), adult and pediatric acute myelogenous leukemia (AML), and some lymphomas. While not the only drug used in the therapy of these diseases, it plays an essential role in the combinations of medications that can be curative. In the case of pediatric ALL, cure rates as high as 85 percent overall can be achieved and the integration of cytarabine into the complex regimens of multiagent therapy is a major component of this approach (Pui, Mullighan, Evans, and Relling 2012). In AML, the outcomes are not nearly as good as with childhood ALL, especially in adults, but remarkable improvements have occurred over the last twenty years and once again, cytarabine has contributed significantly to this success (Lichtman 2001; Lange et al. 2008; Tsukimoto et al. 2009). These diseases generally present with a rapid clinical onset with patients being acutely ill and often needing intensive care; treatment must be initiated as soon as a diagnosis has been established. Moreover, cytarabine is used not only in the initial treatment of AML, ALL, and lymphoma (the "induction" phase), but throughout the treatment plan, which, in the case of childhood ALL, can last up to three years. Thus, we would need a constant and reliable supply of this drug to treat new patients we expected to come in as well as those currently in treatment.

At a meeting of pharmacists and many of the oncology physicians who took care of patients with these disorders, we were informed that our remaining stock would last no more than ten days if we continued to use it at the rate we had demonstrated over the last year or so. There was no information about when the ordinary commercial supply of this intravenous generic (or brand-name) drug would resume; it was thought that it could be a matter of months at a minimum. While we were fortunate in having our own compounding pharmacy and could thus formulate cytarabine ourselves, we would still need to bring in the raw material from England, and for this we would need a special waiver from the Food and Drug Administration (FDA). Furthermore, the strict standard we followed to ensure the sterility and stability of the compounded drug required that the formulated preparation be observed and tested for fourteen days to guarantee its safety. Thus, the earliest we could expect to have the cytarabine available for our patients would be in two to three weeks (with luck and assuming the FDA would grant us permission to import a supply of cytarabine precursor material). And, of course, the situation was made even graver by the fact that all of this was occurring right before the Christmas and New Year's holidays when life seems to slow to a crawl, but people still get sick with startling regularity. What should we do in the interim? How should we allocate the small amount of cytarabine we had remaining?

This is a classic rationing problem. Drug shortages are seemingly a relatively new phenomenon but they have been occurring with increasing frequency over the past ten years or so. The causes are complex, probably interrelated, and to date stubbornly immune to simple structural remedies. Thus, healthcare organizations, doctors, pharmacists, and patients have been faced with an intractable challenge with little to no guidance from almost any source. While it is true that the American Association of Health System Pharmacists (AAHSP) has waged an often-lonely battle over this issue, publishing some suggestions and guidelines on how pharmacies may cope with shortages, these have failed to gain wider acceptance (Baumer et al. 2004; Fox and Tyler 2003; Kaakeh et al. 2011). Unlike the long-standing national and universal system for allocating solid organs that has been in place (and evolving) with extensive publicity and reasonable transparency, methods for rationing suddenly scarce medications have been rare or nonexistent. And, except for occasionally alarmist news reports describing the potentially catastrophic and heart-rending effects of desperate patients not receiving life-saving drugs, these problems have pretty much stayed under the radar.

Fortunately, I had started examining these very issues several months before this event and had come to some conclusions about how we might fairly and effectively prioritize patients (Rosoff 2012b). However, we had neither tested this approach nor discussed how we could generate a consistent institutional procedure. This was a secondary high-priority issue that would demand our attention once we figured out how to deal with the cytarabine shortage, especially since unpredictable and potentially long-lasting drug scarcities looked to be with us for some time. Indeed, one of the first major shortages had occurred thirteen years earlier (there had been many more in the interim) with a human serum–derived product called intravenous immunoglobulin (IV IgG), demonstrating that this was by no means an isolated incident or a new problem (Boulis, Goold, and Ubel 2002; Jensen and Rappaport 2010; Gehrett 2012; Kaakeh et al. 2011).

The framework we developed was based in large part on Daniels and Sabin's "accountability for reasonableness" approach that I discuss in greater detail in the next chapter. It was vetted and approved by the various hospital committees that need to authorize these things, but importantly, the community members of the ethics committee also reviewed it. While there are only two such individuals and they can hardly substitute for a widespread canvassing of opinions and views of the local, regional, national, and even international populations served by our institution, we decided that they could serve this function (as they had in the past with other policy reviews). One additional point deserves notice now and I will discuss it again in greater detail in later chapters (especially chapters 3 and 4). We prioritized patients to receive scarce drugs on the basis of scientific evidence for efficacy, eliminating eligibility for those "indications" that were unsupported by reasonable and statistically significant clinical data. Surprisingly, in a medical system that permits—indeed often encourages—the almost unfettered liberty of physicians to prescribe what they want to whom they want for whatever they want (Rosoff and Coleman 2011), this approach was accepted without controversy or objection. It was not viewed as an abridgement of the practice of medicine. We have recently published our initial experience using this procedure, which was largely favorable (Rosoff et al. 2012).

However, there are some significant caveats. First, this was a policy developed for a single institution, and was not even applied at the two other hospitals in our health system, one a large and the other a small community hospital. There was virtually no coordination with other institutions in the immediate geographic area, not to mention the state (this has not necessarily been for lack of desire or effort). Thus, there was no attempt to pool resources or share essential information, as there is in a better-developed rationing approach, like organ transplantation. Of course, there was (is) no reason to suspect that this approach could not be implemented more broadly in multiple facilities.[21] Second, there were substantive challenges that have not yet been encountered, but undoubtedly will be, and for which a comprehensive decision-making process has not been developed. Examples include a so-called tragic choice of having a single dose of a critical drug and two or more patients who could benefit from receiving it (this is the kind of situation facing organ transplanters every day). Or whether the young should be prioritized over the old(er), an approach that satisfies an inherent moral intuition held by many (Emanuel and Wertheimer 2006; Cropper, Aydede, and Portney 1992, 1994; Eisenberg et al. 2011; Li, Vietri, Galvani, and Chapman 2010). As a third example, should preference in access to scarce medications be given to patients who live in traditional referral areas or close to the institution rather than farther away? In this last case, attention must be paid to what we might term "pharmaceutical tourists," those patients who have acquired information on the availability of the drug(s) they need and have the means to travel to an institution they have reason to believe possesses sufficient quantity to treat them.[22]

Some problems were less issues of individual patient-centered decision making and more at the institutional level. We made a strict decision to not access the so-called gray market in drugs because of the inability to verify the chain of custody or provenance (manufacturing origin) of the material.[23] We could also not address the issue of "hoarding" by which some hospitals would try to stockpile much more of a drug than they could use (for instance, generic intravenous chemotherapy agents that could possibly become scarce). If the entire supply available to all were limited, then overaccumulation by some would necessarily restrict how much was accessible by others. This asymmetrical (presumably geographic) maldistribution of a scarce resource could have the potential to disproportionately affect rural and less wealthy institutions and hence their patients. In the absence of some form of organized and collaborative system among hospitals, pharmacies, independent physicians and practice groups, and others, it seems pointless to make up rules for each institution by itself. They could easily differ in major ways, leading to large inconsistencies in application that could in turn yield crucial differences in potentially life-saving interventions.

Almost all of these matters most likely could be resolved by an appeal to a comprehensive, nationwide approach. (Indeed, the piecemeal and uncoordinated methods employed throughout the country underscore the significant obstacles associated with rationing done in this way.) Of course, it is highly implausible that the federal government (specifically, Congress) would grant the FDA the power to "nationalize" the drug supply to prevent shortages from occurring in the first place. But there are other ways they could create incentives for generic manufacturers to devote more resources to minimizing the chances of unexpected scarcities, or ways they could encourage more companies to go into the business, thus creating fewer single-source producers of drugs that leave patients extraordinarily susceptible to disruptions in the supply chain.[24]

As Callahan (2009, 144) has noted: "Our first and most fundamental challenge is to understand the way the value of individual self-definition makes the larger task of system reform all but impossible but also why that value cannot be changed without a simultaneous organizational change." He is describing the primacy of individualism in American culture, in which we get to define what we want and what we need for ourselves. This is a relatively recent phenomenon in healthcare and can be associated with the sharp decline in physician paternalism (in which decisions were made for patients by their kind and benevolent doctors) and the primacy in medical education of the principle of patient autonomy. This has often been interpreted as minimizing the advisory role of the physician

and empowering the role and clout of patients (and their surrogate decision makers), not infrequently with unfortunate consequences (Quill and
Brody 1996; Lantos, Matlock, and Wendler 2011; Sutrop 2011). Furthermore, Callahan is using this observation to highlight the ways patients
view their needs with respect to medical technology. Curiously, though, it
is relatively absent from situations in which rationing is not a choice but a
requirement because of absolute resource constraints; patients (and their
doctors) cannot define what their needs are.

In summary, while I cannot empirically address whether our experience
at a large academic medical center could be widely applicable throughout
the country on a more systemic level, we have been gratified to observe
that our rationing approach has been well received. This is particularly
significant in that the audience that must endorse and embrace this approach for it to be successful is both large and exceedingly diverse, composed as it is of physicians, nurses, administrators, pharmacists, and most
importantly, patients and their families, all of whom represent widely heterogeneous constituencies, backgrounds, moral viewpoints, and biases.
The fact that this rationing method has been accepted by this population
and has also been adopted at some other institutions suggests a large degree of agreement with a situation and a method of dealing with it that
necessarily entails the possibility of winners and losers, analogous to that
in organ transplantation. So, once again we have an example (imperfect,
perhaps, but close enough) of explicit rationing that people have found
tolerable *as* rationing. But, as is the case with organ transplantation, this
affirmation owes a significant debt to the fact that it is unavoidable.
However, it is reasonable to think that at least some of its acceptance by
stakeholders is due to its inherent fairness in application.

Oregon

I have briefly introduced and discussed the rationing system in Oregon
in the prior chapter, but now I wish to present it in greater depth as an
example of an accepted and explicit rationing plan (albeit imperfect).[25] In
the late 1980s the state of Oregon saw the conjunction of several otherwise unconnected events. First, like most states, their population of marginally poor people without medical insurance was expanding (a sad fact
that has continued to this day both locally and nationally); these were
individuals and families who could not otherwise qualify for coverage
in their Medicaid program. Second, John Kitzhaber was the president
of the state senate. A physician by training, he was keenly aware of this

problem and also possessed an acute moral sense that this was wrong and ill-served the people and state of Oregon. He also saw that it would be possible to include many, if not most, of the uninsured people and control the spiraling costs of the Medicaid program (like healthcare costs in general, it experiences annual inflation rates well above that of the general rise in the cost of living) by limiting (i.e., rationing) what Medicaid would pay for by restricting coverage to the most beneficial interventions medicine had to offer. This way, two primary aims could be met: the ranks of people without access to healthcare could be dramatically reduced at the same time that a broad array of basic healthcare services were made available to the newly expanded patient population. However, the only way to accomplish this goal would be by capping the total Medicaid budget up front and controlling the kinds of medical and diagnostic interventions offered.[26] Therefore, the primary limited resource would be money, because they took the "budget-first" approach I introduced in chapter 1.

Kitzhaber was very successful in persuading both his legislative colleagues and the governor to enact this legislation. There are two signature aspects of the Oregon Health Plan (OHP). First, it was and remains a unique experiment in "top-down," population-wide rationing: a funding body (in this case the legislature) decided how much to spend on healthcare for the poor and near poor for a given budget period, and an independent review board was constituted to figure out the most cost-efficient and health-efficient way to buy the greatest amount for the greatest number of patients. This is an excellent model of reasonable, planned rationing in its purest form. Second, it is the primary example of up-front budgetary rationing that determines what healthcare is available, as opposed to letting the amount of healthcare delivered determine the total cost.

One of the initial obstacles to implementing the OHP into actual practice was how the Oregon Health Services Commission went about constructing "the list" of what would be covered once the finite budget was set. In other words, as soon as the legislature decided how much the state (and they) were willing to spend on comprehensive healthcare for poor people, it was left to the commission to figure what could be "bought" for this amount of money. This is in contrast to the way the American health system works for most people, where services, procedures, machines, devices, salaries, and so on are bought first, with relatively less attention paid to what the final outlay will be (at least initially).

Of course, if one approaches the problem the way Oregon did, then there is a lot riding on exactly how one goes about creating the list; different methods will yield different results, as they found much to their and the public's initial dismay. Not surprisingly perhaps, they started by using a strictly utilitarian strategy—cost-effectiveness analysis (CEA)—which takes a population approach to maximizing the balance between benefit (commonly expressed as "quality-adjusted life years" or QALYs) and unit cost (Eddy 1986; Weinstein and Stason 1977; Eddy 1992a,b,c; Robinson 1993; Mitton and Donaldson 2004; Garber and Phelps 1997; Acharya et al. 2003). There are many advantages to this technique, not least of which is that it is relatively straightforward to apply (assuming that reasonable effectiveness data are available) and it is quantitative, permitting a simple rank ordering of medical interventions from more to less beneficial (for the cost). When coupled with known epidemiological and demographic data on the incidence and prevalence of various medical conditions in a given population with a known age distribution, one can reasonably calculate what can be "bought" for a given amount of money.

Strictly applied, this calculus can end up concluding that relieving suffering or pain for a large number of people for relatively little cost per unit of relief is better than saving the life of one person, especially if the latter is very expensive. So, as Peter Ubel put in the title of his book, this approach is a method of "pricing life" or costing out how much a life is worth, not to the individual whose life is in question, but to everyone else considered as a whole. It is a summative calculus of welfare, advantage, or utility, and not any isolated benefit accruing to one person (Ubel 2001). However, there was a major problem that the commission did not account for: *individual* people get sick—mothers, fathers, sons, and daughters—who together comprise anonymous populations, but separately are identifiable and evoke what Jonsen (1986) has called the "rule of rescue."[27] Furthermore, even a superficial analysis of how conditions were ranked demonstrated how a strict adherence to CEA can violate our intuitive understanding of the relative value and importance of particular life-saving treatments (although not necessarily *all* life-saving therapies). For example, surgery for acute appendicitis, a potentially life-threatening emergency, was considered less cost-effective, and hence listed lower, that certain dental procedures or treatment for temporomandibular joint pain.[28] It was the story of a single child's plight that also threw a major wrench into the plan to use CEA by itself to construct a viable list of covered conditions.

Briefly, the rule of rescue recognizes a psychological empathic impulse that all humans have (presumably excepting those with psychopathy) to feel compassion for people who are identified, usually with a face and name. We find ourselves overwhelmed when confronted with the enormity of the tragedy of the Japanese tsunami of 2011, with thousands dead and even more thousands homeless and affected by the spreading radiation. But we feel a general and moderated form of sympathy, not the kind of strong, internally wrenching reaction we have when we hear about a toddler who has fallen down a well or an intellectually disabled teenager who has wandered off into the woods and cannot be found. Think about how the story of the trapped Chilean miners held the attention of millions as the world awaited word of their rescue in 2010.[29]

And it was this irresistible, instinctual, and highly emotional sense that was aroused in Oregon when the story of Coby Howard was splashed all over the front pages and the 6 o'clock news (Hadorn 1991).[30] As I noted in the previous chapter, Coby was a seven-year-old boy who had been diagnosed with acute lymphoblastic leukemia in the mid-1980s. At that time the chance of a cure with standard therapy for newly diagnosed disease was about 70 percent (Novakovic 1994). However, if it recurred, the only hope for a cure would have been a bone marrow transplant, but this therapy was not one of the condition-treatment pairs that made the final list of covered services in the OHP, the insurance that Coby and his mother had. From here, the story continues:

In the autumn of 1987, seven-year-old Coby Howard's leukemia came out of remission. A bone marrow transplant would give the Oregon boy a 20 percent chance of surviving, but Coby's mom was unemployed and on welfare, and Medicaid would not pay for the $100,000 procedure. The Howards' friends and neighbors tried to raise the money through bowl-a-thons and garage sales. The local press ran regular "Coby Howard updates." Amid all the attention, Coby Howard became an unwilling celebrity. The patrons at a restaurant even pressed him to get up on stage and sing "Rudolph the Red-Nosed Reindeer"! By the scheduled date of the operation, November 25, the Howards had raised enough money to go ahead with the surgery, but leukemia cells had spread through Coby's bone marrow.[31] The operation was postponed, the cancer never went back into remission, and Coby Howard died in his mother's arms on December 2. Several other Medicaid patients were also affected by Oregon's new policy. Donna Arneson needed a liver transplant. Her 14-year-old son Evan appeared before the state legislature, pleading with them to "save my mom." This spurred the "Save a Mom" campaign, complete with posters and videos, which raised enough money to pay for the operation. Two-year-old David Holladay needed a bone marrow transplant. His mom packed the entire family into a pickup truck and moved to Washington State, which pays for organ transplants and has no minimum residency requirement for Medicaid. Another woman needing a liver transplant went to San Francisco, where a hospital performed it free of charge. (Dranove 2003, 120–121)

Not only do these heartrending stories stimulate our rescue "instinct," they also show how this sometimes-overwhelming emotional state can be manipulated to obtain something for someone that may or may not be warranted. Most of us who have worked in large hospitals can tell stories of patients who have been denied some form of diagnostic test or treatment (by their insurance company or the institution) and have threatened to "go public" by contacting the local newspapers and TV stations. Most of the time this form of pressure by publicity is a very effective means of obtaining what they want and the insurance company or hospital relents rather than undergo trial in the court of public opinion.[32] This strategy takes advantage of the rule of rescue for individuals and groups to single-mindedly advance their own agenda, irrespective of other considerations. And indeed it had this effect in Oregon, which went on to revise its list, partially in response to the furor over Coby's story and the heartless OHP. This could prove a significant obstacle for any kind of future rationing, although it is important to note that the organ transplant system seems to have mostly avoided this problem.[33]

An interesting point arises from the manner in which the final list of conditions and treatments was constructed. After the initial fiasco, it was modified to not take cost into primary account (that came later when the legislature had to decide how much money to devote to the program). Rather, it was an exercise in assessing relative benefit to individuals, and that in turn was at least in part based on scientific evidence (when available) in support of efficacy. Unfortunately, if one were willing to stretch one's definition of what constitutes evidence for effective therapy, this could endorse many interventions that offer only marginal or very minimal help or relief to people.

Obviously, as I have considered previously, one of the main reasons we are discussing general healthcare rationing is that we do not have enough money (or don't want to have enough money) to pay for everything that could conceivably be of some benefit to some people. Therefore, we have to draw the line somewhere (this is part of the "cutoff problem" I discuss in chapter 4). With a limited budget, we will inevitably confront the issue of the financial value of a life or of some forms of human suffering. This unavoidably raises the difficult questions of how little benefit is too little, or how much is too much to pay for a life? This can be answered in two ways. First, there are some interventions that can't benefit anyone (i.e., that are physiologically or medically futile), and it seems clear that we shouldn't pay for these; this is relatively noncontroversial. Second, there are those that are of such questionable or minimal or marginal benefit to anyone or to only a small number of people, that under plausible rationing conditions, it would be reasonable (or not unreasonable) to seriously consider not paying for these: any benefit that might exist would be too small for too few people to matter (except, perhaps, to them).[34] It is the latter that would require careful public scrutiny and (democratic) discussion to figure out where to draw the line (Fleck 2009).[35] Of course this will not be easy, especially in America.[36] However, in Oregon, due to the limitations of the budget and the way the "list" was constructed, even those condition-treatment pairs near the very bottom would undoubtedly be considered more beneficial than those interventions that would fall in this latter case.

Another interesting and relevant point is that the main force behind the law, then State Senator Kitzhaber, viewed this program as a start to create a basic minimum of healthcare for all Oregonians, and then the nation. This worried many people, especially in the private sector, who saw it as an attempt to socialize medical care and a demand that they expand the coverage of their employees. The assumption was that whatever was on the "list" would be a de facto definition of a "basic minimum of health care" (Fox and Leichter 1991). On the other hand, since the amount and kinds of healthcare that would be available from the list would in large part be contingent on the generosity of the budget passed by the legislature, the system could expand or contract depending on who was voting during any given budget period. Indeed, since state senators and representatives come and go, especially at the whims of voters who may have widely divergent opinions on how their tax dollars are spent, it is possible—if not probable—that the amount of money used to fund the OHP could fluctuate widely. So whether the fundable condition-treatment pairs go down to number 600 or 500 or even 400 would in large part be determined by politics.[37] It seems that this is an incoherent way to define what constitutes essential healthcare for the poor citizens or Oregon, or anywhere else for that matter.

A cogent lesson from the Oregon tale is that the process used to construct any priority list will be challenging and will undoubtedly require careful review, analysis, and revision to reflect both impersonal population (public health) and individual benefits, costs (both financial and intangible), and tolerability. This last will also have to merge with a consideration of societal justice (see chapter 6). The Oregonians affected by the OHP had limited ability to voice meaningful objections since they are essentially voiceless: they are the poor and powerless. They are Mitt Romney's "47%."[38] They did not have a significant impact on either how much was spent or the way it was spent. If they wanted health insurance (and most people do), they must accept what they got. The coverage decisions were made by people who by and large were not affected by those decisions.[39] While it is true that state law required all meetings of the OHP administration to be open to the public, thus enhancing transparency, it was reasonable to assume that attendance at these events was not appreciably greater than at similar gatherings of other government commissions.[40] This erodes legitimacy and diminishes the broad public warrant for this program. Thus, this could not work as a general program for the entire country. But it's a decent starting point. Moreover, even though Coby Howard revealed one of the major flaws in the system, he and his mother did take advantage of the media, which is occasionally a great leveler between rich and poor, offering a voice to the often voiceless. And these events occurred well before the advent of social media that provide even more venues for people to make their perceived injustices known. Nevertheless, the frequency of Coby Howard–like cases has been quite low, which could suggest that the recipients of the OHP insurance are reasonably satisfied (or possibly that they have no choice but to acquiesce).

One final point should be made. Not surprisingly, anything as enterprising and novel as the OHP is going to have both its critics and advocates. In addition, it would be naive to think that everything could have worked out the way it was supposed to, seeing as the economy and politicians have their ups and downs and come and go, so the degree to which the plan would adhere to its original expectations could vary depending on the generosity or stinginess of the state legislature funding the plan, among other factors. For some time Jonathan Oberlander has been a vocal critic of the vaulting ambitions of the OHP. He has argued that those (mostly enthusiasts) who view the OHP as a shining example of unvarnished (and largely successful) comprehensive rationing are in error. He has suggested that the OHP has not saved much money, perhaps because it expanded coverage to so many people who previously were ineligible for Medicaid insurance, because of its susceptibility to a form of gaming by doctors (see chapter 3), and because the list of covered condition-treatment pairs was quite generous (his words). Finally, over time, much of the original intent has been unfulfilled due to a variety of exogenous influences (Oberlander 2007; Oberlander, Marmor, and Jacobs 2001).

That being said, his (valid) criticism doesn't mean that the OHP was/is not rationing, just that perhaps the original goals were a bit too high. More important for the purposes of my argument, though, is that the Oregon experiment demonstrated that it is possible to construct a list that is quite generous, and to do so while keeping healthcare expenditures under control and making the list reasonably publicly palatable (with the caveats that I have already discussed). This should give us some hope that larger-scale experiments of the same type, incorporating the lessons learned from the Oregon experiment, might be applicable elsewhere in the country and in populations that would be trading their current health insurance for something else.

On the other hand, Oberlander's analysis of how the OHP was so susceptible to shifting political and budgetary whims, as well as to the overly optimistic calculations of presumptive beneficiaries' behavior, should be taken as a warning for future planners of healthcare overhaul systems. Somehow something as integral to human well-being as basic healthcare should be made to be reasonably immune to the vicissitudes of local elected officials or even members of Congress. Finally, as Oberlander also points out, even if the OHP worked perfectly, it would have had no impact on medical inflation, because it was still based on a fee-for-service payment plan that rewards doctors and institutions when they do more stuff. Until healthcare delivery is attacked from multiple directions, and restraints imposed on some of the perverse incentives that encourage doctors and hospitals to order more operations, tests, expensive drugs, and the like (all of which reap more income and profit for the sellers and prescribers), rationing by itself may not be capable of limiting the costs of healthcare, unless it is so harshly restrictive in what benefits it offers that no one would endorse it. A point I stress throughout this book is that one of the key circumstances that would permit rationing to be broadly acceptable in the United States would be its generosity, coupled with reasonable limits. An analysis of the benefits of the OHP experienced by its most vulnerable recipients suggests that it did quite a bit of good, which is encouraging to those who argue (as I do) that rationing does not have to be a bad thing (Baicker and Finkelstein 2011).

Conclusion

It has become accepted wisdom in the United States that our ever-escalating healthcare costs must be controlled in some fashion. Planned rationing is a commonly discussed approach to reining in the unrestrained healthcare budget. At the same time, rationing could have the associated beneficial effect of restricting access to treatments, diagnostic tests, and other interventions that have been shown to be either ineffective or of so little advantage to patients that they cannot and should not be offered. Since a significant percentage of total healthcare costs are spent in the last six months of life in the pursuit of mostly hopeless cures, it seems reasonable to look there (and elsewhere) for ways to limit some potentially futile therapies (Angus et al. 2004; Jox, Schaider, Marckmann, and Borasio 2012; Scheunemann and White 2011; Zhang et al. 2009; Kravitz and Feldman 2010; Riley and Lubitz 2010). But one of the main obstacles to open discussion of rationing has been the common understanding that rationing could never work in the United States because people would never accept or even tolerate it, especially when it is explicitly labeled as rationing. Commentators have even been warned to refer to rationing using less emotionally laden terms, such as priority setting or other such euphemisms, because of the negative reactions that instantly arise once the topic is broached (Matas 2009; Truog 2009b).

In this chapter, I have presented two well-known and one less well-known examples of explicit rationing systems that are ongoing in the United States—systems that are tolerated and even accepted as necessary and reasonably fair. Even though all three have some problems in application (several of which are significant), they are by and large considered satisfactory responses to widely different and very challenging conditions. As long as we continue to be successful with organ transplants and expand the possible clinical indications for these procedures, the number of potentially eligible patients will also continue to increase, making rationing inescapable. While unpredictable drug shortages may be thought to be a relatively recent problem, they are not, and it is unlikely that the market and other conditions that are the most common causes of shortages will be altered any time soon, making rationing once again inevitable. Finally, the OHP is an explicit rationing procedure with the dual goals of controlling Medicaid costs and expanding the number of patients covered, and it was moderately effective in accomplishing these aims.[41] All three approaches use rationing as a way of solving problems (but are perhaps more successful at revealing the difficulties and challenges of designing and implementing such a program).

Even though the effect of not receiving organs is almost certain death, the risk of not being treated with a vital drug could be similarly catastrophic, and poor people in Oregon have had to accept limits on the availability of some types of treatments, these three methods have become part of our healthcare landscape, integrated into the mix of patient care with relatively minimal objections. Unlike the explosive public debate about rationing in general, these unambiguous and transparent rationing schemes have raised little rancor or anger. The obvious question is why. What is it about existing explicit rationing systems that has instilled trust and reliance on the part of patients, their families, and doctors, even under the most trying and frequently tragic circumstances? What was it about the proposals for allocating scarce initial supplies of influenza vaccine in 2009 (in anticipation of an expected worldwide pandemic) that engendered confidence that the vaccine would be given out fairly?

One answer might be that at least some of the populations affected by these rationing plans—organ-failure patients and poor Oregonians—are unique in that they really have no choice in the matter. In the one case, if they want a chance of having a transplant, or in the other, if they want any healthcare at all, they must participate in the system. Their desperation makes them uniquely susceptible to enforced rationing, which doesn't seem to be a particularly admirable way of imposing a reasonable and morally defensible system on people. In the other situation I have described—that of allocating scarce drugs—the population is potentially desperate and, to a certain extent, they are similar to transplant patients and poor Oregonians, in that their choices are limited in the extreme, but the prioritization procedure is newer and has yet to be implemented in the wider healthcare system. Even so, these people are more or less at the mercy of those who control the supply of available drugs. So, one trivial response to my questions is that the fact that these patients accept what is offered in terms of rationing is only because the alternative is to go without.

But all three systems have also gone to great pains to design allocation and priority methods that are as fair as they can make them. Indeed, in Oregon, one of the motivating factors behind creating the OHP was to define a basic minimum of healthcare, not only for the poor, but presumably for everyone. Now a minimum is perhaps not what we should be satisfied with, and no one would argue that a more equitable and fair distribution of healthcare dollars to everyone in a wealthy country like the United States would leave people with a minimalist version of medical care. Indeed, it is likely that if we just spent what we do now in a more rational way, or even what many comparable European countries spend per capita, we would be able to deliver considerably more than some minimum (actually, very much more). Both transplant specialists and the state of Oregon are continually attempting to make access and allocation more transparent and more just, within the constraints of what they have to work with. And, as far as we can tell, recipients are credibly and reasonably satisfied with what they have, even when they have not necessarily gotten what they wanted. Admittedly, the Coby Howard story grabbed headlines, but it is arguably an outlier, one that we know about solely because of the publicity surrounding the events. While it may be unfair to accuse desperate patients or their relatives of gaming the system, there no doubt will always be people who will take advantage of the system, by preying on our rule-of-rescue sensibilities to obtain what they ordinarily would not be eligible for (and even poor people can call the newspapers and TV stations or engage public sympathies via social media; indeed, some might argue that this may be the only method available to the weak and powerless). That should simply strengthen our resolve to make the system more resilient and less vulnerable to being taken advantage of in these situations. In truth, the organ transplant system seems mostly immune to these kinds of strategies, although as I will discuss in chapter 3, it still has a way to go before it becomes immune to being gamed (but it has made significant progress over the last twenty years or so).

Even with these caveats, I think that these three examples demonstrate that very different kinds of rationing systems can be designed to be reasonably fair and actually work in a way that is mostly fair, or at least fair enough. And while we can quibble about whether the sole reason they are accepted so well is due to the captive populations they affect, I suspect that is not the sole reason. After all, most people with private health insurance are covered under some sort of rationing scheme as well; they can only use some doctors and not others, some hospitals and not others, some drugs and not others, and so on. And while surveys suggest that most insured people are satisfied with their healthcare, these questionnaires rarely ask about the details of the plan (or the fact that very often people are happy just to be covered at all). Furthermore, if these surveys are performed in an atmosphere in which many believe their insurance is threatened with being taken away (by the Affordable Care Act, for example), people only naturally want to hold on to what they have (even if they could possibly do better), in the spirit of "I may not like it, but at least it's mine." People can accept rationing if it is done openly, if it is done with their input, and if it is seen as fair and hence legitimate. I have discussed three examples of just that, and there is no reason to think that a nationwide system could not be similarly designed and implemented *given the will to do so.*

In the chapters that follow I introduce some important features that should be components of any sensible, generous rationing scheme that could be applied more broadly in this country. These characteristics are drawn from deeper conceptions of the moral foundations of what would be reasonable to attempt to accomplish with a comprehensive healthcare system. They also represent the limits of what can be achieved in a pluralistic democracy, with a widely diverse population in which many different views of what should be offered and to whom are expressed. More important, they represent attributes of rationing that would be essential to make it palatable to a skeptical public. First I consider the singular importance of fairness in any approach to rationing. Fairness is a central tenet of all existing rationing systems, including the examples I have given in this chapter.

3
Fairness

In the previous chapters I have introduced some general concepts about healthcare rationing and several of the challenges, especially psychological, that would be potential barriers to overcome in any attempt to convince people that embracing rationing would be in their best interest. However, since the reaction to discussions of rationing are often laden with fairly distraught emotions, often stoked by interest groups who believe they stand to lose something of significance should a universal healthcare system with rationing be implemented, it is also important to discuss other features of any plausible rationing scheme that would help make it palatable to anyone who is sufficiently open-minded to consider the possibility. I began this process in the previous chapter with my presentation of the organ transplantation system (and several other rationing frameworks) that is clearly endorsed by a wide portion of the public (at least by those who could conceive of themselves or a relative or friend becoming an organ recipient). Of course, if one wants an organ one has no choice but to accept the way they are distributed. However, I would suggest that it is not simply the presence of what might be described as a Hobson's-choice situation that could lead to a false affirmation and trust in the system;[1] it is not a veneer of allegiance that undergirds the system's acceptability in the mind of the public and the physicians, nurses, and others whose participation is vital for the structure to function. Rather, it is a true trust in the integrity of the allocation methods and the way they are created and modified (as I discuss in more detail later in this chapter) that endows it with the legitimacy that it has. Indeed, if the circumstances surrounding organ transplantation access and allocation truly were a Hobson's choice where, unlike the eponymous Mr. Hobson's stable where the only penalty for refusing to abide by the coercive rules was the lack of a horse to rent, not accepting the strictures of organ transplant (whatever they may happen to be) results in death. Hence, the temptation to simplify the regulations and governance—perhaps to openly favor the socially well connected or the wealthy at the expense of others—could be considerable. But such is not the case. In point of fact, as I have described, a great deal of effort is devoted to attempting to reduce disparities and enhance fairness for fairly laudable and praiseworthy reasons: not because they must, but because they want to. I would suggest that the lesson(s) to be learned here can be applied to a more general healthcare rationing plan.

However, this is not to say that the forces arrayed against the implementation of such a system would not be formidable. One has only to look at the firestorm of negative advertising and publicity by various groups launched against the Affordable Care Act, or go back to the 1990s and the massive opposition mounted against the previous attempt at reform of the healthcare system by the Clinton administration, to reflect on the potential obstacles that loom ahead (Goldsteen, Goldsteen, Swan, and Clemeña 2001). Nevertheless, the ACA was enacted and withstood a Supreme Court challenge (albeit not intact).

There are intrinsic features of any rationing system that would be essential for it to move forward. Supreme among those would be fairness. Clearly the essence of any distribution scheme must be some sense of fairness. People will ask what the system offers to them and their neighbors or to the strangers in the clinic: Will they all be treated as equally deserving? Will the rich guy or the politician who is "connected" be able to shove others aside and buy his way to the front of the line? Even if the system is extremely generous, people will not accept it if they feel that other people are getting more than they deserve. I will begin my discussion of what could (or should) constitute fairness in a practical and acceptable healthcare rationing system with a more in-depth analysis of the features of existing systems that make them equitable (at least equitable enough). I will also call attention to some significant gaps or holes that still remain that permit the systems to be gamed, or that permit some individuals to take advantage of the allocation algorithm or method to undeservedly advance their own interests before others similarly situated. The persistence of these flaws tends to diminish the legitimacy of these systems and erodes trust that all will be treated alike. I will argue that the essential features of fair distribution of goods, combined with a generous provision of those good to satisfy reasonable needs, will contribute substantially to making a rationing program tolerable, even acceptable. But I will start with some history.

In 1962, the noted journalist Shana Alexander published a long article in *Life* titled "They Decide Who Lives, Who Dies." It told the story of what was arguably one of the first (if not the first) hospital ethics committees in the United States, a group of seven non–healthcare professionals appointed as the "Admissions and Policies Committee of the Seattle Artificial Kidney Center at Swedish Hospital." Its job was to decide who of the large number of medically eligible candidates would be granted the opportunity to be hooked up to one of the institution's few kidney dialysis machines, and thus have the chance to live. Prior to this time one of the major limitations in hemodialysis was the inability to maintain stable and long-lasting arterial and venous access, a prerequisite for long-term treatment. But in 1960, Dr. Belding Scribner of Swedish Hospital in Seattle (along with Dr. Wayne Quinton) invented what went on to be eponymously called the Scribner shunt, an indwelling Teflon catheter device that linked a vein to an artery and hence provided secure and enduring vascular access (Quinton, Dillard, Cole, and Scribner 1962; Clark and Parsons 1966). With this development, almost anyone in renal failure could be made anatomically technically qualified for dialysis. No longer was this a choke point for patients who would otherwise die. The only problem was that there were insufficient numbers of the very expensive machines compared to the large number of patients who could presumably benefit from them. And of course, this presented the committee with a classic rationing dilemma, so much so that Alexander applied the sobriquet "Life or Death Committee" to this group.[2]

For decades *Life* was a large-format, magazine that millions of Americans read each week. A glossy heaven for photojournalism, each week's issue contained a combination of hard news, gossip, and social "fluff," all accompanied by gorgeous black-and-white and often color photographs. In some ways, this article represented a significant departure from the generally lighter fare that was a staple of the magazine. When Alexander's piece appeared and she quoted verbatim from the deliberations of the committee, literally deciding who would live and who would die from kidney failure, it was probably the first time that most readers ever thought about such things, except for those who had some familiarity with battlefield triage. But even the latter did not consider some of the factors that the committee felt were relevant to the kinds of decisions they made, such as whether the patient was supporting a family, was a lawyer or a longshoreman, single or married, and so on. Social worthiness (in the committee's estimation and the society they presumably represented) was a major component in the recommendation of whether someone was dialyzed. Since the consequence of not being dialyzed was almost certain death, the gravity of the deliberations and the judgments being made—and most important, how they were made, who was making them, what the source of the committee's authority was, and what reasons were given in support of these decisions—all combined to generate a national debate on the ethics of rationing (Blagg 2007; see also Sanders and Dukeminier 1968, Rescher 1969, and Childress 1970).

The solution offered to the dialysis problem was relatively simple and straightforward: buy more dialysis machines and avoid having to make difficult decisions. This was accomplished in 1972 with the passage of amendments to the Social Security Act that created the End-Stage Renal Disease Program guaranteeing government-funded dialysis for all who could medically qualify.[3] Of course this solution, even if dollars were unlimited (which they are not, and cannot be), can only be applicable for situations in which you can buy your way out of a scarce-resource predicament.[4] For solid organs for transplant, all the money in the world won't buy more livers or hearts.[5] How should decisions be made when they cannot be avoided?

What rules should govern the distribution of healthcare interventions and resources—vaccines, devices, doctors, medications, or even dollars—in a society that nominally places a premium on fairness? One might argue—possibly convincingly—that the main reason the organ transplant system (or the Oregon Health Plan) enjoys general support, might be due to the fact that desperate patients with little choice must cooperate if they wish to live. True enough. But this would not explain why such great efforts have been expended to make the process both publicly transparent and remarkably fair. I don't believe this is just for show. Moreover, people who do not receive organs either wait patiently (those on dialysis waiting for kidneys or on left ventricular assist devices waiting for a heart) or die; they and their families sadly accept their fate, but generally do not protest that their deaths were a result of unfair treatment. Rather, the fairness of the system, and the frequent tinkering to make it more so, are integral to its being acceptable to potential donors and recipients alike. The features that make it fair enough are what we need to explore.

What Is Fairness?

Fair play, fair division of the spoils, fair and square, fair rules, fair judgment—most people have a reasonably good notion of what we mean when we describe an activity as fair. It designates a situation in which decisions are equitable for those who are equally deserving, or where any distribution of goods ("stuff") is equitable for people who are similarly situated. No cheating or bribing is permitted. Likewise, jumping to the head of the line in front of those who honestly got there first is not allowed, unless (and this is a big "if") there are good and acceptable reasons for allowing this.[6] Importantly, the regulations and procedures governing how the distribution should proceed, or how the game should be played, would be evaluated and appraised as fair ahead of time by those who would be affected by those rules and no arbitrary decrees from on high would be recognized.[7] When whatever it is that has to be divided up or apportioned fairly is mostly unlimited, deciding who will receive something and who won't or how they will or will not receive it doesn't raise much of an issue; in this case it is more a matter of timing or determining the rank order of the receipt of the goods. But when the amount of stuff has limits or there is not enough to go around when it's something people want (or think they want)—or more important, need—it brings into stark clarity issues of fairness ("Why does she get X and not me?").

In this chapter I want to introduce some general notions of the features that must be present (and those that must be absent) in order for us to judge a situation as fair. And more pertinent to my overall goal of describing socially and morally acceptable healthcare rationing, I want to discuss whether the same characteristics that contribute to situational fairness can be applied systematically to an overall resource allocation scheme. In some respects my description of situational fairness is superficial or simplistic. After all, I will not delve into any of the deeper philosophical complexities of justice, but I do not do so for a reason. I assume that almost all of us have an intuitive understanding of what fair play is, or what constitutes even-handed treatment by others. Most also probably have a pretty good grasp of what fairness demands of us in our dealings with friends, colleagues, and strangers. However, it is at the institutional level that things get considerably more complicated. By this I mean both the nature and derivation of the process by which the rules are created and enforced to regulate the fair distribution of goods or manage the ways we go about the business of obtaining those goods.

What is our general understanding of a state of affairs that stimulates us to judge whether it is fair or not? There are clearly features of a situation—whether it is a clinical situation or one from everyday life—that commend it as fair or not. To try and tease out those attributes that contribute to a widespread view of fairness, I begin this discussion by presenting two very different clinical scenarios that will demonstrate the challenges that fairness can demand.

Case #1

University Medical Center is a large, academic teaching hospital affiliated with a major medical school in a moderate-sized city in the United States. It has a stellar national—even international—reputation for patient care, research, and teaching. It not only serves its local community, but many patients come from hundreds, and sometimes thousands, of miles away seeking the best that American medicine has to offer. Its firm policy is never to turn anyone away, regardless of their ability to pay, even though the U.S. recession has made this more of a challenge in recent years. Fortunately, UMC has been very successful in attracting a stable of wealthy donors who share the hospital's vision and mission and have continued to be generous in supporting it during its current financial difficulties.

Like other hospitals throughout the country, UMC has also had to cope with the ongoing problem of sudden, severe, and unpredictable drug shortages. Affecting mostly intravenous, generic medicines, one week it could be an important diuretic that is unavailable (for which there is fortunately a similar substitute that can be used), the next a vital chemotherapy drug for which there is no alternative. The hospital's administrators, lawyers and risk managers, pharmacists, chief medical officer, and ethics committee have been meeting for months in a so-far fruitless effort to develop a policy to distribute scarce drugs when there are more patients who need them than can be treated with the available supply.

One Sunday two patients are admitted to the hospital, both in their fifties and both seriously ill. They are each diagnosed as having acute myelogenous leukemia (AML), a rapidly progressive and fatal disease that must be treated very quickly with aggressive and high-dose chemotherapy in an attempt to put the patient into remission, an absolute prerequisite for a cure. One of the irreplaceable medicines used in the initial treatment of AML is a drug that has been available for decades, cytarabine. Unfortunately, two weeks before these patients were admitted, UMC was notified that there was a severe national shortage of cytarabine due to manufacturing problems, and it was not known when a new supply would be available. Based on past patterns of use, UMC would have a stock sufficient for about fourteen days. Attempts to obtain cytarabine from other hospitals or other sources were unsuccessful, because they, too, were faced with the same problem. Now there were two patients who desperately needed cytarabine and there was only enough to treat one of them. Each of their doctors pleaded with the hospital leaders to release the drug to their patient, but a careful analysis of the medical records showed that they were clinically indistinguishable. There was only one difference between them that several people noted: one patient was the wife of a prominent man in the state and a member of a family that had donated millions of dollars to UMC over the past ten years. The other patient was a local man who supported his family by working in a convenience store. Who should get the last remaining doses of cytarabine and thus a chance at life?

Case #2
In 2025, the United States is nearing bankruptcy due to the continuing escalating costs of healthcare. Prior attempts at reining in expenditures have been unsuccessful. Due to the desperation of the situation, Congress, and the president agree that the inconceivable must be accomplished: a single-payer, national health insurance plan, similar to Medicare and the Oregon Health Plan devised in the 1990s, will be instituted. There will be some significant differences, though. It will apply to all residents of the United States, and there will be limitations on the availability of interventions based primarily on the probability of efficacy in both populations and individuals. After many public discussions and tweaking of the plan, it starts on January 1, 2026.

One year later, an eighty-three-year-old man, a resident of a nursing home, is admitted to the local hospital because he has a fever. He has moderately severe and progressive dementia and is unable to make his own healthcare decisions. He must be fed by others and is frequently incontinent. He is diagnosed with both aspiration pneumonia and a urinary tract infection.[8] He is also noted to have several very deep decubitus ulcers (bedsores) on his buttocks. He is treated aggressively with antibiotics and wound care. His family—a son and daughter—want "everything done." When questioned about what they mean by this, they say that they want him to have all treatments possible to save his life, no matter how little chance they have of being successful or how much he may have to suffer. This would include full cardiopulmonary resuscitation, with possibly the risk of broken ribs and breastbone, and intubation with mechanical ventilation. His doctors and nurses state that under the new healthcare limitation law, this patient meets the criteria for not being transferred to the ICU should he get sicker and for not having CPR performed should he have a cardiopulmonary arrest. His children are furious and again demand that everything be done for their father. Several days later, the patient develops another fever, hypoxia, and hypotension. He is made as comfortable as possible and dies peacefully. However, his son and daughter remain very angry that their father was denied the treatments they requested. They state that "in the old days" he would have received what they demanded. The doctors reply that their father received excellent care and met the publicly debated and accepted criteria for withholding CPR and ICU care, according to the new national health insurance plan. His children mutter that they hadn't agreed to this plan and are considering hiring a lawyer.

Analysis of the Cases

The first case is an example of rationing under strict- and finite-resource scarcity, where some must do without a drug that could definitely help them; there is little doubt that both patients "need" cytarabine to get a chance at a cure, and if there were not an acute shortage of the drug, there would be little doubt that they both would receive it. But the situation, albeit sudden and hopefully temporary, is very similar to what happens everyday with solid-organ transplants: there are never enough livers, hearts, and kidneys for all those whose lives could be saved by a transplant. Decisions must be made and some patients will inevitably and inescapably have to go without. The only question that needs to be answered is how to go about deciding who lives and who dies. That question must be preceded by one that addresses the process of deciding: What rules should govern the decision-making procedure (and thus the decision makers) for allocating drugs or organs? Should the wealthy benefactor's wife receive preferential treatment over the convenience store clerk simply because of who she is? Should her family and social history make her life more valuable than that of the other patient, so that she should receive the scarce drug? One could argue that the donations the wealthy patient's family members have made to the medical center have undeniably contributed to its ability to weather the poor financial conditions and thus enable them to continue to fulfill their mission of providing significant amounts of charity or unreimbursed medical care to indigent and uninsured patients. Isn't that worth a life as a "fair" trade-off? Should (or can) allocation decisions permit these kinds of factors to count?

Conversely, is it reasonable for a publicly available and accepted policy that restricts life-saving therapies to those who can sensibly benefit from them to permit an older, cognitively disabled man to die without access to the ICU when his children demand it? The second case reveals an admittedly hypothetical, perhaps illusory, futuristic portrayal of what could happen should universal limitations on healthcare be enacted in this country. As I discuss in greater detail in chapter 4 (and have already introduced and will continue to consider throughout this book), it is highly likely that in a wealthy country such as the United States, any reasonable national insurance plan would have to offer a wide array of services and treatments available to all, subject to some publicly debated and agreed-on limitations, including (I assume or would hope) curbs on the availability of interventions that offer only marginal benefits, if any at all. That would be an acceptable price to pay to be able to deliver everything else and to gain acceptance by the public. I speculate that most people would agree to this as reasonable and probably fair since the public already agrees to considerably more draconian restrictions in other rationing situations. Furthermore, when questioned about their preferences for end-of-life care, few people prefer life and death in the ICU without a reasonable chance of recovery with some acceptable level of mental functioning (McCarthy et al. 2008).

The overwhelming majority of rational and reasonable people, which presumably includes all of us who are either not suffering from severe cognitive or intellectual disability, want to be treated fairly by others. This is not a controversial assertion because most, if not all, cultures or systems of morality devote a significant effort to outlining how fair exchanges between people should operate. Even in dictatorships, some attention is paid to a minimal form of justice, though it may not seem so to observers from less autocratic societies. It would be difficult to imagine how a cooperative social arrangement composed of persons with widely different capabilities, desires, and interests could possibly function stably over time without some sort of structure that regulated interpersonal conduct in an equitable manner. Indeed, recent discoveries in neurobiology and evolutionary biology strongly support the notion that human beings are "hardwired" to both generate and respond to fair states of affairs.[9]

As Adam Smith noted more than 200 years ago,

Beneficence, therefore, is less essential to the existence of society than justice. Society may subsist, though not in the most comfortable state, without beneficence; but the prevalence of injustice must utterly destroy it. ... Justice, on the contrary, is the main pillar that holds up the whole edifice. If it is removed, the great, the immense fabric of human society, that fabric which, to raise and support, seems, in this world, if I may say so, to have been the peculiar and darling care of nature, must in a moment crumble into atoms. (Smith [1759] 1969, 125)[10]

This is not to say that there are uniform conceptions of fairness or justice. Rather, people easily sense when they are being taken advantage of, when the system is rigged, when they are being treated unfairly, or when others seem to have disproportionate access to the benefits society can bestow (assuming they have access to full knowledge about the relevant facts of the situation). And, if given a choice between distributive systems that are more or less fair, most rational people would choose to participate in the former.[11] These observations lend support to the proposition that the public acceptability of allocation schemes affecting everyone would be strongly correlated not only with the degree to which these schemes are perceived as fair, but with the degree to which they actually are fair.

What do I mean by *fair, fairness*, and related terms? The *Oxford English Dictionary* approaches this quite broadly:

Fairness: Equitableness, fair dealing, honesty, impartiality, uprightness.

Fair: Of conduct, actions, arguments, methods: Free from bias, fraud, or injustice; equitable, legitimate. Hence of persons: Equitable; not taking undue advantage; disposed to concede every reasonable claim.[12]

Superficially, these definitions point to a general way in which people treat each other equitably. This plays out in daily living in a variety of ways, revealing that this is an ideal to be aspired to, but often is not fully achieved in real life. For example, we would hope that the poorest defendant in a criminal trial accused of say, burglary, would be treated the same way, and have the same chances of a given result, as a defendant who is wealthy. But of course that is not the way it actually works. This is due to the fact that the criminal justice system is an example of imperfect procedural justice (Rawls 1999, 74–77). This means that as set down on paper, the rules (if strictly followed) would dictate absolute fairness in an ideal world, such that juries (for example) would always and unerringly find the guilty as guilty and the innocent would go free. But there are many ways the rules may be manipulated so that some may gain advantage to obtain skewed results (hence, the "imperfection").

Likewise, if the transplant system were strictly fair, we would expect that solid organs would be allocated according to a rigorously equitable system in which the determining factors of eligibility would have to do with how sick patients are or how well they might expect to do postoperatively. How these factors were weighted relative to each other would presumably be worked out beforehand in a public discussion to garner comments and engender buy-in and trust. While the system has improved over the years, there are still instances in which it can be gamed, as I will describe shortly. The fact that these cases exist can erode confidence in the system as fair and thus its overall legitimacy with those it is designed to serve.

There are two aspects of fairness that I wish to consider. First, what does it mean in general when we describe a state of affairs as fair (this includes interpersonal exchanges and transactions of goods of one form or another)? Second, what procedures or rules can be put in place or enacted that would ensure—to the fullest extent possible or practical (I will discuss this latter problem in chapter 6)—that undertakings that followed these rules could be judged by impartial observers as fair? And even more important, what approaches would be judged by those affected by the outcomes as fair? I will begin this part of the discussion with some actual examples of weaknesses in rationing systems that detract from their overall structure of fairness, and thus tend to undermine their legitimacy.

Examples of Unfairness: Gaming the System

Apple's Steve Jobs lived in northern California and after the progression of his rare form of pancreatic cancer with metastases to the liver, his doctors believed his only hope for survival and a cure was a liver transplant. He was placed on the long waiting list for a transplant, knowing that he might not receive one before he died from his underlying illness; this is a risk that all transplant candidates must run since there are many more patients than there are organs. Jobs was successfully transplanted, but not in California, and not because there are no transplant centers nearby (Stanford University Medical Center, one of the biggest, was just down the road from his home). Rather, he temporarily moved to Memphis, Tennessee, where the wait time was considerably shorter, and thus his chances of receiving a transplant much higher.[13] Was it fair for him to take advantage of his wealth and connections to afford himself a better chance of obtaining a liver? Is this an example of gaming the system? Of course it is, because his affluence and position in society made it possible for him to profit from these regional differences. Other patients without his resources would not have been able to move someplace else, and so most of them would have died waiting for a transplant. One could hold Jobs accountable for this outcome, but it really was the transplant system itself that permitted this type of allocation of organs.[14]

Another instance of what appeared to be abuse of the organ allocation arrangement occurred in California. As initially reported by CBS News in a segment on *60 Minutes*, one of Japan's chief organized crime gangsters, Tadamasa Goto, was granted a visa—apparently by the FBI—to come to the United States for a liver transplant at the UCLA Medical Center.[15] He received his transplant within six weeks of arriving, evidently jumping to the head of the list, although it was unclear if he did so legitimately by being very sick. What is more to the point is that he paid cash for his medical expenses and also made a $100,000 donation to the hospital.

While his gift may not have been a quid pro quo exchange to shorten his waiting time for a liver, it certainly gave the appearance of inappropriate influence. Furthermore, his somewhat socially unsavory past and foreign residency raised questions about the fairness of the transplant.[16]

These stories tend to raise our hackles for a single, common reason: they reveal an apparent unfairness of the organ transplant system (at least as it existed at the time). In both examples a wealthy person—one a role model of a successful entrepreneur and innovator, widely admired throughout the country if not the world, the other a reviled figure from another country who entered the United States under suspicious circumstances and seemed to move to the front of the line perhaps influenced by a generous donation—received a life-saving transplant. Both men possessed financial resources that were used to manipulate the system in their favor, resources not available to most other desperately ill patients waiting for livers.[17] And of course when they received a liver someone else did not. It is the essence of unfairness when people who are otherwise equal (medically) to others can exploit loopholes in the allocation system to their own advantage and to the disadvantage of others who are no less deserving. Indeed, the existence of the loopholes themselves is the issue, because one cannot necessarily fault people for benefiting from a situation under such desperate circumstances. All they did was capitalize on rules that permitted such exploitation, despite the fact that the vast majority of people who need an organ transplant do not have the financial and social resources to follow this strategy. What seems unfair about these cases is that the only reason these men were able to have their lives saved was due to their ability to pay extra, which has nothing to do with their medical qualifications or ability to gain from a transplant. But there are other actors in this complex drama: doctors.

It turns out that not everyone thinks that gaming the system (or what some might call cheating for personal advantage) is inherently wrong. Indeed, a recent essay suggests that under certain circumstances doctors "ought to lie for their patients" in order to best advance their (the patients') interests.[18] This view is worth examining for several reasons, the most significant of which is that in general we trust our doctors to have our personal well-being as their primary objective. Another is that fairness demands that the participants in an exercise governed by rules that are in place to ensure a level playing field obey those rules. If some people are considered (or consider themselves) to be above the rules, then the system cannot be fair to all and is inherently corrupt (or corruptible). Moreover, doctors are the gatekeepers for entry into the system and they wield enormous discretionary power over the dispersal of a wide array of medical resources, ranging from prescription drugs to permanent surgi-cal implantable devices (Chandra, Cutler, and Song 2011; Sirovich, Gal-lagher, Wennberg, and Fisher 2008; Hu et al. 2012).[19] Finally, rules that are flexible or even capricious—that is, those that can be applied in an undependable and unpredictable manner or at the behest of powerful individuals—are emblematic of a system that some participants can take advantage of and others cannot. Typically, the former are those who al-ready enjoy disproportionate advantages in life such as wealth and social position. Doctors who misrepresent facts to insurers or others to game the system, even if this is done out of the best of motives, are a special case because of their stature in the community.

The legitimacy of any healthcare delivery system that will distribute a limited supply of resources must be granted not only by the vast popula-tion of patients who will be intimately and directly affected by the kinds of allocations permitted, but also by the physicians (who of course are also patients in a different role) who will—in many senses—be making and administering resource allotment decisions. To minimize the problem of gaming and cheating, almost everyone must buy into the system and accept judgments and conclusions as reasonable and legitimate. Other-wise, we will have made little progress over what we currently experience, with anywhere from 11 to 39 percent of physicians either participating in or finding the practice acceptable (Werner, Alexander, Fagerlin, and Ubel 2004; Wynia, Cummins, VanGeest, and Wilson 2000).[20]

We expect that physicians will ignore any conflicts of interest they may have, and do whatever is necessary to ensure that we receive the required care to achieve the goals that we have agreed are worth pursuing.[21] In-deed, if my insurance company refuses to pay for a test or procedure or drug that my doctors say is important, I am relieved and happy when the doctors do whatever they must to change the company's mind, even if it means that they will bend the truth a bit. The problem arises when everyone's doctors do this. A lot of little lies add up quickly to a bunch of big ones. And not all doctors tell little lies or tell them occasionally. There could easily be a competition of lying to ensure that specific patients get what their doctors believe they deserve (independent of whether this is actually justifiable). And just as some lawyers are more skilled advocates for their clients (especially rich ones) than others, some physicians may be more persuasive or carry more clout because of who their patients are and not because of what ails them. This is not to say that one's doctor may not be correct and that the insurance company denial was not a mistake, just that it's unlikely they are mistaken all the time.

It is easy to see how this could be intensely corrosive to any sensible rationing system because it would undermine its very foundation of fair play, assuming the system has been set up to work reasonably fairly.[22] For the system to function, the overwhelming majority of participants must agree to abide by the rules. Only a very small or minimal number of free riders can be tolerated.[23] Given our general antipathy toward health insurance companies, we might tend to give a pass to doctors who are manipulating the truth on behalf of some unfortunate soul, trying to extract what they think may be due their patient.[24] However, if we had a national health insurance plan that was reasonably fair and generous, then it would be more obvious that the doctors who are gaming the system would be taking from all of us, rather than just the anonymous gigantic and faceless insurance corporation ("and they can afford it anyway").[25]

I will make only one more point about gaming the system in a way that may not often be interpreted as such but to which I alluded earlier. It is not uncommon for desperate patients, often aided and abetted by their equally determined doctors, to make public their plight in order to bring pressure to bear on insurance companies, hospitals, and so on to provide treatment they believe they have been denied unfairly. To a very great extent this was the genesis of the Coby Howard story I presented in the previous chapter. These tales take advantage of our "rule-of-rescue" emotions, and stimulate us to want to help that individual obtain what he or she wants (and ignore all of the nameless and faceless patients whose equally tragic stories and dire predicaments were not publicized).

For example, a California graduate student used the Internet to advertise her case. She had been diagnosed with a rare and aggressive tumor—a paraganglioma—and was denied coverage for proton beam radiotherapy, an accepted form of radiation treatment, but one that had not been shown to be any more effective than standard types of radiation and is considerably more expensive. Furthermore, only a few institutions possessed these costly machines, and she would have had to travel and live near the hospital for the duration of the treatment, which could last many weeks. Her public appeal went viral and in a short period of time her insurance company relented and paid for the therapy.[26] Or consider this unfortunate woman's story:

Danni Gilbert wants another season. She wants to see the leaves change, to return to Mountain Home High School to meet a new class of students, to possibly watch her 5- and 7-year-old daughters open presents under a Christmas tree or to blow out the candles on another birthday cake. But she needs some help. Cancer has made its way into her 39-year-old lungs and liver. Her oncologist, Dr. Dan Zuckerman, knows what to do: administer a biweekly cocktail of chemotherapy complete with Avastin, a drug designed to rob a cancerous tumor of precious blood cells. But Gilbert's insurance company, Blue Cross of Idaho, won't pay for the Avastin, ruling that the drug doesn't meet what it calls a "standard of care." So instead, Gilbert is faced with shelling out $3,300 every other week for a drug that her physician says is her best bet to prolong her life.[27]

Both of these patients resorted to publicly proclaiming the unfairness (by their definition) of their situation. The adverse publicity, as it so often does, persuaded the insurance company to change its decision. While there is a superficial difference between this form of manipulation and doctors lying to an insurance company, they share a conceptual base, because their purpose is to obtain something for a patient that may or may not be reasonable or that they may or may not deserve outside of the established rules. And the only way they have of getting what they want is by exploiting loopholes or taking advantage of companies' aversion to negative publicity, rather than making a principled appeal to either change the decision by reasoned argument or alter the rules by which decisions are made. This is not to say that there are always accessible, sanctioned, and just options to pursue appeals through legitimate channels or means, simply that desperate or angry people often pursue desperate or ill-tempered choices. And, if everyone went public to get what he or she wanted (and especially if most of these sympathetic appeals were granted), it would wreak havoc with the insurance system as well as dividing patients up into two pools: those who were savvy enough to know how to game the system and those who were not, potentially exacerbating existing inequities and disparities in access to healthcare interventions.

Finally, disease advocacy groups abound, such as those for heart disease, diabetes, cancer, and especially so-called orphan diseases or very rare conditions, and they have been extremely effective in attracting publicity and money for their individual causes. Since they are all competing with each other for a piece of the funding pie, they necessarily draw attention and thus dollars away from needs that might be less conspicuous but more significant from a public health point of view. In this way, they are also manipulating the system to potentially disproportionately affect stakeholders' interests in one area without necessarily engaging in a public debate about the merits of their case. All of these examples demonstrate ways that people have discovered to exploit loopholes in a disorganized and polyglot healthcare system that is often viewed as intrinsically unfair, especially to ordinary people. This state of affairs is believed to justify employing maneuvers to avoid arbitrary and capricious decisions that ignore the plight of suffering patients. The irony is that these strategies, while often successful on an individual level, contribute to perpetuating and even expanding the inequities in the system.

Other Cases of Unfairness

Other examples of unfairness are common in everyday life. They illustrate a fundamental feature of unfair situations: people who are more or less similar and comparably placed in a given set of circumstances are treated differently for unacceptable reasons. Of course, there is a gray area. An example might be a commercial airplane trip in which some (very fortunate) people get to sit in large, comfortable seats with ample legroom simply because they or their companies have enough money to pay for a business-class or first-class seat. If we assume that the manner in which their money was acquired was itself fair (i.e., they didn't steal it or obtain it by cheating), then we may grumble a bit with envy, but we have to admit that the fact that some people can afford fancy seating and we can't is a feature of life and if not exactly fair, is not unacceptably unfair. On the other hand, if I have the sudden onset of crushing substernal chest pain that radiates down my left arm along with profuse sweating, and an ambulance takes me to the local emergency department with the suspicion that I am suffering a heart attack, and another man my age with the same symptoms arrives ten minutes after me and they treat him first solely because his brother-in-law is the CEO of the hospital, that is patently unfair (to me, and anyone else who could be in my situation).

The reason the second example is unfair is due to the fact that in a liberal, decent, and democratic society we generally accept the proposition that persons are inherently morally equal and that they should be treated as such. Individuals as well as organizations or institutions should respect this equality in their dealings. The former expect reciprocal fairness and the latter should be structured in such a way that the rules by which they operate are fair and are administered in a fair manner. If the emergency-department doctor tossed a coin to choose between the other patient and me, that could be understood as fair, but to prefer him merely because of his relationship to the hospital CEO seems to be a gross ethical abuse. If he were sicker than me, or arrived ten or twenty minutes sooner, or there was any other reasonable distinguishing feature that could provide sufficient grounds for taking him first, fairness would be preserved. By the same token, if Steve Jobs had stayed in California and waited in line along with other patients with bad liver disease—even if he also gave a huge donation to the hospital or to UNOS—that would also have maintained the fairness of the system, so long as his gift did not influence his standing on the transplant list.

Another consideration is the general fairness of society. We are often led to believe that America is at heart a nation in which people are equal before the law and have equal opportunities in life for education, careers, life prospects, and so on. But of course that is far from true. Admittedly, conditions in the United States may be considerably more just and equitable than they are in many other places in the world, but they are also not as good as in some others. There are significant departures from the ideal, as any cursory examination of the existing inequities and disparities in a variety of social settings will easily reveal (for instance, in the healthcare system). There are vast differences in the opportunities a person has in life based on a number of features over which he or she has little to no control (so-called morally irrelevant facts). Examples include traits like race, ethnicity, gender, country of origin, who one's parents are and whether they are educated or wealthy, and finally, the genes one possesses and the kinds of phenotypes they predispose one to developing (including diseases). All of these life circumstances amount to what is often labeled "brute luck" or the results of the "natural lottery." Both terms imply that one is—to a great extent—stuck with these states of affairs or preconditions. This is not to say that people cannot break the bonds of their birth and social circumstances, just that it is more difficult for some than others. Furthermore, society itself may be arranged such that some people have greater opportunities or chances for a better life than others, solely based on morally irrelevant characteristics. Finally, it is obvious that even if all things are otherwise equal, people are born with and develop a wide array of different capabilities, which clearly can influence their prospects in life: people come with diverse intellectual, physical, and athletic abilities, as well as varying propensities to be stricken with disabilities or illnesses, all of which can exert enormous influence on how their lives turn out.

By itself, there does not appear to be anything inherently unfair about the range and distribution of what are often labeled "natural" abilities and features. Short of some sort of utopian fantasy where everyone is exactly equal in his or her social and biological circumstances, it is not surprising that a normal society is so heterogeneous. Indeed, that heterogeneity can also be viewed as a significant advantage because it would be both boring and unproductive if everyone were alike in these (nonmoral) characteristics. However, when social arrangements are such that people are prevented from taking advantage of opportunities that should be available to most, if not all, members of society simply because of these morally irrelevant features, it reveals an intrinsic inequity in the system.

In healthcare this plays out in a number of ways. For example, in order to see a doctor or a nurse, one has to have relatively easy access, and not everyone does, often because of poverty. Next, once someone gets in the clinic door, they should also have the same access as anyone else to the entire range of medical care and technology appropriate for the condition they have. For instance, if the system were fair, we would not expect to see significant disparities between white and African-American recipients of certain cardiac procedures or cancer treatments, but both have been demonstrated for years (Bickell et al. 2006; Farjah et al. 2009; Farmer et al. 2009; Fedewa et al. 2011; Gregory, LaVeist, and Simpson 2006; Jha, Staiger, Lucas, and Chandra 2007; Shippee, Ferraro, and Thorpe 2011). These differences in the kinds and amounts of interventions available to members of some groups inevitably lead to variations in patient outcome.[28] They are also inexplicable using any form of medical or scientific reasoning, and therefore raise the suspicion that the system is more or less unfair to African Americans for no other reason than their skin color, which is prima facie unfair.

When deciding who can have access to what (and why), it should be a matter of justice (fairness) in dispensing healthcare to consider issues of equality between similarly (medically) situated people. Of course, no two patients are ever *exactly* alike, but many people are similar enough to not make a substantive difference. After all, when we speak of prognoses for a given disease when treated with a specific therapy, we refer to statistical populations, in which membership is earned by fitting into (more or less) a specific diagnostic category or group. Being a population, it tends to smooth out small differences between people, who are represented in the middle of the curve. Others, when compared to those in the middle (i.e., the mean or median), are perhaps quite different by virtue of their locations in the tails of the population distribution. Where in the population of expected outcomes a given patient falls may be difficult, if not impossible, to predict. Nonetheless, while individual doctors and their patients may notice and attend to the small differences between people, when allocating resources we may not be able to permit so-called microdifferences to matter. Naturally, they could matter to the patient's supposed benefit (gaining access to something he or his doctor thinks he needs) or to his detriment (being barred from gaining access for any of a variety of medically—or morally—irrelevant reasons).[29]

Healthcare Rationing and Fairness

Not surprisingly, health and healthcare have been major foci of attention and concern for those interested in fairness. Topics such as whether there is (or should be) a human right to healthcare, the equity or inequity of healthcare delivery and its receipt, and various ways of financing national or regional medical systems have demanded the most consideration. In particular, the recognized need for healthcare rationing of one sort or another has generated a number of proposals for approaches by which it can be done fairly. It is believed—and I think correctly—that the legitimacy and acceptability of any rationing scheme will largely depend both on its perception of fairness in application and on how just it actually is in principle. How fair it should be and how that should be achieved is the challenge. Up to this point I have described various kinds of unfairness, all of which tend to cluster around unequal treatment. Although it may be true that if we treated everyone equally badly, this would have the appearance of fairness, but if the resources to do otherwise were readily available, not taking advantage of them to alter life's circumstances in a positive way would itself be immoral.

In this section, I want to narrowly focus on the features of a rationing method that would enhance its acceptability to a skeptical public. These cardinal attributes center on fairness, and must concentrate not only on foundational tenets ("the system must be just") but also on how to implement these doctrines in actual practice. The feasibility project calls for creating rules that people could accept as legitimate and therefore embrace and follow.

Caplan, citing a 1993 report of the Swedish Ministry of Health and Social Affairs about setting priorities for restricted access to healthcare services, noted that the Swedes set out three bedrock principles that should guide any allocation decisions they make. These principles would form the framework from which would emerge more granular recommendations and judgments about the sorts of diagnostic tests, treatments, technologies, and so on that should be offered and to whom. Significantly, two of the three principles stressed the singular importance of fairness and equity. In Caplan's words, "Any scheme for prioritizing must accept three core principles: that all human beings are equally valuable; that society must pay special attention to the needs of the weakest and most vulnerable; and that, other things being equal, cost-efficiency and gaining the greatest return for the amount of money spent must prevail."[30] By emphasizing our shared susceptibility to disease and disability,[31] as well as our equal desert of caring and a proportional share of the available resources required to relieve that burden, the report underlines equality of concern and treatment. While the third principle indicates that efficiency or utility is a worthwhile consideration, by joining it with the first two, the Swedish approach avoids the charge of a strictly utilitarian focus, with its tendency to diminish the importance of the individual versus the collective.[32] However, the central priority remains fairness.

If we possessed the amounts of money, personnel, facilities, and equipment that could be devoted to healthcare and the will to use these resources in a manner in which anyone could get whatever they wanted, then the issue of imposed limits on availability would be moot. We still might wish to discuss whether there should be limits on what was reasonable for people to want, but conceivably, if money and other necessary supplies were no object, even treatments that could only help someone in theory would be conceivably offered (or at least not denied a priori), so long as it wasn't physiologically futile.[33]

The challenge is to devise a strategy or strategies that can account for two parts of any rationing plan or scheme for distributing resources, while at the same time maintaining enough fairness that it would be acceptable to the overwhelming majority of the population.[34] The first would be how to decide what is or should be available to divide up. To a great extent that will be dependent on how much money is to be devoted to this enterprise. As I have suggested on several occasions, in a rich country like the United States it seems difficult to imagine that we would be anything other than generous to ourselves (perhaps too much so), if for no other reason than to lessen the perceived pains in making the transition from a poorly regulated free-for-all to a rationing system, and the probable fact that the American people would not tolerate anything less than a system with fairly ample benefits. However, no matter how lavish the services, they would have to be less that what we permit now (at least in some cases).[35] Since we spend so much more per patient that anywhere else in the world with outcomes that are mediocre for the money, we could conceivably spend less if we cut out waste, useless treatments, huge administrative and overhead costs, and other unnecessary expenditures.[36] Thus, it is reasonable to think that most people would be able to receive what they want and need because of our wealth and our willingness to spend it on healthcare. How could we decide how much money is sufficient to fund a magnanimous (perhaps even reasonably lavish) healthcare system?[37]

Fleck (2009) has argued that democratic discussions and tempered arguments would be an approach that could be used to reach consensus on what would be available and to whom and under what conditions. While this might be a plausible and sensible method for small communities, it seems to me to be cumbersome and probably unworkable in a country of over 300 million people. On the other hand, one could imagine a state of affairs in which we elected delegates to a broadly representative commission charged with determining distribution schemes, the rules, and so on, subject to amendment in public debate (alternatively, we could have Congress appoint outside members to the panel, but the widespread lack of trust in the House and Senate would not bestow much confidence in the outcome).

The second challenge is to devise a system than can fairly administer the distribution of resources, adjudicate disputes, and supervise alterations to the arrangement. One of the best-known approaches is that proposed by Norman Daniels and James Sabin, which they call "accountability for reasonableness" (Daniels and Sabin 1997; Daniels and Sabin 2008, chap. 4). It assumes that most rational people, given the right set of circumstances and rules or regulations, would accept restrictions or limitations on the availability of or access to certain healthcare services as legitimate, even if they happened to be austere, so long as several initial provisos were fulfilled.[38] Daniels and Sabin list four conditions that would have to be met in a substantive manner in order for people to substantively accept such a state of affairs:

• *Transparency*: The rationale and allocation scheme should neither be crafted nor applied in secret; all must be open to public scrutiny save details that would breach patient confidentiality in individual cases.

• *Relevance*: Unbiased, neutral observers must be able to view the allocation scheme as relevant to the situations for which it has been devised and applied.

• *Appeals*: There must be a process by which those who feel that they have been dealt with unfairly can appeal. This process must be both timely and have the possibility of reversing the original decision—otherwise, it would be mere window dressing.[39]

• *Enforcement*: The institution or body responsible for administering the system must have the means by which it can ensure that the first three conditions are implemented in an effective manner. This means that the rules must have the backing of an effective and powerful authority to warrant that they are both imposed and followed correctly, demonstrating that the rules are not a mere facade.[40]

In my adaptation of this method to the rationing of critically scarce drugs within a healthcare institution, I added a fifth condition that I believed served to recognize a significant feature of how bureaucratic organizations—such as hospitals and healthcare systems in general—work. I called this condition *fairness* to recognize the fact that people from all backgrounds present themselves to doctors and hospitals for care (Rosoff 2012a; Rosoff et al. 2012). To avoid confusion with the overall concept of fairness with which this chapter is concerned, we might label this condition as "small-f" fairness, covered under the umbrella term "big-F" Fairness. Rich, poor, well-educated, illiterate: the entire panoply of life at some point in time gets sick and needs medical care. The institution and the people who work there can view some people differently from others, and this can influence the kind of care they receive. One of the best-known examples is the case of "very important people" or VIPs. VIPs come in a variety of different stripes, including relatives or friends of the staff, major donors to the hospital, community leaders, or politicians.[41] Almost any feature or characteristic can be used to distinguish an individual as one "deserving" of special consideration. Conversely, there are morally irrelevant facts about people that can and are employed to make them into what we might call "very unimportant people" or VUPs. For instance, race, ethnicity, immigration status, and insurance status may all signal to the organization that a patient is not as significant as someone else.[42] This can result in overt discrimination (although it may not always work to one's advantage to be a VIP).[43] When patients are vying for a scarce resource that is insufficient to meet all their needs, it is clear that desperation will generate attempts to use whatever advantages they may possess, including VIPness (see the discussion above about Steve Jobs and the Japanese gangsters). However, if the institution hews to a view that people are inherently morally equal, it must declare that VIPs have no more claim to scarce drugs, ventilators, or livers than VUPs who are clinically similar, thus eliminating these artificially designated categories as significant factors in medical decision making and allocation judgments. A similar adherence to the principle of fairness or moral equality should exist in any kind of national or universal rationing scheme where most healthcare resources would not be expected to be absolutely limited.[44]

The conditions of transparency, relevance, appeals, enforcement, and fairness ensure that Fleck's criteria about democratic debate are met, along with the criterion of a lack of secrecy. And since not everyone has equal access to the political process, significant effort would have to be expended to maximize the opportunities to engage people in the process described here. Respecting these five conditions will do most of the work required to bestow and maintain legitimacy and conformity to whatever rules are created. Of course, even if these guidelines are followed and a plan emerges that conforms to the reasonable demands of justice, there will undoubtedly be people who cry foul or who disagree with the end product. Work would have to be done to attempt to attract their support, because the more people who endorse a plan, the more secure its legitimacy will be. Ultimately, no one should anticipate that even a well-deliberated and reasonable plan would be ideal. The goal should not be perfection in fairness, but rather something that is "just enough."[45]

Finally, one more essential element of a fair allocation scheme must be stressed: individuals vested with the responsibility and power to make the rules should themselves be bound by them. Such a criterion would necessarily temper the enthusiasm on the part of some designated rule makers to craft exceptions for themselves or those like them. While I have not accused the Oregon Health Plan of being unjust, it could have been viewed as such in this sense, because most of the people composing the rules were doing so for others and not themselves. While this point may seem obvious to people accustomed to participatory democracy, to many others who are more familiar with a less representative system or even those whose position in life is so far removed from the locus of power that it may appear unapproachable, it may look very foreign. However, it would be naive to think that rule makers on a scale necessary for something as gargantuan as wholesale universal healthcare reform with rationing would completely avoid the temptation to grant themselves special privileges or exemptions.[46] Though one could possibly construe this requirement as subsumed under the fairness principle, I think it is actually different. One could have a rule requiring fairness of the kind I have described, but some people could still figure out a way to portray themselves as exceptional. For example, some of the plans preparing for pandemic influenza suggested that members of Congress should be in the first tier of eligibility for a scarce vaccine, similar to healthcare workers and first responders. The rationale for this was never exactly clear, because the necessity for functional federal legislators even under normal conditions sometimes seems questionable. It is conceivable that this principle might be one of the more challenging to accomplish in a society with existing significant inequities of power, influence, money, and other factors. Those at the top could be expected to resist any attempt to level the playing field if they interpreted this as a lowering of their benefits rather than a raising of those for everyone else.

What makes "accountability for reasonableness" more fair (or if not more fair, at least easier to apply and possibly implement) than other approaches that might be used? To answer this we might briefly review some other options. For example, a less representative group of "deciders" could be convened that would have the power to determine what services would be available and to whom they would apply. There is nothing about this method to say that it is inherently unfair and their conclusions not the "correct" ones or similar—if not identical—to those that might be chosen by a more democratic process. However, it is not only the decisions that are made, but how they are made that contribute to the credibility and legitimacy of the outcome. Indeed, one of the charges leveled at the failed Clinton healthcare reform initiative was the initial opaqueness of the deliberative and decision-making process (Thomas 1995–1996; Yankelovich 1995). Moreover, to be truly fair, the process actually has to *be* fair and not just appear that way. In these days of spin doctors and manipulative public relations, the only effective way to combat disinformation, disingenuousness, and distortion may be to ensure that the publicity and transparency conditions are always made an integral component of every decision.[47] People must know not only the substance of a rule but why it came about and how it could be subject to amendment with appropriate, reasoned argument. Some of the biggest complaints about insurance companies concern the enigmatic or Delphic manner of their decision-making methods, yielding judgments that are sold as benefits but often appear as coldly restrictive.[48]

One could also discuss the actual way that rationing schemes prioritize the allocation of resources when there is true competition (such as when there is a finite scarcity). In this case, some people are privileged over others in any one of a number of approaches, including sickest first or most likely to survive first (emblematic of traditional battlefield or emergency-department triage); first come, first served (those waiting the longest or who managed to get in line first have first crack at the supply); age (usually younger privileged over older); and in some rare cases that "regular" people take seriously and think important but ethicists shun, social "worthiness" (or lack thereof). Each of these methods, or combinations of them, may have a role to play in any rationing scheme, but all have their drawbacks, some of them significant. Nevertheless, one would have to accord them very careful thought if surveys of the public revealed that they should be given precedence (assuming they were provided with complete information about both advantages and disadvantages, both logistical and ethical).[49] While these allocation systems are most obviously problematic when the good to be rationed is tangible and scarce and has minimal interchangeability with other resources, it is straightforward and simple unlike when money is the limiting resource, because money is fungible. True, there are certain things money cannot or should not buy (livers, for example), but there are many more goods available for purchase and therein lies the challenge. With unlimited choice comes the difficulty of choosing. We could either set a predetermined limit on funding (like Oregon) or decide what we wanted to buy and for whom and that would dictate how much was needed, or—more realistically—some combination of the two. But no matter how this conundrum is approached, if it lacks the elements of fairness, its credibility for those who must abide by its rules would be questionable or even absent.

There is ample evidence of the effect of mistrust on the functioning of a rationing scheme. Almost all of this is due to the perception of either past or present injustices or unfairness. All one has to do is examine the solid-organ transplant system. Many consider this an example of a system whose integrity and fairness people generally trust, and this trust is certainly warranted, but only when one looks at the *allocation* part of the methodology. This is what we might refer to as the "demand" side of the equation. When one examines the other half—the "supply" side—a different story emerges. It is there that one butts up against other issues of suspicion of and doubt about the motivations of the entire medical apparatus, of which organ transplantation is a small part. For instance, there is ample evidence to show that African Americans are willing to donate (and actually do donate) their organs for use in cadaveric transplantation at rates significantly below those of other groups in the population, such as people who self-identify as "white."[50] Studies have repeatedly demonstrated that one of the major factors contributing to this disparity in donation rates is the lack of trust that African Americans have in the American medical system (Minniefield and Muti 2002; Minniefield, Yang, and Muti 2001; Russell et al. 2011). Of course, one has to die first in order to donate a liver, kidney, heart, or other organ; this is in accord with the dead-donor rule. Many members of this historically medically and socially marginalized and exploited group of people feel—rightly or wrongly in the present day—that doctors eager to transplant their organs will not do all they can to save their lives, and even may actively work to shorten them, so that their organs can be harvested to save the lives of others. Ironically, this applies to all organs, including kidneys, even though African Americans are disproportionately overrepresented in the end-stage renal disease population.[51] Indeed, it is the perception that the "system" is unfair—that people will be treated differently based on medically or clinically irrelevant facts about them, such as race or ethnicity—that fuels wariness, skepticism, or resentment, leading eventually to a complete lack of trust. A healthcare system deficient in or bereft of trust on the part of its users is bankrupt and could never ask its users to willingly embrace change. As I have suggested earlier, the effort devoted to enhancing and ensuring basic fairness in the allocation of organs in the national transplant system is a distinctive feature that, despite its deficiencies and occasional lapses, contributes substantially to its legitimacy and, hence, its acceptance by the public.

It is a fact that sick people are vulnerable, especially to exploitation by others, be they doctors, unscrupulous salespeople, or even those who purport to love them such as friends and relatives. Physicians can prey on the sick for their own gain, financial or otherwise, such as to enhance their reputation or for academic advancement, fame, publicity, and the like; salespeople can try to sell the sick insurance policies they don't need or want or other goods and services they would not purchase were they well; and loved ones can either inadvertently or maliciously take advantage when they try to help or are pressed for surrogate decisions on what is the best course of action to take. Importantly, for our purposes, we should note that this vulnerability could be enhanced in a rationing setting because, unlike the situation where access to a resource or service is absent, there is a real chance that patients might have to forgo something that could conceivably make them better. However, as I argue in the next chapter, a generous health plan—that is, one that might have a chance of acceptance in the United States—would probably limit these to marginally beneficial and/or unproven interventions. This could induce a form of desperation that, together with illness, might increase the susceptibility of patients to being the victims of those who would prey on the weak. The inherent defenselessness of the sick, the prevalent asymmetry of information and power (that no amount of Internet data gathering can possibly eliminate) and the overwhelming desire of people who are ill to get better are more than sufficient reasons for fairness and justice to be the elemental, foundational basis for any rationing plan that pretends to be anything but dictatorial and autocratic.

Finally, it would be instructive to consider one of the more radical, perhaps outlandish, proposals that has been made to distribute scarce resources, and whether it meets any of the Fairness criteria I have described. John Harris proposed his "survival lottery" in the mid-1970s (Harris 1975). I have never been quite sure how serious he was about this idea, although he did repeat it several times in different published venues, including a chapter he contributed to an edited collection (Harris 1994). In perhaps an expression of utilitarian (or consequentialist) excess, Harris suggested that all individuals be provided with a lottery number that could be chosen at random (with a few exceptions) when his or her organs were needed to save two or more people's lives. The rationale was that it is better that two people have the opportunity to live than one person, hence justifying killing the one to save the many. While the numbers add up, no one would ever think this was fair, although it should be pointed out that Harris does argue that the dying potential transplant recipients would hold that their lives are just as valuable as the healthy person's, and thus he "reasonably" argues that the latter should count for more (in the aggregate). Although this sounds logical, it would violate one of the cardinal principles that I and many others suggest are necessary for public legitimacy of any sort of allocation scheme.

The only reason to mention Harris's idea is that these are the types of proposals that are taken seriously by some people (at least in the academy as an intellectual exercise) but that horrify almost everyone else as perhaps emblematic of what planners, deep ponderers, (and heaven forbid) medical ethicists are thinking about when they consider how to reform healthcare in the United States. While the survival lottery may be at the far end of the "thought-experiment" spectrum, it is by no means unique. As I discuss in the next chapter, it bears at least a passing emotional and conceptual resemblance to Daniel Callahan's call for people over a certain age to renounce any claim on expensive medical resources on the grounds that they have lived a full life (their proverbial "three score and ten," as he puts it) and should forgo access to interventions or treatments that would only extend their lives for a short bit while shortchanging that available to younger people (Callahan 1987, 1998, 2009). Respected thinkers and experts discuss these kinds of suggestions seriously. But they are exploited mercilessly by the mass media and others in order to shock and terrify less knowledgeable and sophisticated people (which is pretty much almost everyone) about what could happen with healthcare reform and rationing. Fairness is what should be emphasized, not radical schemes.

Nevertheless, Harris does raise the question of the redistribution of resources and how much leveling of the playing field will be tolerable to as many as possible. To a certain extent this is an empirical question that could be approached by surveys of the public and other research. To a lesser degree this objection may be met by a modified form of the lottery as proposed by Øverland (2007), who would restrict the pool of people to be liable to the lottery to those in need of an organ themselves and thus likely to die waiting for one. Although even this approach, while perhaps meeting the legitimacy objection if we assume that this demographic group would buy into the idea and participate, remains troubling from a societal point of view. That is, would we want to live in a community that tolerated the attitude that people could be killed for their organs, even under carefully controlled conditions? After all, we do not permit people to consent to sell themselves into slavery, even if it might benefit them (or their loved ones) in some way. The point of bringing up Harris's idea was simply to note that any deliberation on the distribution of resources would need to consider a variety of proposals, some more idiosyncratic and impractical than others. Harris's plan does possess the virtue of imaginatively considering a situation in which there is a dire need for life-saving organs due to a finite scarcity. In contrast to general healthcare resources to fund a comprehensive healthcare plan—even one in which there is a cap on the total amount of funds to be expended—it is implausible that any rationing plan in the United States that could be accepted by employing "accountability for reasonableness" or some similar method, would be as draconian as resorting to a "survival lottery" to make limited supplies go further.

Finally, it is worth considering the following question, because it is bound to arise in some form: Can or should a distribution scheme that adopts fairness as a foundational principle accept trade-offs as in the first hypothetical case I presented, where a member of a prominent and wealthy family was competing for a scarce, life-saving drug with a less fortunate individual? Should her family's prior generous donations to the medical center earn her the right to jump ahead of the other patient who is competing for the drug? Or is this a form of "selling" that should be prohibited? It would be easy to imagine a wealthy individual offering a large amount of money to receive a scarce resource. This would be no different than offering to buy a kidney or a piece of a liver. What about more quotidian resources that are not so precious? Many institutions have so-called VIP service for patients who have already donated or from whom they wish to solicit more donations; should this practice be continued? Should some patients be more equal than others, to paraphrase George Orwell (1996)?

Undoubtedly some would argue that the money supplied in the form of a true gift, with or without an implied or overt quid pro quo, could be used for a variety of beneficial purposes, ranging from reimbursing the institution for charity care to upgrading existing facilities or perhaps even building new ones to reduce overcrowding. However, there is no guarantee that the hospital or medical center would use these funds to relieve deficiencies or reduce destitution. Indeed, it is not uncommon that many affluent people who donate money to nonprofit institutions do so with a memorial of some sort in mind, either to themselves or others, and nothing says that better than a plaque on a brand-new building. It is true that some individuals could require that their donation only be used to mitigate the needs of the poor in an unrestricted fashion, so that the hospital would have the discretion to spend the money as conditions warrant. But in my experience, this is not very common among the "big leagues" of fundraising. However, there is certainly no reason to believe that hospitals couldn't offer priority consideration for a scarce resource in exchange for donations to the institution's charity fund; desperate patients and their families would probably leap at the chance to evade the strictures imposed by rigorous fairness procedures. Be that as it may, unrestricted monies are loved for their lack of constraints, and there is also no reason to assume that the hospital's administrators would not use some or all of the money to give themselves raises, redecorate their offices, or have a lavish meeting for like-minded administrators in a plush tropical resort.

Finally, the moral and practical disruption and destruction that such a practice could exert on the legitimacy of the allocation system in the minds of those who could not afford to buy their way to the front of the line would be terminally corrosive. As both Satz (2010) and Sandel (2012) argue in their respective books, some things should not be for sale, and in this category I would include the ability to evade the responsibilities, limitations, and rules of fairness.

However, this does not mean that we should necessarily eliminate all avenues for obtaining what might be called "special treatment" for those who can afford to pay for it (just not for those resources that are absolutely scarce). For example, even though I have been suggesting that any rationing scheme that would have a ghost of a chance of being implemented in the United States would have to be quite generous in its benefits (in addition to being fair, as I have described above), it must restrict access or eliminate some resources or services, or else the justification for rationing would be incoherent. Like conditions today, it seems implausible that a universal healthcare plan based on rationing would cover treatments such as elective cosmetic surgery. But again, as is the case at present, it would be reasonable to permit these activities to continue to be available in the private sector, obtainable by anyone with the means to do so. In the same way that we have public and private schools, we could plausibly have public and private hospitals, so long as the latter were supported by private dollars that did not subtract from the overall support for the former. (That is, "private" patients would not get a break or relief from the taxes used to fund the general healthcare system; any care they sought outside of it would have to be paid for in addition.)

The more difficult issue arises for interventions or treatments that are more questionable, such as those for marginally beneficial care or unproven therapies (outside of a clinical trial). Currently, doctors prescribe these treatments in the same clinics and hospitals where more conventional or effective therapies are employed and patients and their families are none the wiser. In the same way that it is often obvious where the sequestered "special" patients are located (they are the ones with the single rooms, the bigger rooms, the VIP service, etc.), it may similarly be easily apparent who is getting treatments proscribed for the majority of patients who do not have the means to purchase them. This would be especially noticeable in intensive-care units (it may be more practical to have a separate VIP ICU in the same hospital if one wanted to really go after this "business"), rather than a mixed unit where families of both "plebian" and "patrician" patients are not sequestered from each other and can compare notes for treatments their sick relatives were receiving. However, the undisguised availability of some things for money for some people in the same location might again add to a deterioration of trust in the intrinsic fairness of the system. Thus, careful consideration would have to be given to how to physically manage a dual healthcare system in which the overwhelming majority of patients would receive all their care from the national plan in which rationing (and fairness) would be an integral component.

In this chapter I have emphasized the importance of fairness as the basis for establishing trust in any rationing scheme, be it for resources that are both scarce and in finite supply (like livers), or for a more total allocation system for all of healthcare. In a rich country like the United States, it is highly likely that most of what would be restricted in an attempt to rein in costs and more equitably distribute healthcare to more people would be interventions that would offer marginal or limited benefits.[52] This would still result in a system with extremely generous benefits, but one in which that generosity would be extended to all. Even so, an attempt to say no to people, no matter how justified I or people like me may think that decision may be, undoubtedly will anger some who disagree. To convince them, or for them to make me change my mind, there must be a structure and a procedure by which fairness is understood as an essential and inherent guiding force in allocation decisions, both at the overall system level and at the bedside or in the medical office. Without that, people will mistrust the system and not endorse or participate in it or even feel bound by its rules. There will be no way to persuade people to accept any decision as reasoned and reasonable and just.[53]

While by no means perfect, the organ allocation schemes mostly adhere to the principles of Daniels and Sabin and most neutral observers would judge them as reasonably just, or fair enough. Significantly, organ transplant candidates and their families, including those who die waiting for a transplant, endorse this view, which itself is a powerful indication that a vital constituency affirms the basic equity and legitimacy of the system. There is no reason to believe that a similar approach could not be applied to a much larger and more complex structure—namely the health system itself—to achieve similar validity. In the chapters to follow I discuss some aspects of how one might go about deciding what would be reasonable to include and exclude in the range of health benefits offered, creating a system that could plausibly be supported by most people.

4

The Cutoff Problem, or Where and How to Draw the Line

In the previous chapters I have argued that rationing applied to the entire healthcare system could potentially be acceptable and not especially onerous. Both claims are based on the premise that if it were fairly and justly applied and thus bore some resemblance to existing well-tolerated rationing systems, such as that for the allocation of scarce organs, then it could be similarly well accepted. Indeed, compared to this system, in which there is an absolute shortage of livers, hearts, lungs, and kidneys and where the failure to obtain a transplant is most often certain death, it is doubtful that any kind of realistic, organized rationing plan would have as severe consequences for those denied something they might think they need or want. This is related to the second claim, which is grounded on the assumption that a wealthy country such as the United States would be generous in its healthcare funding system, even though there would necessarily be limitations.[1] If there were no limits, then changing how healthcare is delivered in the United States based solely on economic factors would be hard to justify. Moreover, it is inconceivable that the American public would permit the imposition of any form of rationing that resulted in a significant loss of benefits they deemed meaningful when it was feasible to do otherwise. Indeed, the trade-off or compromise—for both political and social reasons—would undoubtedly have to entail a package of benefits sufficiently generous and wide-ranging to quell the most vociferous public dissent.[2]

However, the very fact that there must be a ceiling on the budget means decisions must be made on where to draw the line on services—in other words, on what or what not to include. While there clearly would be a major challenge to "selling" rationing to a suspicious public due to the fear provoked by a wide variety of interest groups who might stand to lose something should this form of reform be instituted, I suggested in chapter 1 that a good deal of this trepidation may be due to concerns about what might be lost or absent should comprehensive healthcare rationing come to pass. And since this in turn is based on where the cutoff in benefits would be placed—how generous and extensive the coverage would be—it is vitally important to consider how this might be accomplished. I suspect that some straightforward changes that could accompany a national healthcare system, such as a vast decrease in the administrative needs and overhead (and hence, costs), could be relatively painless to patients, doctors, nurses, and presumably hospital and clinic management. It is unlikely that any of these people would complain about less paperwork and fewer bureaucratic layers (however, pain would be felt among the thousands of people who would stand to lose their no-longer-necessary jobs).

There are a number of methods that could be used, all of which have their virtues and faults, but all have the same goal: identifying the lines of demarcation between interventions (broadly construed) that would or would not be included. In this chapter I will discuss the challenges this presents and some constructive ways we might think about addressing them so as to make them widely acceptable. Importantly, cutoffs are inextricably bound to other considerations, including that of fairness, which I discussed in the previous chapter. I will begin by recounting a real-life episode from several years ago.

In 2009, infectious disease experts, epidemiologists, and public health authorities around the world were preparing for what they feared could be a massive pandemic of a virulent strain of influenza A. There were projections of enormous numbers of dead and dying people, which had the potential to be similar to the 1918–1919 influenza pandemic, in which around 50 million people (perhaps many more by some estimates) died in a time frame of just two years (Barry 2004). However, unlike the situation that existed a century ago, we now had all of the diagnostic and therapeutic power of modern, scientific, technological medicine, including the ability to produce an effective vaccine against the virus. Presumably, one would wish to offer everyone the opportunity to benefit from a vaccine, but it would take time to produce the quantities needed to protect all those who could benefit from it, and this raised the question of who should receive the initial batches. This was a classic rationing situation with an absolutely scarce resource, and one that necessarily involved drawing lines or imposing cutoffs.

Many allocation schemes were proposed. Surveys were performed that asked members of the public who they thought should receive the limited supplies available and in what order. Interestingly, they gave top priority to healthcare personnel (doctors, nurses, etc.) and first responders such as police, firefighters, and National Guard members. That they listed the former as first in line was not all that surprising, but the latter choices were unexpected and differed from those initially proposed by public health authorities. Many people who were queried said that they wanted to protect those people who would be needed to take care of the legions of anticipated patients sick with the flu as well as those who were charged with protecting public order, life, and property. The federal government (via the Centers for Disease Control, which was coordinating the preparation and response) altered the priority list in response to these expressed preferences. The outcome of these surveys provided a significant lesson: in a society where the will of the people is held to be important and often decisive, it would be wise to consult the public prior to making any momentous recommendation that can affect their welfare in such a vital manner.[3]

The next big question concerned how to distribute the succeeding batches of vaccine to the general public. There still would be insufficient amounts to vaccinate everyone. Another dilemma that arose somewhat later involved a related question: how to allocate relatively scarce ICU beds and ventilators for those patients who were sick with severe acute respiratory distress syndrome (ARDS) secondary to influenza. (In chapters 2 and 3 I introduced a different aspect of this issue when I discussed the ECMO dilemma.) In both cases, there clearly would not be adequate quantities of vaccine or ICU beds for everyone who could conceivably benefit. Therefore, the challenge was to develop a method to prioritize recipients. Presumably this would be primarily based on some form of scientific calculus of medical risk and advantage. But there were additional considerations that took into account our feelings about what might be called just deserts. This is somewhat different from the kinds of social worthiness that I discussed in chapter 3 as morally irrelevant facts about people that should not generally enter into prioritizing decisions.

One of the most widely publicized ideas was that proposed by Emanuel and Wertheimer (2006). They suggested that vaccine should be preferentially given to the young over the old. This idea was based on a concept that has been called the "life-cycle principle," which was related to Harris's notion of "fair innings" (Harris 1985; Williams 1997). There was also evidence to suggest that young, healthy people with strong immune systems might have a much higher likelihood of being sicker than older patients who could not mount such a robust immune response to the virus (Ma, Dushoff, and Earn 2011). Both views privilege younger versus older persons because the former have not yet had the opportunity to achieve those experiences and landmarks we associate with a reasonably full lifespan, such as schooling, work, marriage, and parenthood.[4] Even though Emanuel and Wertheimer's approach was both clever and thoughtful, it, like all others of this type, suffered from the cutoff problem, the inevitable and inescapable dilemma associated with attempting to arbitrarily impose distinctions between people or create and separate out groups where there may be none to be found. In their proposal for the distribution of influenza vaccine, there had to be sharp demarcation points that marked off those who were at the front of the line from those further back, the latter being individuals with a lower likelihood of getting vaccinated. Any method that attempted to discern perceptible and significant differences—either medical or moral—between synthetic categories of people based on an ordinal quantity such as age necessarily imposed a substantive difficulty. By using the variable of age, they confronted the challenge of breaking a continuous variable into discrete components by arbitrary means.

This is an obstacle that will confound any attempt to differentiate people on the basis of attributes that differ continuously from lesser to greater, be it age, weight, height, annual income, and so on. While some continuous variables are "lumpier" than others and many also demonstrate so-called bell-shaped distribution curves (more appropriately labeled Gaussian distributions), the challenge lies not in discerning palpable and meaningful differences between individuals who reside at the far ends of the scale and thus great distances from each other. Rather, it is being able to distinguish two (groups of) people who lie on either side of the imposed cutoff line. For example, if the cutoff between receiving and not receiving some good or resource is set at age 55, it would be implausible (if not impossible) to assert that there is a substantive difference that is both practically and morally meaningful between someone who is 54 years and 364 days old and another who is 55 years and 1 day old, such that it justifies favoring the former over the latter. Other than having the good or bad luck to be born on the right or wrong date with respect to the arbitrary cutoff line, the two are identical, assuming all other things are equal. This is not to say that reasonable and ethically defensible cutoffs are impossible to achieve; they are just problematic.

The pertinent point is that any rationing scheme involving either fixed, finite resources that are absolutely scarce or those that are relatively scarce must involve the application of cutoff lines that require decisions about where to place them (and why) and how to successfully and ethically manage borderline cases. I suspect that this last matter will prove to be the most vexing, because it is unlikely that there will be a major chasm between conditions, cases, people, and so forth that makes obvious the differences between those situated on either side of the borderline. This problem will demand the most comprehensive and careful examination.[5]

Most important, if the claims I (and others) have made in chapter 3 are both true and relevant to the successful creation of any kind of rationing plan—especially one that embraces democratic input to give the plan legitimacy and win the support of those affected by it—one has to be able to convince people that these distinctions are reasonable, especially people whose lives could be materially influenced by the imposition of cutoff lines. In the discussion that follows I will first consider some common types of cutoffs in healthcare and present a more complete examination of age as an arbiter of where a line could be drawn (I do this mostly because it has been the focus of much discussion about the merits of rationing over the past couple of decades). Finally, I will mention the peculiar problems that arise when a fungible resource (such as money) must be limited, and consider how we might think about cutoffs involving expendable funds. This will require a discussion of marginally beneficial interventions and some of the advantages of using this approach as a metric for cutoffs. I will advance a tentative conclusion that focusing on this latter case may be a worthwhile place to begin determining when certain amounts and kinds of healthcare are too much. First, let us consider why we have a cutoff problem in the first place.

Why Do We Have a Cutoff Problem?

Let us assume for the moment that the overall goal of any universal healthcare rationing plan would be to deliver as much effective medicine to as many people as possible within whatever budget constraints are set. Therefore—short of completely uncontrolled spending in which everything is made available to everybody (which is, of course, not rationing)—cutoffs of some sort must be made. Any attempt to control spending necessitates saying no to some people; they can't have something they may want or think they need. Whether it is an operation they and their doctors believe will help them, or a new and expensive drug that may offer them hope of one sort or another, or continued intensive care for pneumonia in an elderly person who also has advanced, metastatic cancer, these cases all involve decisions that some medical interventions will or will not be reasonable to cover. That doesn't necessarily prevent individuals from obtaining what they want on their own with their own money, just that the "system" won't pay for it. In many ways this is no different from what private insurance policies do all the time: if you want elective cosmetic surgery, then you will most likely have to fund it yourself because the insurer has drawn a cutoff line.

Most people in the United States with any kind of health insurance, be it public or private or some combination, are subject to a wide variety of cutoffs. For example, in an effort to control costs, in most states, Medicaid has a formulary that lists the names of the drugs doctors are permitted to prescribe. Most of the time when there is a generic alternative to a higher-priced brand-name drug, the former will be included in the formulary. This might seem a somewhat trivial instance of a cutoff, but it is one nonetheless. Another is the common practice of insurance companies imposing annual or lifetime caps on paid benefits per beneficiary (although this practice is greatly curtailed under a provision of the Affordable Care Act). And, to a certain extent, any time an insurer decides that it won't pay for something (say, a radiology test) because it is "experimental" or the data supporting the indications for its use are not strong enough, a cutoff is imposed, in this case involving the standard of evidence required to validate a proposed use.

If we are talking about systematic rationing, then the question is how to draw lines ethically and how to best distribute the benefits and burdens of what can and cannot be bought and paid for. How to create the classifications and distinctions between various interventions when the scientific data that supports their use (or not) may be good, but far from exacting, is a major challenge and will undoubtedly contribute to much of the concern over the fairness of any approach to making cutoffs. As I just mentioned, health insurance companies are constantly faced with patients and doctors disputing their rationale for denying coverage for a proposed treatment in which there may be a fundamental disagreement over the meaning and value of the existing scientific literature. Where there truly is controversy, resolution may be very difficult to achieve, thus causing cutoffs to appear even more arbitrary.[6]

To a very great extent, the Oregon Health Services Commission was charged with creating a mechanism for imposing a cutoff by establishing a series of condition-treatment pairings. They initially rank-ordered them using pure cost-effectiveness analysis data and then amended the list by the application of other methods (see chapter 2). How far down they went on the list was determined by how much money the legislature voted to spend on healthcare for the poor and near-poor, together with how many of these potentially eligible people there actually were in the state. The largesse of the legislature and the status of the economy would then dictate who got how much. So the cutoff was determined by the legislature and the budget it passed to fund this program. Whether the line was drawn at condition-treatment pair #699 or #700 or somewhere else depended on the cost-estimate projections and the total amount allocated to the OHP.[7] When times were flush, more people would get more, and when the economy faltered or the resolve of legislators to devote sufficient tax money to indigent healthcare weakened, fewer people would be covered and/or the remaining people would receive less. Or, if the legislators were stingy or generous, poor people would receive less or more healthcare.[8] Nevertheless, rationing required a cutoff. The kind of cutoff was dictated by the way the funding decisions were made. For example, they could have decided beforehand that condition-treatments, say, #1 to #733 were reasonable to pay for because the current medical evidence suggested that these were disorders that caused significant suffering and for which effective therapies existed. Accordingly, condition-treatments #734 and below affected either too few people or the efficacy data were scant and hence it was reasonable to exclude them. However, decisions were made the other way around. Thus budgets dictated the quantity of care rather than the reverse, making a relatively arbitrary cutoff inescapable.[9]

The main point I wish to make at this juncture is that if we decide to limit the amount of money we spend on healthcare, no matter how we arrive at the final total, it will still be a limit. This requires the setting of some sort of cutoff. Some number of patients who may have access to something now may no longer do so. On the other hand, many more patients who don't have much or anything at present would gain enormously. The question is how to determine where to draw the line. It would be sensible, if not optimal, to do so in such a manner that anyone who could reasonably be helped by healthcare would receive that help in the future. That would be both generous and fair (not to mention, of great practical significance, because it would contribute enormously to the palatability and therefore public acceptability of any plan). However, it then means that we have to decide what is reasonable. Most of the characteristics that have been discussed or proposed in the literature as possible targets for cutoffs are those that are quantifiable in one way or another. These include age, cost-effectiveness, comparative effectiveness, and money. This brings us up against the challenge of continuous variables. I introduced this topic earlier when I referenced it with regard to using age as a cutoff. I now want to discuss this problem in more detail, because it plagues most kinds of measures that might be used to determine cutoff points for rationing healthcare when one of our goals is to control costs.

There's an important point to note here. Many people—with or without health insurance—are under the illusion that their doctors have unfettered freedom to give them whatever treatments or diagnostic tests they think they should have. As I've mentioned frequently in this book, that's a complete fallacy. There are myriad limits, restrictions, qualifications, and constraints on what an individual patient may be offered. Therefore, neither the idea nor the actuality of cutoffs can be considered novel; to hold otherwise is either disingenuous or deceptive. However, it is accurate to assert that the existing state of cutoffs is variable, often arbitrary or capricious, and habitually inexplicable.

Continuous-Variable Problems

Most proposals that aim to ration healthcare resources try to do so either with characteristics of individuals (when viewed as members of one or more groups) or stuff of various types (like money), almost all of which vary continuously, and it is this attribute that generates both the difficulties and the controversy over the cutoff problem. The purpose of doing this is quite simple: to attempt to identify traits that people possess intrinsically that are easy to measure and quantify, and hence that can be employed to describe differences between individuals based on their numeric representation, whatever that may be. This approach also makes it quite straightforward to lump people into groups with similar quantities of the characteristic of interest. Common examples of continuous variables in populations include traits like height, weight, age, intelligence as measured by IQ tests, and the like. The fact that they are continuous does not mean that their distribution has to be on a straight line from lesser to greater values. Indeed, many of these characteristics have normal or Gaussian distributions, meaning that their dispersal is such that some values are more common than others.[10] The critical point is that if the population is big enough, its constituent members will occupy points continuously along a distribution curve as shown in figure 4.1, which displays height among adult men and women in the United States. Contrast this with the data in figure 4.2, which shows the heights of a small group of unrelated men, demonstrating discrete differences between those measured.

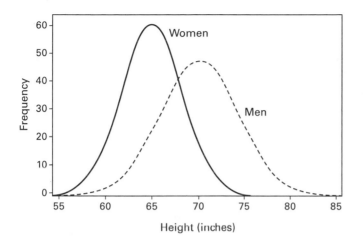

Figure 4.1

Height distribution for adult men and women in the United States. (Used with the permission of Jeff Sauro, from http://www.usablestats.com/lessons/normal.)

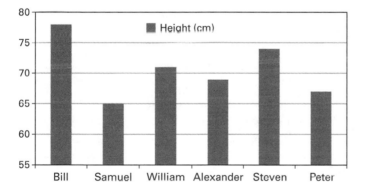

Figure 4.2

Height distribution of six unrelated men showing discrete and easily separable differences between them.

The key consideration to take away from these figures is that the greater the number of data points contributing to the population characteristic being quantified—in this example, the more people whose heights we measure—the smoother (more continuous) the curve. When we just wish to analyze these data mathematically, there is no difficulty at all distinguishing two points on the distribution, as long as they differ in some measureable amount, even if it is infinitesimally small. But when we transform this numerical information into chunks we have problems, especially when we want to relate them to differences between the groups. Another way to look at it might be to see it as "reverse reification" in which a concrete entity (say, height or weight or age) is transformed into packages or constructs that we then label as "tall" or "short," "obese" or "skinny," and "young" or "old." Conceptually (and mathematically), differences between the arithmetic means of these group measures are quite stark; the problems arise at the boundaries that are used to define the borders between them and that then permit us to bestow these names on them. The names represent broad descriptors in which quantities are transformed into qualities.[11] Not all "tall" people are the same height and not all "slender" people weigh the same. Within each arbitrarily defined group there is also variation.

Most important for all of these scalar, measurable qualities is the understanding that the difference between smaller and larger magnitudes is relative. While we readily see and evaluate the height difference as significant between someone who is 155 cm tall (about 5 feet, 2 inches) and one who is 193 cm (about 6 feet, 4 inches), it would be very challenging for us to make the same calculation and assessment if we were trying to distinguish an important difference between two people whose height varied by less than 1 cm. Age works the same way. Most of us would have little problem saying that there is a major contrast between a 5-year-old and an 80-year-old: it's not even close. And we could probably agree that there is a substantive dissimilarity between two people whose ages were separated by as little as 25 years.[12] But when the two hypothetical individuals get closer in age, it becomes much more difficult—if not impossible—to distinguish between them. There are statistical methods for accomplishing this, at least by computational means, but that doesn't help us appreciate a *practical* (as well as moral) difference between people whose ages differ by 6 months or heights by 1 cm. Nevertheless, even though it is increasingly criticized for statistical shortcomings, the analytic technique of separating items that exist on a continuous scale (like age) into dichotomous variables remains a fairly popular method to bring sense to measurements that are difficult to distinguish by other means.[13]

However, significant conceptual issues with this approach remain. They are far beyond the scope of this book to discuss in detail (not to mention vastly exceeding my level of mathematical competence), but suffice it to say that many experts in this area are quite critical of its application in just the manner I am discussing. To state the main problem with this up front, I can quote from an editorial in the journal *Medical Decision Making*: "Misclassification tends to be most extreme near the split, as subjects who are similar are treated as being in completely different groups. For example, splitting age at 70 years assumes that the 70th birthday is a dramatic event, directly affecting the risks of outcomes" (Dawson and Weiss 2012, 225). The basic challenge is how to mark distinctions among people when we have a commitment to all persons being morally indistinguishable, at least for the purposes of distributing benefits and burdens. For the moment, at least for the purposes of this discussion, I will ignore the very real and practical import of the limits of tolerability for this idea due to societal constraints that are subject to deeply held (and sometimes unjustifiable) prejudices and biases (see chapter 6 for a more detailed discussion of this topic). However, we cannot avoid the need to establish some forms of cutoff if we accept the fact that resources—in whatever form they occur—are not unlimited. An undeniable characteristic of the distribution of scarce resources, whether done well or poorly, is that there are those who must do without something they might want, and that entails the creation of a cutoff.

Examples of Cutoffs

One way to think about cutoff problems in healthcare rationing is by grouping them into general categories. These classifications are separate from, but certainly dependent on, the structural problems I just described, such as those inherent in using measures of continuous variables: this will be obvious in the examples I present. The first major group contains cutoffs that are episodic or situation-dependent. These would include the types that are confronted when dealing with an absolute shortage of a specific resource or resources, such as influenza vaccine, critically scarce drugs, solid organs for transplant, or other items. The number or quantity of the good to be distributed is fixed and hence determinative of the number of patients that can be recipients. What remains to be decided is who among the world of possible beneficiaries should be eligible and how many of them can be served. In these contexts, one has to decide how to prioritize patients (recipients) in order of importance, which in turns entails establishing measureable or quantifiable criteria to employ as determinants of primacy. This could be a parameter as simple and straightforward (and hence less vulnerable to exploitation) as laboratory values that are surrogates or indicators of the severity of a patient's illness, such as the MELD score for liver transplantation (Avolio et al. 2011; Bonney et al. 2009; Dutkowski et al. 2011; Moylan et al. 2008). The most significant feature of this category is that the resources with which it is concerned are relatively inflexible in their application, meaning that their uses are limited and usually indivisible. Livers can't be cut into pieces so as to make a single organ help many potential recipients. Moreover, one could think of the nature of these decisions or judgments as "first order": since little can be done to increase the supply of the resource, the necessary determinations first and foremost concern how to distribute the finite quantity available. The cutoff point is dependent on the number of organs available; if there were more, then the program would presumably be more expansive and thus permit more patients to be transplanted (the line would shift). But, so long as the quantity of patients with organ failure who could truly benefit from a transplant exceeds the supply, the latter will establish the cutoff point (leaving aside for the moment what we might mean by "truly benefit," which of course itself implies a cutoff).

In contrast, the second category applies to a resource that is perhaps the greater challenge simply because of the kind of resource involved: money. Money is fungible. It can be used to purchase many different things (although not all) and is therefore maximally adjustable and versatile depending on the priorities, desires, and choices of the individuals who control the purse strings. Except for the obvious (and occasionally ambiguous) exceptions of things money cannot and/or should not buy (Sandel 2012; Satz 2010), the difficulty encountered in making decisions here involves both first- and second-order rankings. In this case, the first-order decision again involves how to spend the money that is designated for this purpose. The second-order decision concerns the debate and then verdict on how much money should be spent, or the total budget allotted to whatever the pursuit might be. Of course, the two must be highly interrelated, if not integrated, because it can be presumed that a body endowed with budgetary authority would not endorse a financial plan without having some idea of the details of what they would be paying for.[14] For the most part, rationing decisions that would govern an entire healthcare system would belong to this group. We have a great deal of experience working with rationing of the first type and we have found this approach both acceptable and fair (i.e., organ transplants). The challenge remains with the second group.

That is where the big decisions lie: how much money to provide to determine where the cutoff should be. And presumably, because we are a wealthy and (hopefully) generous country, the cutoff could be similarly generous. But assuming we have a choice about where to draw the line, where should it be? If we are discussing what to pay for, perhaps it should be up for debate what quantity and kinds of interventions are worth funding. For example, how marginal (or too little) a benefit is too marginal (or too little) for it to merit public support? Would it be reasonable to declare some kinds of patient desires or wants illegitimate (for the purposes of funding under rationing)? Following the template I proposed in chapter 3, what would a reasonable and informed public discourse conclude are the limits of attempts at curative care? Or, if we wish to prioritize certain kinds of people for access to certain types of care or resources over others—such as using age as a determinant—how would this look and is it something that would be acceptable to people in general?

To illustrate some of the very real challenges associated with creating cutoffs that are meaningful (by "meaningful" I want to specify those that would be taken seriously by others in a manner that they would respect if applied to themselves or those they care about, and that would result in appreciable savings), I wish to discuss some criteria that have been proposed to serve as a basis for drawing a line for benefits (i.e., for rationing). I will examine some of the real problems associated with dichotomizing a continuous variable, such as age (it is actually the creation of multiple categories or groupings rather than just two, but this is the term most often used). To do so I will return to Emanuel and Wertheimer's 2006 suggestion to use age cohorts to prioritize the allocation of a scarce influenza vaccine to combat the spread of an anticipated influenza pandemic; this idea was expanded in a paper (with Persad) in which they described this approach as an integrated "complete lives system" that incorporated moral values and considerations from several different, more restrictive views such as utilitarianism (Emanuel and Wertheimer 2006; Persad, Wertheimer, and Emanuel 2009). In contrast to this, I will also discuss the concept of marginally beneficial care and how one could choose to establish a cutoff point at some minimal level of expected benefit for restricting medical interventions.

Age

Why would age be an attractive objective for establishing cutoffs for access to certain kinds and amounts of healthcare interventions? A patient's age has long been thought to be a ripe target for healthcare rationing because it is a characteristic that we all possess and that may have a reasonably relevant relationship to resource utilization. Age also triggers reactive emotions that activate certain moral intuitions to which many are susceptible such as viewing serious illness in the young as deserving of more sympathy than when it occurs in the old.

It is well known that older people on average have more chronic health conditions than younger people and thus use more healthcare resources. In the United States, people over the age of sixty-five consume up to 20 percent of the total annual healthcare budget (in 2010, the most recent year for which complete data are available).[15] Moreover, a significant proportion of these expenditures is devoted to care in the last six months of life, especially to exceedingly costly intensive care (Riley and Lubitz 2010; Thorpe, Ogden, and Galactionova 2010; Kwok et al. 2011; Morden et al. 2012). And, with the overall aging of the population due to a combination of increased longevity, a low birth rate, and the looming retirement of the baby-boom generation demographic "bubble," this figure is likely to grow even larger. Since we know that much of this kind of treatment is devoted to very expensive and possibly marginally beneficial interventions that rarely cure anyone, why not simply say that everyone over some arbitrary age should be limited in the kinds and amounts of healthcare they can receive? Presumably this would save enormous sums of money that could either be diverted to other important government projects, or could be used to be more generous in funding healthcare programs for the poor and uninsured populations.[16]

A major proponent of this view has been Daniel Callahan. He has suggested that people who have lived a full life (he seems to define this as something greater than seventy years, often lyrically basing this on the biblical "three score and ten" that defines a complete lifespan) have had the time and opportunities to undergo most, if not all, of the things one might wish to encounter in a reasonably satisfying and rich life. (These include such experiences as education, work, marriage or its equivalent, and childrearing, which have contributed to the completeness of the lives of people who have lived to, say, seventy and beyond.) Callahan proposes that such individuals should not have an equal claim to healthcare resources that may be in short supply (like organs) or expensive technology, medicines, intensive-care beds, and the like. He assumes that there is a competition for the healthcare dollar with younger people who have not yet had similar chances to accomplish these milestones (Callahan 1990, 2009). In making this claim he does not assert that people who have led impoverished or otherwise unfortunate lives should be treated differently than others who have been luckier in attaining goals and goods, although some might criticize his view for this.[17] Rather, he is simply stating that in an environment in which resources are not inexhaustible, older people who have reached some agreed-on—but reasonably arbitrary—age, and who have reaped the benefits of living to that ripe seniority, should renounce any entitlement to expensive technology and other medical interventions in favor of those who have yet to achieve their longevity and fulfill life's benchmarks (as he lists them).

Importantly, he does not say that we should abandon the elderly as in the often-apocryphal stories of aged Inuit, who, knowing their time has come, sacrifice their lives so that the rest of the community could benefit from them no longer draining resources.[18] As I understand his argument, it does not appear as if he is asserting that old people never have a right to high-priced care near the end of their lives, simply that this is an approach that needs to be considered as a response to ever-escalating healthcare costs and the need to restrain them, given that older individuals use a disproportionate share of medical resources with a diminishing return for the money spent (in terms of years gained and suffering relieved). Rather than limiting the availability of medical care for all, better that it should be restricted for those least able to benefit from it by virtue of their age and the fact that this population has already experienced most of the rewards life has to offer. However, as I will discuss further in the next section, one could reasonably ask if certain kinds of care for certain kinds of people, irrespective of age, should be restricted, rather than assuming all old people are the same. The blanket assumption that eliminating access to costly interventions for everyone over some arbitrary age cutoff would benefit many (everyone else) and burden few (those immediately affected by such a policy) may be mistaken.

In some manner, this belief about preferring or privileging youth for receipt of goods and services over older people (when competition must occur and choices must be made) fits well with our moral and social intuitions that—as many have put it—the death of an older adult is sad, but that of a young person (especially a child) is a tragedy. This is particularly true in industrialized, wealthy countries where the historical causes of mass death in the young were infections. But, due to modern public health measures, vaccines, antibiotics, good nutrition, and so on, death before adulthood is unusual, unexpected, and more painful to both loved ones and the public than in prior eras. This reaction is not just a subjective impression, but is also supported by empirical data.[19]

Ronald Dworkin has poignantly expressed our intuitive feelings about the tragedy of early death (associated with youth):

> We believe … that a successful human life has a certain natural course. It starts in mere biological development—conception, fetal development, and infancy—but it then extends into childhood, adolescence, and adult life in ways that are determined not just by biological formation but by social and individual training and choice, and that culminate in satisfying relationships and achievements of different kinds. It ends, after a normal lifespan, in a natural death. It is a waste of the natural and human created investments that make up the story of a normal life when this normal progression is frustrated by premature death or in other ways. But how bad this is—how great the frustration—depends on the stage of life in which it occurs, because the frustration is greater if it takes place after rather than before the person has made a significant personal investment in his own life, and less if it occurs after any investment has been substantially filled, or as substantially built and is anyway likely. (Dworkin 1993, 88)

It is important to note that Dworkin is making a distinction by demarcating the significance of lives lived (to the individuals living them and those who grieve at their loss) based upon a calculus of investment. Babies, who have not yet had the opportunity to expend substantial personal energy and time into preparing for their futures, may be viewed as "worth less" on this scale of tragic loss than older children or adolescents who have made more meaningful investments (equated with time) in preparing for the years to come. How one delineates boundaries among these categories is left unsaid.

This is not to say that death at an older age does not affect us emotionally; it does not imply that we do not grieve the loss of our ancient loved ones, but that loss tends to be much more personal, confined to those who knew and cared for the dead person. It is tempered by the knowledge that the older person has mostly lived a full extent of years for our species, and this is irrespective of what that individual accomplished in life. When we read the obituary of an eighty-year-old who was not a friend or a relative, it does not have the same impact as reading that of a six-year-old who died of a brain tumor or a seventeen-year-old killed in a car crash, even if we had never met him or her. Dworkin and others also argue that when we are comparing the depth of our feelings about premature mortality, the death of infants—who have yet to mature to a point where much besides love has been invested by others in them or by them in themselves—provokes less feeling of loss than that experienced for an older, more established, life. Now simply because we all react more deeply at the deaths of children than we do for the aged should not form the basis for creating healthcare policy. On the other hand, it would be unwise to ignore these sentiments and the role they may play in influencing public opinions.

Another strategy that could justify denying equal resources to older adults might be to attempt to incorporate some modification of Daniels's principle of fair equality of opportunity as he applies it to the aging process. In this view, normal functioning—given the fact that even under the best of social and public health circumstances the natural lottery will endow some with greater talents and skills than others—offers the wherewithal to take advantage of a range of available, acceptable, and reasonable opportunities as individuals endeavor to fulfill their life plans (which are themselves contingent on there being a range of accessible opportunities of which one can take advantage). Naturally, the kinds of preferences and desires that one might have and express would change throughout life as one ages and experiences the successes and failures that are a normal part of any life. As Daniels (1983, 509) notes,

Life plans, we might note, have stages that reflect important divisions in the life cycle. Without meaning to suggest a particular set of divisions as a framework, it is easy to observe that lives have phases in which different, general tasks are central: nurturing and training in childhood and youth, pursuit of career and family in adult years, and the completion of life projects in later years. Of course, what it is reasonable to include in a life plan for a stage of one's life reflects not only facts about one's own talents and skills, tastes, and preferences, but also depends in part on social policy and other important facts about the society. These qualifications already are present in the notion of normal opportunity range itself.

To the extent that effective healthcare can successfully intervene so as to further these pursuits and life plans, it should be encouraged and provided. And it stands to reason that the kinds of healthcare that can contribute more to those who have had fewer opportunities to develop or achieve life plans such as the young (and perhaps also the socially or economically disadvantaged or marginalized: see chapter 5) versus the old or more accomplished should be more available. Daniels refers to this changing personal aspiration as the "age-relative opportunity range." This approach can offer a justification for our intuitive notion that often favors youth over the aged in a competition for scarce resources.[20] A major point is that looking at life in this way and the kinds of things that might be offered to people throughout the progression of their lives does not discount age per se (especially with respect to healthcare that may be available under resource constraints). It simply acknowledges that the range of accessible or possible options should be in some way predicated on what one has been able to obtain or achieve in the past. As an example, many jobs come with mandatory retirement ages that may only be loosely linked to declining abilities with age. Thus, many people who retire at age sixty-five or seventy may still be perfectly capable of doing their jobs, but there is some belief that "making room" for younger workers is a good thing both for them and society.

Think how this approach might be applied to organ transplantation. First, we acknowledge certain incontrovertible facts: there are many, many more patients whose lives could be potentially saved if they could get a liver, heart, or kidney than there are organs to transplant. Hence, most must go without and almost all of those patients will die of their underlying organ failure. Second, we can reasonably posit that to most people a quantity or length of life with reasonable quality (i.e., the kind that might be offered should a sick person receive an organ and do well) is worth more or less the same amount to persons of various ages assuming they are not depressed, suicidal, or the like. Finally, it seems plausible to hold that the expected non-organ-dependent lifespan of a patient should not be shorter than the average or median amount of time that a transplanted organ is predicted to last. For example, if the median survival time after heart transplantation is about eleven years, one would not wish to transplant a heart into someone with say, metastatic cancer, who is expected to die from that disease within a year or two (Stehlik et al. 2011). That would make little practical (and certainly utilitarian) sense and could be viewed as a "waste" of a valuable organ if there were another patient better situated to take advantage of the full range of extra years granted by the transplant. Following this analysis, we could then propose that in many types of rationing situations, be it organs or dollars that require prioritization decisions, in general those individuals whose life plans and opportunities to advance those plans have a greater chance of coming to fruition or who have not yet had the opportunity to experience them, should have greater access to these resources than others. For organs, this certainly fits with what the public seems to endorse (Eisenberg et al. 2011; Cookson and Dolan 1999; Johannesson and Johansson 1996; Nord 2005; Stahl, Tramontano, Swan, and Cohen 2008; however, for a different survey result see Diederich, Winkelhage, and Wirsik 2011).

There are two important caveats I must inject at this point in my argument. First, even if we accept the proposition that we can deny expensive and technologically advanced healthcare resources to older adults (and what age qualifies as "older" can be determined at some other time; for now it will simply serve as a placeholder), this does not mean that we offer no care at all to them. They should be provided with all that medicine can offer to relieve suffering and ensure as reasonable a quality of life as feasible. But they should not have access to interventions that are both expensive and have little chance of restoring them to a satisfactory level of functional health. Second, we justified denying an organ to an older person with an expected limited lifespan because another recipient could potentially benefit more from receiving this public resource. We could apply similar reasoning with the money saved by withholding say, ICU care, from an older sick adult or a desperately ill and extremely premature infant, both with dismal prognoses, and transfer it to a need that helps others or society in a more substantive way. However, as I pointed out previously, money is fungible (and as a result highly flexible) in a way that livers, hearts, and kidneys are not. Therefore, in order to justify this restriction, there must be a credible reason to believe that the funds saved would be put to good use, similar to the organ that is diverted to another candidate.

Nevertheless, as attractive as age might be to serve as a cutoff measure, there are several substantive problems with using age itself as a surrogate marker for "too old to benefit" (especially if we stipulate "no matter what"). First, while it is certainly true that chronic diseases (and more of them) are heavily concentrated in older adults, it is by no means a rigid rule, and not all people of a given age, say seventy years old, are physiologically or clinically the same. Some are extremely healthy and use very few medical resources, while others have multiple chronic illnesses and as a consequence consume an enormous amount of healthcare. It would be grossly unfair to lump the two groups together and treat them as if they were the same. There are large numbers of older adults who are vigorous and could be expected to live reasonably healthy and active lives for a number of years, and it would be unjust and in fact cruel to deny them access to effective medicine that could contribute to maintaining their quality and quantity of life. It is also reasonable to assume that if efforts to encourage more wholesome and health-promoting lifestyles were successful, a generation of older adults with a much better performance profile is to be expected, negating even more any contention that old age equals decrepitude and that the medical care used by them is wasted. If, as I argued in chapter 2, any limited-resource distribution plan (rationing) is going to be even minimally acceptable to the public that would be affected by these kinds of decisions, the plan cannot resort to seemingly arbitrary discrimination such as this. Furthermore, the proposal to limit access to certain kinds of healthcare would have to be tolerable and justifiable to both those people who would possibly bear its (nonfinancial) costs or burdens in the future, and those individuals currently situated so as to be affected by it. This relates to the fact that the majority of younger people hope to grow older, and most will do so. While I assume that nearly all of us want to age with both good health and dignity, it would be unrealistic to think that this rosy prospect will be everyone's fate. And since we cannot often predict with any certainty what will happen in the future—whether we will get sick or be injured—it would be a great comfort to know that our society and healthcare system would not abandon us in our time of greatest need and vulnerability.

Second, as with all cutoff problems with continuous variables, we are confounded by what we might call the "borderline issue." In the abstract it may seem perfectly acceptable to relegate anyone over the age of seventy to palliative care (or pick your age; it doesn't really matter if it's seventy-five or eighty for my point), unless you happen to be about to celebrate your seventieth birthday and worry about what kinds of treatment would be available to you when you cross the age Rubicon. While these conclusions may comport well with comparisons of patients separated by many years as generically "young" and "old," they do nothing to help us distinguish between more or less "deserving" people who are closer in age to each other—that is, they don't help us establish a cutoff point. And separating people into cohorts of age groups, such as zero to fifteen years, sixteen to thirty, and so on, does not solve the boundary quandary. So we may seem to be stuck with an irresolvable problem. How could we decide who is old and who is young for purposes of allocating resources? One way might be to simply say, as appears to be attractive to many, including Daniels and Callahan, that once a "normal lifespan" has been reached, anything beyond that is gravy, meaning only if we can afford it and want to pay for it, and while these people are not old, they may be too old to have a claim on significant resources.[21]

As I have noted, it is difficult, if not impossible, to create an absolute cutoff that is finite because those closest to the border and on either side of it would be virtually impossible to distinguish other than by the numerical and quantifiable characteristic used to create the line. Almost any method of determining a finite cutoff has the taint of arbitrariness. Why seventy? Why not seventy-two or seventy-six? And, of course, what is the difference between two people who are on either side of the line that separates the "haves" from the "have-nots"? Even making the flexion point "fuzzy" or blurry by say, changing it to seventy-three or seventy-five years, does not avoid the boundary problem. I can find no method of dodging this obstacle in a way that would be plausibly acceptable to the large number of people who would have to buy in to the plan, either the older adults to whom it would apply at the time of implementation or shortly thereafter, or those it will affect in the future (or whose parents, grandparents, etc., fall into the former group). Lastly, we must ask ourselves what we should do with people who are receiving ongoing care and then reach the age cutoff point: Do we continue giving them what they have been accustomed to or would they be removed from the list?

Third, while it may seem reasonable in the case of some absolutely scarce resource like livers to show preference for people whose expected longevity exceeds that of the transplanted organ (one wouldn't want to transplant an organ that could be expected to last for ten years into someone whose actuarial life expectancy is only two or three years), one cannot extend this case example to the more general allocation of healthcare budgets where the total amount is flexible and any cutoff point is adjustable. Moreover, in the transplant scenario, the result of not receiving an organ is very often death. (The exception is kidneys when dialysis is a reasonable alternative; it is a technology that can preserve a patient's life, albeit with many downsides.)[22]

This is exactly the problem ignored by virtually everyone who has proposed these various kinds of age categorizations or groupings. For example, I previously introduced a proposal by a prominent group of bioethicists to allocate scarce influenza vaccine on the basis of age, privileging the young versus the old (Emanuel and Wertheimer 2006; Persad, Wertheimer, and Emanuel 2009, 2010). The justification for this kind of distribution was similar to that which I discussed above, assuming that older individuals would have had more opportunity to experience the pleasures, pains, and accomplishments that only time can provide, compared with much younger people. And this certainly accords with our intuition to favor the young when forced to make a choice of this sort. But it failed to consider the boundary issue that is entailed whenever one artificially imposes cutoffs in continuous variables. Unfortunately, ignoring this issue will not make it disappear, and it inescapably accompanies all measures of characteristics of this type. We would run into the same problem if we were to substitute weight or height for age. In the abstract, it makes sense, but in practice the solution is wanting.

In summary, age is an attractive and convenient metric to target for establishing a cutoff point for rationing purposes. It is easily quantified, there is ample data demonstrating that older adults use more healthcare resources on average (and thus are more costly to care for) with less benefit as a group than younger patients, and it fits well with our moral intuitions that the young should be privileged over the old in prioritizing the allocation of scarce resources *when there is no choice*. But there is a choice and the scarce resource to be conserved is not livers but dollars. Unlike livers, which can be reassigned to others who might be better able to benefit from transplants and there is little likelihood that an organ will be wasted, dollars are fungible. Moreover, there is no assurance that the money saved by denying certain interventions to older people will be used wisely and prudently to benefit others in the system, or for that matter, diverted to other worthwhile funding goals for which the government is customarily thought to be responsible (such as education, infrastructure construction and maintenance, and the like). Finally, age is a continuous variable and there is no viable method for imposing a cutoff or dividing line between those who are eligible for resources and those who are not. Try as we might, we cannot transform age into a discrete entity that would be amenable to applying a simple solution.

Marginal Benefits
Marginally beneficial treatments or diagnostic tests are healthcare interventions that offer some limited benefit. They can be distinguished from those that offer something more (thus raising a cutoff problem) and those that offer no benefit whatsoever.[23] These interventions could be either cheap or costly, although the latter are those that concern us the most on the basis of the very large ratio of expense to benefit. Nevertheless, from the patient's perspective, ineffective treatments remain ineffective and a source of false hopes and wasted time and diverted effort, irrespective of the cost. There are a number of ways of analyzing this ratio, one of the most popular being cost-effectiveness analysis or CEA (Eddy 1983, 1991, 1992a,b,c; Gray, Clarke, Wolsetnholme, and Wordsworth 2011; Ubel 2001). This approach saw its greatest real-life application in the development of the Oregon Health Plan (see chapters 2 and 3). But no matter what yardstick we employ to decide what counts as marginal— CEA, a percentage of efficacy irrespective of cost, and so forth—it still involves drawing a line or cutoff that needs to be justified, both to those who will be affected now and in the future. CEA is sometimes viewed as a somewhat heartless way of gauging the value of a given intervention, seeing as how it calculates a quantitative relationship between price or cost and a population-based estimate of efficacy or benefit. Thus, it can

be considered a method to evaluate the monetary worth of trying to save a life (for example), an effort that many might regard as uncaring toward the sick and suffering. However, it does offer the advantage of being a relatively straightforward way of applying budget limitations (with the real-life caveats and pitfalls as noted in the discussion of the Oregon Health Plan in chapter 2). The funding cutoff point would then determine what counts as too marginal a benefit to deserve support within a rationing plan. How to do this and what can be deemed reasonable and acceptable to most people is a challenge in many ways no different from that for age cutoffs, or any other for that matter.

As Young (1994) pointed out twenty years ago, Americans have come to blur the distinction between what they need and what they want. Although we may not always want what we need, we definitely want what we want but don't necessarily need what we want. Enormous effort is expended by people to satisfy their desires and preferences (i.e., their wants): they get second jobs to earn more money or go into debt to buy the latest gigantic flatscreen TV or the fancy car they can probably not afford (but that they "must" have). The consumer advertising industry, now including ads for all sorts of prescription drugs, stokes this lust for more stuff. They use clever psychological ploys to make us believe we cannot do without something that we previously never thought about, even if we knew it existed. The same is true with healthcare "stuff," and not simply the latest expensive wonder drug just approved by the FDA (especially for "lifestyle" improvements like anxiolytics, impotence relievers, and the like), but technologies including exorbitantly priced diagnostic tests and interventions such as ICU care. Many people have lost or at least obscured the difference between healthcare needs and what we think we must have.[24] And of course this includes treatments that can have little or no benefit for individual patients, and occasionally for anyone at all. We have also bought into the idea that modern medicine offers a treatment or cure for almost everything, including such fatal diseases as advanced heart failure or cancer (Weeks et al. 2012). Anyone can be healed and medical miracles happen everyday; the next breakthrough is just around the corner, if only we can hang on a little bit longer. It is undoubtedly true that the marketing campaigns of hospitals, health systems, and individual physicians all touting the latest discoveries, cures, advantages, and the like also feed this fantasy (not to mention driving up the costs of medical care by increasing the amount purchased). And while many doctors complain bitterly about patients or their families/surrogate decision makers never "giving up," refusing to "pull the plug," or wanting "everything to be done" when all there should be is a peaceful death, they have difficulty refusing to provide interventions that many see as a right.[25]

The other side of the cutoff-problem coin is the attempt to reestablish boundaries or definitions between desires and necessities. At first glance this looks like it should be simple, and perhaps it is for the low-hanging fruit of interventions like childhood vaccinations (needed) and elective cosmetic surgery (not needed but instead a "want"). But as treatments or diagnostic tests become more questionable in terms of their significance and efficacy, or hold out the promise of benefit for fewer and fewer patients, it can become a very debatable point about whether they are necessary or not. Indeed, to a very great extent, the test for the planners in Oregon was to figure out a way to draw this line. Their answer was a preset budget, and perhaps that may be one approach to how to proceed.

Treatments and diagnostic tests that offer little or no benefit are not a trivial matter in the U.S. healthcare system. Berwick and Hackberth estimate that a minimum of 20 percent of the entire annual healthcare budget expenditure is a waste.[26] Of course, incorporated in this total are a variety of wasteful items, including a bloated administrative overhead apparatus in private insurance plans. But they also consider system failures and over- and undertreatment. Others have offered estimates in the same ballpark (Baicker, Chandra, and Skinner 2012).[27] Nevertheless, in a health system that spends more than $2 trillion per year, 20 percent of that total is a lot of money that could be saved. The important point is that there is general agreement that American healthcare is grossly inefficient, and the relative lack of uniformity and regulation of what is permitted to be paid for exacerbates this situation. But what metrics can we use to establish the approximate amount of benefit bestowed by a specific test or treatment? And, assuming that such an endeavor is both feasible and fruitful, what do we do with the information? How do we then establish how little benefit is too little a benefit to support? Where do we place the cutoff?

The Affordable Care Act passed by Congress and signed into law by President Obama in 2010 (and passing Supreme Court muster in 2012) mandated, among its many provisions, the creation of a new agency, the "Patient-Centered Outcomes Research Institute," or PCORI (Kamerow 2011).[28] It was established, after significant political wrangling, to both sponsor and initiate research into comparative effectiveness (CE). But because of the various constituencies that demanded, and won, a place at the table, its board represents a broad range of interests who believed that they might receive short shrift if their (loud) voices were not present to help guide the kinds of research performed, the questions asked, and how the results would be interpreted and used. Roughly speaking, CE is expected to investigate various interventions—mainly therapeutic—and compare and contrast their relative efficacy for a given condition. Unlike CEA, the agency was forbidden to consider cost in their evaluations. In its simplest form, the randomized, placebo-controlled clinical trial would be the gold standard against which other research would be judged.

However, such a trial (or trials) that demonstrated therapeutic benefit for a given treatment compared to a control intervention (this is the comparison part) would present prima facie justification for supporting (i.e., paying for) that treatment unless equivalence was demonstrated. The problems arise from the small-print details of these trials; it all depends on how one defines "benefit." For example, statistical benefit can be defined in a number of ways and using a variety of measures, including so-called surrogate markers (usually some form of laboratory test) instead of some parameter that is either too difficult or too time consuming to measure. But not all surrogate markers really tell us what we should be interested in, such as people getting better from whatever ails them as a result of the treatment they received (Moynihan 2011; Walter, Sun, Heels-Ansdell, and Guyatt 2012). However, in an ideal world, comprehensive CE data would provide a guide to the best and most effective medical interventions available, as well as indications of where future research should be aimed. Unfortunately, this lofty, perhaps quixotic, goal was felt to be threatening to a variety of people, ergo their presence on the board.[29]

Why should reliable clinical information about effective forms of diagnosis and treatment frighten certain people (Carman et al. 2010)? It may be simplest to understand by using an example of a pharmaceutical company product. Over the last ten years or so, it has become increasingly common for the FDA to approve anticancer drugs for advanced disease that do not cure anything and only offer a few to several months of life extension for the average patient at enormous expense (sometimes more than $100,000 per patient). Since these drugs are routinely approved and paid for by Medicare, and oncologists who prescribe and administer these drugs make significant portions of their income by doing so, it would seem as if many people might have much to lose if such a practice were curtailed on the basis of the limited effectiveness of these treatments.[30] Nevertheless, this only makes the problem of choosing among the openly available options that much harder, if for no other reason than that the criteria for entry of therapies and diagnostic tests or devices into the clinical marketplace and practice are so low. Moreover, it makes the definition of what should qualify as a marginal benefit exceptionally difficult. Even so, effective implementation of CE research could go far toward saving a considerable amount of money (Basu, Jena, and Philipson 2011).

CE is by no means a new idea. During the height of the craze for managed care as the holy grail for reining in healthcare costs more than 20 years ago, Schwartz and Mendelson proposed that this could not occur without some form of explicit—meaning overt and centrally planned—rationing. They suggested that CE could be a way to approach this by stressing the importance of relying on evidence of efficacy in choosing which types of interventions to endorse versus those to consider as experimental or, worse, ineffective or even harmful. They believed that the practice of medicine is so rife with unproven therapies and diagnostic tests that significant savings could be achieved by limiting access to those that fit this definition, hence the reliance on CE to help inform these types of decisions (Schwartz and Mendelson 1992). There is no reason to believe that the cost problems and overuse or abuse of interventions that have minimal to no evidentiary justification are any different today than in 1992 when Schwartz and Mendelson wrote their paper. Indeed, it is likely that the situation has become worse, because of the greater availability of expensive technologies and drugs today.[31]

Where does this leave us with marginally beneficial interventions? Where should the cutoff be that separates acceptably small, but favorable, effects? Buyx, Friedrich, and Schöne-Seifert (2011) have proposed placing the cutoff at marginally beneficial treatments and suggest that exactly how they should be defined (i.e., where the cutoff should be) could be determined by open, public debate.[32] However, I suspect that such deliberations would be highly charged, as a quick review of congressional testimony by disease interest groups would quickly reveal. Indeed, it was due in no small part to an especially poignant appeal by a witness actively receiving dialysis in the hearing room that Congress decided to create and fund the End-Stage Renal Disease Program in 1972 as a component of Medicare (Blagg 2007). This is not an exceptionally effective or efficient way to determine where a cutoff point such as this should be placed.

Buyx and her colleagues go on to argue that "rationing by clinical effectiveness" would avoid the pitfall of doing so by pure (or even moderated) cost-effectiveness analysis—that is, the cost of an intervention that is minimally helpful does not enter into the calculus, only its efficacy does. This has the consequence that both expensive and cheap, but always marginally effective, treatments fall under the same ax, hence distributing the pain or loss evenly, assuming that patients who are affected are also more-or-less randomly apportioned. For example, very expensive new cancer drugs that offer at best only a few extra months of life to anyone (on average) might not be covered, but the very costly enzyme replacements for some rare genetic metabolic disorders would be because they are truly life saving for most patients with these diseases.[33] However, while these authors claim that this approach is immune to the arbitrary decisions that value some types of people over others (such as young over old), it would not be surprising if the public continued these kinds of preferences when trying to decide where to draw the marginal benefit line. For instance, it is conceivable that a treatment that had a median survival advantage of six months might be considered to be below the threshold if it affected patients over the age of eighty, but might be appraised differently if the target patient population was, on average, six years old. In other words, a one-in-a-hundred chance of a cure may be thought acceptable for a child (a chance worth taking and thus paying for) but not so for an older person.[34] What may be tolerable for the former may prove less so or intolerable for the latter. I suspect that if Coby Howard were not seven years old, but had been seventy-seven, very few people (not to mention newspapers and TV stations) would have paid much attention to his plight. It will prove especially challenging to satisfy our need to be consistent and prudent with our healthcare dollars while at the same time coping with our emotional intuition to save or rescue the innocent (such as children).[35]

Finally, one more factor must be considered in this matrix: the role of patient desires independent of needs (also defined as efficacy). Restricting access to beneficial interventions determined by one or more of these methods would necessarily ignore some patient wants. This would almost certainly include such fervent patient and family wishes as continuing treatment or life support in critically ill patients near the end of life to give time for a miracle to occur. It seems highly unlikely that a public health insurance plan that embraces both rationing and inclusivity and that utilizes cutoffs at marginally beneficial care would endorse supernatural interventions as worthy of funding. To appropriate the term coined by Stephen Jay Gould (1997, 16), medicine and miraculous events comprise "nonoverlapping magisteria" and healthcare coverage benefits categorically must reside in the former domain and not the latter. It is to be hoped that the actual number of such frustrated, disappointed, and perhaps very angry patients would be acceptably low, if the cutoffs were placed appropriately with due deference to public debate.

It seems to me that we could approach this in three different ways. First, we could determine how much money we had or wished to spend, and this in turn would govern more or less where the threshold of effectiveness would be. We could call this the budget-determinative method. Second, we could decide what we thought was important or what should be covered and then figure out how to pay for it. We could label this the intervention- or treatment-determinative method. Third, we could utilize some combination of the two. In all likelihood, we would choose the last method. It is difficult to imagine that representative decision makers would put an absolute cap on healthcare spending other than some reasonable target (say, as a percentage of GDP), subject to the public's willingness to pay for it (assuming it was not financed by incurring debt) and subject to what they thought it was important to pay for. It is possible to imagine the citizenry, if they were more closely associated with the costs of medical care by taxes or some other direct funding mechanism (i.e., not subject to moral hazard), turning out to be much stingier than when someone else is seemingly responsible for the bill. If this turned out to be the case, then the cutoff for what would count as a marginal benefit might be much higher than if we decided that we couldn't let the Coby Howards—and others like him—die from lack of attempted treatment.[36] And presumably it would not be some arbitrary number such as greater than a 1 percent chance of efficacy (Schneiderman 2011c; Schneiderman, Jecker, and Jonsen 1990). Of course, it should be noted that we already do a form of marginal effectiveness rationing for organ transplantation.

The underlying primary justification for eliminating marginally beneficial treatments from consideration for inclusion under generalized healthcare rationing is that doing so will save money. Yet, while it is true that a significant portion of Medicare[37] dollars are spent on treatment—especially intensive care, chemotherapy, and so on—in the last six months of life, and thus by definition may be at least considered by some to be of marginal advantage, it is unclear exactly how much money could be saved by this approach, but it is likely to be significant. For example, if we limited access to the ICU to patients who had a reasonable chance of some form of meaningful recovery with an expected lifespan of more than six to twelve months and sufficient cognitive function to appreciate their improved health, it is reasonable to assume that sizable savings could result without serious harm to anyone, and possibly a large benefit if one applies Harris's negative action theory of harm (Harris 1980, chap. 3). However, there is another reason to do this. One could argue that it is the right thing to do irrespective of the costs. To continually offer patients the hope of a cure by providing treatments that are themselves rarely benign and often come saddled with significant negative side effects, seems to be a waste and often precludes giving the kind of effective, compassionate end-of-life care that could really help them.[38]

Hadorn (1991) proposes creating clinical-care guidelines to decide what should be paid for and what should not—that is, where the cutoff point(s) should be. He has suggested that the guidelines should be created by bodies of experts (presumably with no conflicts of interest)[39] who would duly consider the evidence for or against the efficacy of various treatments and then make recommendations. With the advance of medical science constantly testing new ways to treat various conditions, and hopefully demonstrating new or improved interventions, these guidelines would be periodically reviewed and revised to reflect the state of the art. In many ways this proposal is very similar to the current functions of the National Institute of Health and Clinical Excellence (NICE) in the United Kingdom and the U.S. Preventive Services Task Force.[40] However, they would still be confronted with that challenge of public acceptability and the cutoff problem.

There are at least two other significant challenges to eliminating coverage for interventions that offer only marginal benefits. No matter how we decide where the line will be drawn (i.e., how we decide what we mean by "marginal benefits"), by definition, the judgment that an intervention belongs in this class is based on a statistical analysis of populations, either a mean, a median, or some other mechanism of assigning some weighted average to the "ordinary" patient. It is obvious that this statistical patient is representative of a large number of individuals, all of whom, to one degree or another, differ from the mean. Depending on the amount of variation (such as the size of the standard deviation), there could be fairly small or large "tails." This translates into a reality that most patients will derive no benefit from a treatment (and could never derive a benefit) but a few could receive a fairly robust positive effect. Of course, by looking at pooled data we cannot distinguish one patient from another because they all belong to a grouping under some category label, like "middle cerebral artery stroke with dense hemiparesis" or "prostate cancer with metastases to bone and brain." Moreover, at the outset, it is virtually impossible to predict with any accuracy where on the treatment response curve a particular patient might be: Will she be one of the rare individuals who is cured or be in the overwhelming majority who fail to receive any benefit?

This problem is closely connected to the second, which relates to the major effort underway to foster the development of "personalized medicine" (Hamburg and Collins 2010; Guttmacher, McGuire, Ponder, and Stefansson 2010). While I would like to think that physicians have been practicing personalized medicine for thousands of years, this is not what is meant by the newest iteration of this term. Rather it is the ability to use specific genetic, proteomic (the detailed study of proteins), and other—usually laboratory-derived—information about individuals so as to specifically tailor a treatment to their disease process and thus their ability to respond to a treatment. For example, the use of genomic signatures of normal and mutated variants of genes in breast and lung cancer, to mention just two types of disease, are leading to alterations in treatment as well as perhaps outcomes (Chin, Andersen, and Futreal 2011; Ziogas and Roukos 2009; Schilsky 2010; Kwak et al. 2010; Slamon et al. 2001). And the kind of subtype of a key metabolic enzyme may influence the ability to respond to the antiplatelet function drug clopidogrel, which is often prescribed after cardiac procedures (such as the insertion of stents) (Sofi et al. 2011).

But population data is inherently impersonal, and comparative-effectiveness analysis is inescapably neutral to individual differences except as they might skew the mean one way or another or affect the degree of variance. The bottom line is that these efforts appear to be working at cross-purposes: personalized medicine (along with one's individual physician) has the goal of customizing and attuning treatment for a single, identifiable, unique individual with a disease that is a singular example of a general category (*not* an exemplar), whereas population-based information is, by its very nature, reasonably anonymous and homogenized. Can the two somehow be reconciled? Garber and Tunis (2009) certainly think so, as they wrote in a powerful statement published in the *New England Journal of Medicine*. Indeed, they believe that CER can be a robust tool to make singular or small-group disease signatures more clinically relevant by supplying the data that demonstrates what they mean. This can then direct diagnosis and therapy more specifically, which is the hallmark of any consequential personalized medicine. After all, the goal of individualized or customized medical intervention is to enhance the chances for success and minimize the influence of chance outcomes. Regrettably, for efforts to reduce overall healthcare expenditures, this projection holds out the prospect of innumerable small groups of patients who we would have previously lumped together as indistinguishable, but who now would be separable. If each gets a personalized off-the-shelf treatment (such as the controversial BiDil®), then such an approach might not prove to be more expensive (Akinniyi and Payne 2011; Krimsky 2012). However, if it stimulates pharmaceutical companies (for example) to create multiple new (and costly) "orphan drugs" for these small groups of patients, costs could skyrocket (Braun, Farag-El-Massah, Xu, and Coté 2010; Kesselhcim, Myers, and Avorn 2011; Meekings, Williams, and Arrowsmith 2012).

In addition, it is unfortunate for reconciliation that most patients believe that the attention and treatment they receive from *their* doctors is personalized *for them*. Whether this is actually true is irrelevant for the maintenance and perpetuation of these beliefs. Moreover, patients want their doctors to fight for them and what they think they need, even to go to the length of gaming the system, as I described in chapter 3. I suspect that doctors would continue to attempt to portray their patients as "different" and thus deserving of special consideration for something they would ordinarily not be entitled to (unless, of course, they were penalized for doing so).[41] And it is true that there remains a significant obstacle to instituting treatment guidelines as a prototype, because doctors are reluctant to change their practices no matter what evidence exists to support or counter their thinking.[42] Indeed, while the mantra in medical schools, academic medical centers, and professional medical societies has long been that practice should be centered on evidence-based medicine, with clinical practice guidelines, it remains a significant challenge to get physicians to adopt this approach. Doctors don't like to abandon their devotion to what they think works, irrespective of data that may contradict their faith in their customary way of doing things.[43] On the other hand, the views of patients (i.e., the "public") may not be so monolithically opposed to the imposition of guidelines and rules, depending on how they are framed and used.[44]

Examples of unproven therapeutic clinical interventions in widespread use abound. Some of the most popular (not to mention remunerative for their providers) include platelet-rich plasma treatment for bone and joint injuries (De Vos et al. 2010; De Jonge et al. 2011; Paoloni et al. 2011; Griffin, Wallace, Parsons, and Matthew 2012; Sheth et al. 2012), chelation therapy for autism (Davis et al. 2013), and many types of last-ditch treatments for advanced cancer.[45] This is not to say that these treatments are by definition not beneficial or capable of being so, just that they have not yet been shown to be so by accepted scientific criteria, usually randomized, controlled clinical trials.[46] If they just went away under some form of reasonable rationing—barred because of their "unprovenness"—would anyone truly miss them, other than perhaps those who tend to benefit from their use (such as doctors or drug and device manufacturers)? It is difficult to say without data. But perhaps unproven interventions should only be available under the aegis of clinical trials. This would allow some people to receive them, and presumably there would be a great incentive for the most interested patients to volunteer to be subjects in these studies. It would also stimulate the very thing that CE research is designed to do: winnow out interventions that work from those that don't, thus depleting the supply of useless or questionable treatments from the world of possible therapies. The problem that arises from this seemingly sensible approach is that some would view it as violating the sacrosanct tenet of medical practice, that physicians should be free to prescribe and do what they (and their patients) believe to be in the latter's best interest, which may not necessarily be restricted by the relevant scientific knowledge base.[47] Indeed, this is the rationale for justifying the exception to the federal regulation of prescription drug use, that once a drug is approved by the FDA, doctors are free to prescribe it for any reason they feel would help their patients, a practice known as "off-label use." Not surprisingly, such liberality can be both helpful and prone to abuse (Rosoff and Coleman 2011).[48]

Money
Cutoffs for money present an interesting problem and probably the largest challenges. Unlike some of the other resources I have discussed, money is almost completely fungible. This means that money can buy almost anything tangible in healthcare (except perhaps health itself), and it is easily diverted from one kind of purchase to another. Money can buy guns or ventilators, and at least theoretically, governments make these kinds of decisions all the time (except those governments that do not devote any public money to healthcare, and those are quite rare these days). For the sake of argument, let us assume that the U.S. federal government was going to decide how much of the total annual budget to spend on healthcare (this would be analogous to the Oregon legislature enacting a two-year spending plan for the OHP). In effect, this would lead to overt rationing, presumably because an absolute cap or limit would be placed on the total: no matter how generous the final amount would actually be, there would still be stuff that patients, doctors, drug companies, insurance company executives, and others would want for which there were insufficient funds. Now, the government could just say that there are X billion dollars for healthcare in the country for 2014–2015 (for example) and do with it what you will. When it runs out—let us say in the middle of July (the federal fiscal year starts on October 1)—that's all there is, there won't be any more, and tough luck for anyone who needs healthcare before the new budget starts on October 1, 2015. That seems extremely harsh, if

not draconian and cruel and probably foolish as well. Nevertheless, the first cutoff (sort of) is the one made at the top that is contingent on the answer to the question: How much do we want to spend on healthcare? Of course, many components figure into how one addresses this question, including what other things must be paid for, how high taxes should be to pay for healthcare, and so forth.

Alternatively, one could first determine what is important or essential to have as part of the coverage system. Everything else could be considered extras or fluff, available to all who could purchase it separately if they wanted, but not a constituent of a basic healthcare package. I have stated throughout this book that I believe it is inconceivable for both moral and political reasons that a wealthy country like the United States would fail to be quite generous in what it offered to its citizens if a universal, Medicare-like insurance program were enacted. Indeed, if the basic package of covered benefits were sufficiently comprehensive, even those people who might want more but couldn't afford it on their own would receive an excellent range of services. That being said, cutoffs then move to the next level.

I personally believe that we would do best by deciding what a basic (albeit liberal and ample) benefit package available to all should contain and tailoring the budget, within some limits, to it. I think this might be an interesting experiment to undertake as a first try. For example, let us refer back to chapters 2 and 3 and the story of the Oregon Health Plan. Ignore for the moment how the first attempt to construct a list of condition-treatment pairs was done by pure CEA techniques; just assume that we have a way of soliciting the opinions of various interest and expert groups (including patients) about what should be included on the list. We could then have a congressionally appointed panel (perhaps not as laden with industry representatives as the PCORI board, but that can be open to debate) examine the list and remove, say, 10 percent of the least effective disease interventions from each list (heart disease, lung disease, etc.).[49] In this way all interest groups who advocate for their organ or system will lose out equally (nobody should win or lose more than others). But the "loss" they would sustain would be relatively minimal since for the most part only marginally beneficial interventions would be unavailable (outside of clinical trials).

Then the arithmetic comes in: an estimate of the amount it would take to pay for this healthcare for the existing population of the country, taking into account the approximate incidence and prevalence of the various covered conditions and treatments. If this were less than or even equal to what we would currently be paying without any cost controls whatsoever, we could celebrate and call it a day (because this exercise doesn't even consider the elimination of other inefficiencies and waste in the system such as administrative overhead). If the estimate were much higher, we would have to carefully consider whether as a society we would think it worthwhile to pay for all of this healthcare for everyone, which would entail raising the money to pay for it. If not, then we have to start over: maybe fewer things should be covered, such as by drawing the marginal benefit line at 15 percent, not 10 percent. The point to emphasize is that by restricting access to interventions that are of little benefit to most people (or of unproven benefit to anyone), this could probably enable us to modestly control healthcare costs without hurting large numbers of patients (I suspect). Of course, I arbitrarily chose 10 percent as the cutoff for benefit; it could just as easily have been 5 or 15 percent. Approaching setting limits in this way does not avoid the need to draw the line somewhere; it simply seems more plausible and justifiable (as well as practicable) than resorting to such variables as age or money (up front).

Conclusion

I think it is fair to say that people are scared of what may happen to them if a broad-based, explicit rationing plan were put into effect. They are scared that what they might want or need will no longer be provided (even if it isn't now), or that faceless government bureaucrats would be making medical decisions for them and their families. This is irrespective of the fact that faceless insurance company bureaucrats are often making these decisions for them now. Doctors are scared that their incomes and autonomy will be at risk, even if these are threatened now with the existing public-private mélange. Most important, people are worried that when rationing comes, they and their needs will be below the cutoff line.

However, the imposition of planned cutoffs cannot be detached from the general fear of healthcare rationing, because both factors are inextricably linked in the frightened imaginations of those who dread any kind of rationing. Indeed, it can be plausibly maintained that it is an aversion to the arbitrary elimination of certain treatments or interventions (for whatever reason) applied to both populations and localizable, identifiable individuals that is the main source of this apprehension. This should not be casually dismissed out of hand as an irrational belief held by only ignorant or uninformed people. While it may be true that comprehensive and effective education may dispel some people's unease, it won't work with all. To neglect the feelings of the rest—probably a plurality or more of the fearful—and brush aside their opinions would be both demeaning and wrong, not to mention counterproductive, because a rationing plan that is open, honest and fair cannot work if it is not embraced and endorsed by the vast majority of the population.

When there are absolute limits on resources as there are in organ transplantation, drawing the line to make a cutoff is actually quite simple. Once the rules governing the distribution of the resource have been established, the number of livers actually available sets the cutoff point. However, when the resource is money, the cutoff will be determined by how much is devoted to healthcare. I have suggested that for a rich country that wishes to devote a not unreasonable percentage of its wealth to maintaining and improving the health of its people the best initial approach would be to define a sensible (and practical) range of healthcare benefits to offer and calculate the budget based upon this "list." In actuality, this would have to be done by creating a complex amalgam of both efficacy data for healthcare interventions and cost, as well as factoring in what the populace will tolerate. If we cannot solve the cutoff problem, it will be very difficult, if not impossible, to create conditions in which elective rationing, of the sort I describe in this book, can be acceptable to most of the public. Conversely, I think that solving the cutoff dilemma will go a long way toward reducing the perception of loss and unfairness that seems inherent in healthcare rationing.

In the next chapter I take up the thorny problem of what I call "losers." If the essence of rationing, irrespective of how generous it may be, is that there will necessarily be some people who will be dissatisfied with what they have been allocated, be it what they might view as incorrect (I got the wrong stuff), insufficient (I didn't get enough stuff), or even absent (I didn't get any stuff), they very well might view themselves as losers. These are the people who fall on the wrong side of the cutoff line. What I want to consider is whether we (the system) owe anything to those who are so situated.

5

Losers

In the preceding chapters I have discussed various aspects of systematic healthcare rationing, including features that I have suggested would make a rationing plan fair enough to convince people that it is in their best interests to agree to it. I have coupled this proposal with the assumption that healthcare rationing would have to be reasonably to very generous in its benefits to attract significant public support. This argument is based on the premise that the public already tolerates draconian—but fair—rationing in the organ transplant system, as well as episodically for emergencies and disasters. I have also examined the manner in which we could begin to think about establishing where cutoffs should be for what may and may not be sensibly offered.

I now wish to turn to what people often fear most (once we set aside all of the misinformation and negative hype about "socialized medicine," "death panels," and the like). If rationing is applied to all, fairly and evenly in a national program, the kinds and numbers of people who have limited or no access to the healthcare system should be minimized. But a natural result of imposing cutoffs, whether they are liberal or conservative, miserly or munificent, is that some patients will be told "no," irrespective of whether they would or could have received this service before official rationing. Rationing thus implies that there will be individuals who want or need something that they will be unable to receive. If we assume that at least some of them will be angry and feel they have been wronged and denied something of real value to them, how should we consider their situation, and what—if anything—should be done to address their grievances? In chapter 3 I discussed various features of a rationing system necessary to have it judged fair (or fair enough), and presented my adaptation of Daniels and Sabin's "accountability for reasonableness" approach. One of the cardinal principles for a procedural application of this method was having an avenue by which people could appeal what they viewed as an unfavorable decision to deny them something they believed they were owed by right (according to the rules). Some of them will undoubtedly be correct and others not. How we should cope with their grievances and their perceived or actual plight is what I turn to now.

Much of the debate about the prospect of planned healthcare rationing in the United States is not concerned with what people will get under any conceivable scheme, but what they *won't* get (not that the former is insignificant). While few would claim that fears of "death panels" express a justifiable worry about the unavailability or refusal of life-saving treatment to older adults so that they die bereft and medically abandoned, the unease has some basis in reality. As the experience with the Oregon Health Plan has demonstrated (see chapter 2), not everyone who might want or conceivably even need something will receive it, even if it could possibly help them, although as I have repeatedly suggested, any healthcare rationing system that could have a chance of being implemented in the United States would almost certainly have to be quite generous in its benefits. Unless the amount of healthcare services allocated were so limited by restricted resources that some (or many) people would have to do without something that could potentially help them in a significant way (such as with the absolute shortage of solid organs for transplant), a sensible plan in a wealthy, industrialized nation should be able to deliver almost all that people need, if not all that they might want. However, any rationing plan, no matter how generous it may be, will by definition set limits on the availability of some medical interventions. Therein lies the problem.[1] People who don't get what they think they need or deserve may view themselves as having suffered a loss, and may thus judge themselves as losers.

I would like to begin my discussion of the possibility of losers under healthcare rationing (of the sort that I have suggested might be acceptable) with several imagined, but I believe quite realistic clinical scenarios. This kind of hypothetical, envisioned rationing would be both generous and wide-ranging such that very few people would have to go without any medical intervention that could reasonably be defined as beneficial. The cutoff point would be such that only marginally beneficial (and, of course, completely nonbeneficial) interventions would be disallowed. Under these conditions of seeming largesse, at first glance it would appear inconceivable that anybody could truly be considered as having lost a substantial amount. Indeed, since such an imagined system would serve everyone and deliver a fairly lavish range of services, it might strike us as churlish that a patient would be unhappy that he didn't receive something to which he thought he was entitled, and hence saw himself as a loser.

But it is undoubtedly true that you can't please everyone all the time, and I think it almost a certainty that there will be people who believe they have been given a raw deal. The question to be resolved is whether their complaints are in fact reasonable. And, if so, what conditions would have to prevail to convince us that their claims were valid, since it is unlikely that everyone who objects to the manner in which she has been treated is genuinely a loser. We will need to distinguish between the complaints of people who believe they have been truly cheated by the inappropriate application of a fair allocation system and its rules, and those that are grievances about a perhaps sad, but justifiable, and hence, legitimate, denial.[2] The first case is an example of what commonly happens under our current healthcare system; the second suggests what could happen under what I envision would be fair and universal healthcare rationing (see chapter 3); and the third applies both now and potentially in the future. It might also be worth considering how we could treat accusations of inherent unfairness of the entire system, although it may be presumed that a charge of this type would (or should) be dealt with by the formal appeals process that would be a component of any rationing system considered fair (see chapter 3).

Case #1 (the Present Day)

Ms. Smith is a sixty-two-year-old woman who was diagnosed with advanced breast cancer two years ago. She has been divorced for many years and has two grown children. She was treated with surgery, intensive multiagent chemotherapy, and radiation and was considered to be in remission for about eighteen months. At the time of relapse she was offered second-line therapy with single drugs, to which she had a modest response with stable disease for a few months. However, routine CT scans again detected progression of the cancer. At that time she was informed of the existence of a Phase I clinical trial in which she would be eligible to participate; this study was testing the side effects and tolerability of a new type of chemotherapeutic agent. She was told that there was little chance that this treatment would help her live longer, and that she would have to spend considerable time at the clinic as well as in the inpatient unit, getting the blood tests mandated by the study. She was very equivocal about participating, but did so after her children discussed it with her. Her doctor and nurse also mentioned advance-care planning since her prognosis was dismal. However, her son and daughter refused to consider this, because they denied that their mother was that ill and wanted everything done to keep her alive as long as possible, including access to full ICU care; they were praying daily for a miracle for her. (The patient herself was too tired and ill to argue with her children and thus let them speak for her.)

After the first course of the experimental drug, Ms. Smith was admitted to the hospital for shortness of breath, altered mental status, and fever. Her blood pressure was low and at the insistence of her children she was admitted to the medical ICU and resuscitated with fluids, a central venous catheter, a urinary catheter, antibiotics, and eventually medicines to maintain her blood pressure. Her blood oxygen level was very low, which thus necessitated intubation and placement on a mechanical ventilator. The ICU staff told her children that she was actively dying and that life support should be withdrawn so she could die in peace. They disagreed and insisted on "doing everything." The medical team felt they had no option but to accede to their demands. After two weeks of intensive care, with her being unconscious almost the entire time, Ms. Smith suffered a cardiac arrest while her children were visiting her; she underwent thirty minutes of attempted resuscitation to no avail and died. Her children think she received wonderful care and that they have fulfilled their duty to do all that could be done to help their mother.

Case #2 (the Future under Rationing of the Sort Presented in This Book)

The situation is the same for Ms. Smith, except that she has been told that irrespective of whether she agrees to participate in the Phase I clinical trial, she would not be admitted to the ICU or receive anything other than interventions to make her comfortable. She could die at home or at an inpatient hospice facility, but would not have access to the hospital since she was dying. She thinks this sounds acceptable, but her son and daughter are incensed and threaten to sue the hospital and her doctors. They believe she has been denied treatment that is her right.

Case #3 (Anytime)

Mr. Jones is a fifty-five-year-old African-American man. He has been having chest pains with mild exertion for the last several months but has been avoiding going to the doctor. He is a longtime cigarette smoker and is moderately obese. He has poorly controlled type 2 diabetes. He also has long-standing hypertension but only remembers to take his medication about half the time. His wife is very concerned about him and calls an ambulance that takes him to the local hospital emergency department. He is diagnosed with acute angina and cardiac ischemia (low blood flow and oxygen delivery to the heart muscle). The doctors decide to admit him to the hospital, treat his underlying conditions, and watch him for a couple of days. He feels better after receiving nitroglycerin, diuretics, and a beta blocker medication. After he is discharged several days later, his daughter, a nursing assistant at the hospital, does an online search about his condition. She is concerned when she finds out that the standard of care for his degree of heart disease is a cardiac catheterization and intravascular stenting of any significant cardiac artery vessel narrowing (which is highly likely given his clinical and laboratory findings), because not doing so would predispose him to a very high risk of dying. She is angry that he did not receive these interventions and is convinced that it is because of his race.[3]

Analysis of the Cases

The first case represents a situation in which a person is clearly dying of cancer but is demanding (or whose surrogate decision makers are demanding) interventions that seem to be of only marginal benefit, if not actually harmful in that they prolong suffering and the dying process. This is a not uncommon situation in many hospitals in the U.S. today and in many respects is the main driver of the enormous percentage of Medicare (and other) funds expended for patients in the last six months of life. In the second scenario, the same patient, now receiving care as part of a publicly accepted healthcare rationing plan, is offered hospice and palliative care rather than access to the ICU and all that entails, because the cutoff point that had been previously agreed on (by rational, democratic deliberation) was at the level of marginal benefit for aggressive, life-preserving interventions. The final case is one in which a man, possibly because of his ethnicity, receives less than the standard of care. The question I wish to address is which of these three people has lost something of value to her or him—and thus may be labeled a loser—especially under the rationing conditions I have suggested could be acceptable in this country.

What Is Reasonable for People to Receive?

Rationing can be defined as the denial of something that has the potential to be beneficial, usually under conditions of finite or relative scarcity

(Ubel and Goold 1998). Rationing is a necessary byproduct of any arrangement that caps total healthcare spending. It is thus inescapable that some people will not get what they would (theoretically) have received had there been an inexhaustible supply of money to fund medical care with no restrictions on its use. In that case, the only obstacles might be those put in place by physicians to refuse certain types of care to certain people under specified circumstances, such as in conditions deemed futile (Schneiderman and Jecker 1995; Gabbay and Meyer 2009; Moss 2011). Of course, such a situation is pure fantasy, no matter what some people may think about the freedom and open availability of choice in the American healthcare system. There may only be a relatively few very wealthy people who have the financial resources to buy whatever healthcare they might want, irrespective of whether it is reasonable—or rational—to want it; for the overwhelming majority (the rest of us), all sorts of restrictions typically apply that limit our options.[4]

Doctors and their patients routinely make decisions about what medical interventions to use to promote the patients' welfare and advance their health interests. Physicians are constantly winnowing out what should be on the menu of available options from among the myriad of possible things that could be offered to a patient. Not infrequently, the list of potential options may be limited by the type and extent of insurance the patient has, which can also (for example) influence the kinds of drugs available for prescription (i.e., generic vs. brand name). Occasionally, doctors will refuse a patient request for a treatment or diagnostic test that the doctor thinks is either not necessary or even has the prospect of causing harm. Assuming the physician explains her reasoning underlying the decision, the patient can accept the justification or reject it. In the case of something not offered or denied (assuming he even knows that such notional options exist), the patient may feel deprived of something he wants or thinks he needs, but generally would not think he has suffered a loss. Rather, he may believe that his doctor has refused him something, but it was not because someone else got the intervention he thought he deserved. In some situations, he might feel that he has been treated unfairly, but if this were the case he more likely would feel anger (at the physician) at being treated this way rather than mournful for not having received something he believed he was owed. In other words, it is reasonable to assume that the patient would not feel that he had lost out on an *entitlement*, something he deserved as a matter of course or something he *should* have.

By the same token, in a customary clinical encounter, he would not think he had won something if he received what he wanted or hoped for. In cases of extreme disagreement, he may decide to obtain a second opinion or even switch doctors in an attempt to obtain the service or therapy he was refused, but it would be surprising for him to experience a sense of emptiness or privation because the doctor said no. It would seem strange to characterize the patient whose doctor has declined to write a prescription or do surgery or order a specific test, as a "loser." It would be more apt to simply say that he didn't get what he wanted, not that he was defeated in a contest for whatever it was he desired.

Conversely, there are many cases in which doctors meet the demands of patients irrespective of their legitimacy or validity. This may be especially common in circumstances surrounding end-of-life care in the intensive-care unit, such as in the first case presented above (Alpers and Lo 1999; Baily 2011; Davis 2008; Luce 2010).[5] It would probably be incorrect to categorize these patients as winners. However, in both situations the patient may or may not receive some good, but not because of a competition for it as under conditions of scarcity. And that is because the clinical encounter is not normally constructed or perceived as a contest with an outcome in which some individuals receive more of something (be it time, interventions, medicines, etc.) and some necessarily acquire less, or possibly even nothing at all due to the fact that the amount to be allocated is finite in size and/or indivisible (like livers or hearts).[6]

In general, our feelings of loss over the lack of some material object and the manner in which we react to it are magnified when circumstances suggest that another individual received it instead of us. This can be observed in a variety of situations. For example, voters whose candidate lost have a more pessimistic view of the effectiveness and virtues of democracy than those who backed the winner (Blais and Gélineau 2007; Anderson and Tverdova 2001). People in a tournament or contest may feel envy at the success of their opponent when it comes at their expense (as it unavoidably must in a two-person competition) (Grund and Sliwka 2005). Some individuals who lose take it to an extreme and become "sore losers"; they are not just sad or dejected at their plight, but angry and imagine that the contest was rigged or the judges were biased or some form of cheating must have occurred to result in the outcome (Ein-Dor and Hirschberger 2012). This can motivate people to protest the results and lodge an appeal with an authority that is empowered to review and adjudicate these kinds of disputes. But, as I discussed in chapter 3 when considering the requirements of fairness in general and in a rationing scheme, if the "game" was procedurally just and the rules were followed in a reasonable manner, then claims of prejudicial or discriminatory treatment—which if true would invalidate the judgment or outcome of the event—would be false and hence inapplicable. This does not mean that people who lose and believe themselves to have lost unfairly do not have any avenues to register their complaints; rather, if the rules were obeyed and applied correctly, they will have no case.

When people engage in a contest against one another the outcome generally results in a winner and a loser. Sometimes things are not as clearcut as "winner take all" with the loser getting nothing, but often they are. Depending on the stakes of the contest and the rules, the contestants may be more or less pleased or distressed by the results. For "games" in which the prize may be very valuable, the potential anguish of the loser can be assuaged or partially mitigated by the provision of a consolation prize of some sort that to a limited extent can reduce the pain of the loss. Of course, the rules of the game should be known to all participants before it starts, and they will presumably be aware of what the stakes are as well as if there is any provision for second, third, fourth place, and the like. Occasionally, the nature of the loss may be such that a second-place prize (or no prize at all) cannot approach the value of that gained by the victor: nothing can ease the sorrow of a loss or partially substitute for winning. Such may be the case if the competition is for a life-saving medical treatment like an organ transplant: if the patients are competing for a liver, the winner has the opportunity to live, while the loser inevitably dies. However, even in such emotionally wrenching cases, whatever compensation is given to the loser is not done to discharge an obligation. Rather, it is provided out of empathy for his heartrending situation, and compassion for his suffering as a consequence of his loss. Presumably, it is the same kind of compassionate care that would be given to a sick and dying patient if organ transplant technology did not exist at all, but not as recompense.

When healthcare resources are scarce, such as in a sudden disruption in the normal ratio of supply and demand (because of an unexpected drug shortage, a widespread healthcare disaster like pandemic influenza, or a localized emergency requiring triage), even more patients cannot receive the type of treatment they or their doctors think can help them, and this occurs as a direct result of rationing choices. Decisions must be made about who should receive what resources there are, hopefully according to an allocation scheme that is morally and medically justifiable (Rosoff 2012b; Rosoff and Decamp 2011; Daniels 2008; Daniels and Sabin 2008). This state of affairs exacerbates conditions of want and need and increases the numbers of patients who fail to get desired or needed healthcare. Thus, in conditions of scarcity some patients will receive healthcare resources and others will not, all things being equal.[7] Can we characterize the former as winners and the latter as losers, or perhaps more important, would these patients define themselves in this way?

One of the biggest potential obstacles to creating a decent healthcare rationing plan would be the problem of losers: people who believe that they will lose something valuable directly attributable to rationing (something they believe they would otherwise have expected to receive as a matter of course; whether they actually would have or not is a separate question). The size of this problem could be large or small, depending on the number of people who would consider themselves potential losers under any kind of rationing scheme. And, to a certain extent, it is plausible to suppose that the number of people who lose (or think of themselves as losers) will be dependent on the generosity of the system, which in turn will determine where the cutoffs are placed. Whether they are truly losing something of value is an issue worth considering. They could be mistaken; just because one believes that one has suffered a loss (or will do so in the future) does not make it objectively true that a loss has actually occurred (or will occur). In addition, to experience a *real* loss, to actually lose something one possesses or could possess if one had access to it, the thing has to have some *real* value based upon its capacity to benefit one's life in some persuasive and meaningful way. And it is arguable whether the failure to satisfy any desire or preference at all can genuinely be declared a loss.

While most (if not all) scholars and policymakers who write about rationing do not specifically refer to the beneficiaries (and their counterparts) of medical interventions under these conditions as winners or losers (Kamm and Kilner are exceptions) (Kamm 1993; Kilner 1990, chap. 17), there is little doubt that patients and their families would do so. This is almost certainly true if the resolution of "tragic choices" is made using mechanisms such as a lottery or coin toss in which these labels are in common usage (Calabresi and Bobbitt 1978; Kilner 1990, chap. 17). Indeed, it is difficult to imagine a patient not thinking of herself as a winner if she is chosen to receive a scarce treatment that she believes she needs, especially if she knows that not all who want the treatment can get it. Similarly, medical professionals can refer to patients this way (Matas 2009; Weimer 2010). Irrespective of how allocation or rationing decisions are made, since not all patients can get what they want, some will gain access and others will not. While access is not equivalent to receiving the benefit from a treatment, it is a necessary precondition; failing to obtain the resource or worse, not even being deemed worthy of being considered eligible, necessarily defines the loser in these situations of unavoidable choice. The fear that there will be huge numbers of people who think of themselves as losers under any kind of fiscally responsible rationing scheme makes its creation and implementation politically unpalatable, if not impossible. But is this a legitimate concern? In a country such as the United States, a wealthy nation in which any conceivable comprehensive rationing plan would most likely be quite generous to all (if for no other reason than to gain public acceptability), would those patients who do not receive what they want because of rationing be rightfully characterized as losers? In essence, is their fear a rational or legitimate one?

I will first describe the conditions under which I believe we can reasonably label a person a "loser" in a medical (rationing) situation. It will specifically appeal to the intrinsic value of what they have lost due to a shortage, be it a finite or relative scarcity of some resource, and be it planned or unforeseen. I will propose that the only kind of patients who can truly count as losers would be those who lose something of real value and who do so unfairly. I argue that there are patients who currently lose out on access and/or receipt of many healthcare resources, even in the absence of specific rationing, due mostly to existing social inequities, and that any rationing plan could only exacerbate conditions for losers unless it takes specific steps to mitigate these cases of inherent unfairness. Finally, while it is possible to conceive of a theoretical compensation scheme for individual patients who lose unfairly, any such plan would be unworkable in the real world in which we live. Hence, we would be left with attempting to address the structural social causes that create the conditions that make losers possible. Nevertheless, having a robust appeals process as an intrinsic component of the rationing scheme may serve to address at least some of these issues.

What Is at Stake in a Healthcare "Contest"; What Might a "Loser" Stand to Lose?

What one wants and its relationship to what one needs with respect to medical care presents an interesting area for examination. People want all sorts of things, and not everything one wants is needed. In this general sense I want to define *need* as referring to something that one can use to improve one's life, which for some people can simply mean maintaining it at the present level or preserving the status quo. When it comes to modern, developed-world healthcare services, common needs can include various drugs, surgical procedures, diagnostic tests, and a variety of therapies of one kind or another. Indeed, the evolution and growth of scientific medicine over the last 100 years has led to an ever-increasing number of interventions that have the possibility of helping people and hence satisfying needs as I use the term. Of course, needs of this sort are context- or situation-specific: one may need amoxicillin for a urinary tract infection but not for pneumonia or a cold. Many interventions can be beneficial, meaning that they can contribute in a materially significant way to making people feel better, live longer, or be more productive. It may be reasonable to conclude that things that can be of benefit to patients should be things that they would want and, if possible, things that doctors would both want to and are able to provide. Ideally, the connection between peoples' healthcare desires and that which can be obtained that is potentially beneficial, should be concordant (I say "potentially" because a specified outcome cannot be guaranteed up front and people not infrequently don't want treatments that could help them).

Sometimes people desire things that don't exist—such as a cure for incurable cancer—or that can't be provided, such as a liver transplant when a suitable organ is not available. And occasionally they want things they don't need: if you need a car to get to your job, you may earnestly think you must have a Ferrari, but you don't need one, as a Toyota would do just fine. Similarly, you may want an expensive brand-name drug but a cheaper generic form would be just as effective. Or you may want a rhinoplasty (nose job) for nonreconstructive cosmetic reasons, but you don't need one. Generally speaking, it seems correct to say that treatments that have a reasonable chance of success at improving lives should be available to patients and those that don't should not be (although resource scarcity makes this more complicated and challenging, as I will discuss shortly). The level of support or the quantity of some forms of healthcare "stuff"— whatever it may be—will also be determinative in how the term "reasonable chance of success" cashes out (Callahan 1990, especially chaps. 2–6).

For someone to suffer a loss, she must have lost something that she considers to be valuable to her. Whether others would consider it of value and therefore a loss is a debatable point, but presumably some things are valuable to most—if not all—of us. But the amount of value can be relative. For example, if I dropped a penny on the floor when I went to get some change in my pocket to buy a can of soda from the vending machine, I probably would not even bend down to pick it up, and I certainly would not go to any effort to retrieve it if it rolled under the machine. This is because I don't place much value on the penny. If I dropped a quarter or a dollar bill, it would probably be different, but only because I value the larger coins and bills more and calculate that it's worth the effort. Perhaps if I were a multimillionaire, I wouldn't go out of my way to pick up even a $10 bill. But I suspect even the millionaire would say that the $10 bill is intrinsically valuable (to everyone). The point is that the estimation of the value or benefit of an item, including healthcare interventions, is somewhat—but not completely—personalized. One way to look at the difference in both "real" and perceived value of the penny and the quarter or the $10 bill is that the former could be described as having marginal value, both in relation to larger amounts of money and by itself (you can't buy much with a penny). While it is true that the penny does have some intrinsic value, it is so little as to be negligible, or almost equivalent to nothing at all, and this is true no matter who owns the penny. This calculation goes into our thinking when we are deciding whether or not to pick it up off the floor. Conceivably, if I were desperately poor and there were many pennies available to pick up (or not), or if I had nothing else better to do and my time were not valuable, or if I just wanted a penny (and couldn't rationally explain why), I would bend over to grab it. But it would be difficult to argue that I was better off being one cent richer than I was before, even if the alternative was having no money at all. This extended analogy describes the analysis and calculation of benefit for medical interventions: How much better off does someone have to be made by a given treatment or test to make it truly worthwhile to have (to her and/or society), and hence a real loss not to have?[8]

The value of healthcare interventions has both subjective and objective components that entail a complex mix of evidence supporting efficacy in a given clinical situation. Generally speaking, treatments can be divided into three categories, based on what kinds of results can be expected to occur and with what probability. Therapies can be of no benefit whatsoever to anyone (the truly futile and hence irrational to want); they can be of marginal benefit, in which the chances of obtaining a reasonable good are slim but not zero (thus they are unreasonable, but not irrational, to want); and then there are interventions that are truly beneficial, which presumably is an outcome that is anything greater than marginal, and that most of us would desire.[9]

There are some things the worth or value of which nearly all would agree on. For example, we would probably all concur that antibiotic treatment for straightforward, bacterial pneumonia (say, due to the pneumococcus or *Streptococcus pneumoniae*) in an otherwise healthy twenty-five-year-old woman is a good thing that has a high likelihood of making her feel better and probably curing her. On the other hand, we may feel differently about the same therapy for an eighty-nine-year-old woman with advanced Alzheimer's disease and widely metastatic, incurable cancer. Indeed, even if the latter patient were able to make decisions for herself, she may conclude that treatment for this infection is not worth it and will not arguably improve her future, and thus forgo the antibiotics, despite the fact that she could possibly be cured of the pneumonia.[10] If she (or her family) pursued this course, she would have decided that the drugs would offer only marginal or no benefit for her in her particular situation, because it certainly could not cure her cancer (analogous to deciding whether or not to pick up the penny). Conversely, she (actually, her surrogate decision maker) may decide she wants to be treated at all costs (literally). Under current circumstances in the United States, she may very well be granted her wish (see case #1 above). But under formal, consensus rationing conditions she very well might not: she would receive palliative care for comfort, just not curative treatment. And that is because with limited dollars, trade-offs or choices must be made and a cutoff point imposed: in order to pay for interventions of greater net worth to more people, we have to decide not to pay for treatments of lesser net worth. Hence, healthcare of marginal value is likely to be unavailable even in a just and fair rationing plan.[11]

When this reasoning is applied to clinical practice, and especially to the discussion of patients being denied a healthcare intervention, three general situations can be described:

1. The patient is denied a treatment of *no benefit*. This could describe something that is truly futile. (An example might be the patient wanting an antibacterial antibiotic for a viral infection, for which there is no rational or scientific reason for efficacy. Another example might be that of people who demand continued physiological life support for patients who are (whole) brain dead and thus legally dead.) Ideally, the patient would be directed toward more constructive and potentially effective interventions. However, that may not satisfy the patient who may still want a drug to cure his cold. Since this patient has not been denied access to anything of value (to anyone), then it is difficult to say that he has as a consequence suffered a loss, even if he perceives it as such. The patient should receive other routine care and compassion and certainly nothing to make up for the loss or absence of something that was "worthless."

2. The patient is denied something of *true benefit* that could have been given to her. Of course, the interpretation of this condition would have to be made in relation to how we define marginal benefit or where we place the benefit cutoff, because we presume that these circumstances are anything greater than that. No matter how this is addressed, there will have

to be some minimum possible benefits that by consensus (or maybe by fiat for some very troubling interventions) are too small to justify providing the intervention.[12] Therefore, we would only judge someone as losing something—as a result, as a loser—if she was refused or denied a treatment that had the real potential (or a reasonable prospect) for helping her or for providing a genuine, greater-than-marginal, benefit and to which she had a legitimate claim to access. We would feel sorry for her if she couldn't get this treatment, even if she lost because of a coin toss or lottery or because she lacked insurance. In other words, an "impartial spectator" would understand that she had suffered a loss, but this can only occur if, and only if, the resource would have been provided if conditions had been otherwise.

3. The patient is denied something of *marginal benefit* in which there is real disagreement about the potential for effectiveness of the intervention in his particular case. This could be a treatment that offered a relatively minimal chance of improvement or relief of suffering. This could be assessed in real terms—that is, with no reference to its cost—or by figuring the cost of the intervention into the calculus of benefit. The definition of marginal benefit by an individual patient is where things have the prospect of getting complicated. What is one patient's (and doctor's) calculation of marginal benefit could be viewed by another patient as her only chance of a cure or life-saving therapy. The critical question to address is how little chance is too little. Whether one makes the cutoff at less than a 1 percent chance of an intervention working, or somewhat higher or lower, is important but only relevant when placed in the context of a system that does not permit everyone to have whatever they want, no matter how little chance of benefit it has. However, the significant point here is that most "impartial spectators" would tend to regard interventions with marginal benefits as a toss-up with respect to evoking their sympathy for those patients who had to do without. Hence, it is reasonable to conclude that if a patient were denied access to a test or therapy that falls into this category, the loss that he or she would experience would be proportional to the benefit that could be expected—that is, marginal and thus debatable. And, if anything would be a target for restrictions under comprehensive (and fair) rationing, it would be interventions judged to be marginally beneficial.

These three general states of affairs account for most of the plausible scenarios in which there could be disagreements about what should be provided to patients in a reasonable healthcare system. This is a system in which limits have been set on what can be available for use, with those limits preferably being controlled, planned, and fair, and therefore the reference points for determining who is a loser and the depth of his loss. However, people who fail to obtain what they think they need may very well consider themselves losers and view others who receive interventions (especially those they themselves want) as winners.[13] They are likely to feel aggrieved, bereft, even angry and resentful—sore losers if you will—but that is only because the stakes either truly are or are thought to be so high.

In any healthcare rationing plan cutoffs will have to be made, as I discussed in the previous chapter. If the plan was well funded and generous, then the limit would probably be at the level of marginal benefit and the line drawing would, to a certain extent, depend on how much money was available to pay for healthcare. As I mentioned earlier, something like this was done with the Oregon Health Plan rationing method, in which a list was created that ranked medical interventions according to the amount of good they would do for individuals and populations (and their cost). How low on the list they could go—meaning how little benefit they could afford to pay for during each budget period—was based both on demographics (how many people were enrolled and the prevalence and incidence of the various conditions) and on how much money the legislature voted to budget for this endeavor (Daniels 1991; Fox and Leichter 1991; Hadorn 1991; Kitzhaber 1993; Klevit et al. 1991; Lindsay 2009; Mitchell, Haber, Khatutsky, and Donoghue 2002; Oberlander 2007). The OHP has never been so generous as to go all the way to marginal benefit (although this assertion could probably be contested since it does pay for intensive care, including at the end of life, and it has not been accused of turning off ventilators to save money). However, undoubtedly there are people who were denied something they wanted or thought they needed—including potential life-saving measures—and thus considered themselves losers; the Coby Howard story is illustrative of this (Fox and Leichter 1991; Hadorn 1991; also see chapter 2 in this book). The real question is whether these patients, or the postulated patients who wouldn't obtain what they think they need or want during other forms of rationing, truly do count as authentic losers.

Who Should Count as a Loser?

Losing implies (although does not entail) having engaged in a form of competition for a limited and valued resource, whether it is a state lottery prize, a church raffle, the outcome of a baseball game, or (one could imagine) a liver for someone in liver failure. Generally speaking, only one person or party can win, even if there may be some compensation for having come in second. If the rules are just and the game is played fairly according to the rules, and the participants have willingly engaged in the competition, then the results should not be open to question, complaint, or appeal.[14] The winners would be presumed to have won fair and square, and the losers to have lost the same way. On the other hand, if the rules tended to favor one party over another or someone had bribed the umpires before the baseball game to always judge in their favor, or the players were forced to participate, then the result would be tainted, suspect, and potentially wrong.[15] Finally, there are some contests with multiple winners, so not all are arranged such that it is (one) winner take all; a generous healthcare rationing system in which it is dollars that are limiting should enable most patients to "win" with very few losers (with the exceptions I discuss below).

What about losers in a healthcare setting? What conditions would have to prevail to say that someone had suffered a real loss? In the previous section I suggested that the only people we can unequivocally conclude had suffered a real loss would be those who failed to obtain some good that could truly help them (and others like them) such that it would (almost) be irrational not to want it, all other things being equal. I want to analyze the situations in which a sensed or perceived loss occurs and attempt to draw conclusions about the required context and state of affairs that would need be present in order for us (or an appeals panel) to conclude that an individual has truly lost something of value in a healthcare setting. I will describe two scenarios: a justifiable loss and one that is unjustifiable. The difference is that the former would not be owed anything, because a wrong would not have occurred; in the latter, a wrong would have been committed.

In conditions of plenty, or in the semicontrolled chaos of a healthcare system like that in the United States (where rationing happens but it's mostly by accident of circumstance and tethered to patients' financial condition), there are many situations in which patients don't get what they want or need. For example, your primary-care doctor may want you to be seen by a specialist, but your insurance company denies the payment: you can still go, but you will have to bear the entire cost yourself. The company could decide that you don't meet the necessary preconditions to see the specialist (maybe you are not sick enough) or perhaps the specialist is "out of network," meaning that she does not have a contractual agreement with your insurer. Or you get to see the specialist and he thinks you need a certain procedure or test that is performed at the local hospital near your home. But if your insurance company has an arrangement with a different facility fifty miles away you will have to go there if you want the test (paid for). Or your doctor writes a prescription for the brand-name drug because he thinks it works better than the cheap generic equivalent, but the latter is all your pharmacy-benefit provider will pay for. Or you have no health insurance at all and have to decide how sick your child must be before you take him to the emergency room. Et cetera, et cetera. These are all descriptions of types of narrow, focused rationing, and of course our sympathy lies with the patients and families who have to deal with these denials, rules, and restrictions. They certainly have all lost something of value, even if it is only convenience or their time. But this is not the kind of rationing system I really have in mind, and hence not the kind of loss associated with it in either depth or gravity.

First, let me consider a planned rationing scheme in which there is a real, absolute scarcity of resources. For instance, this could be where people are denied access to a treatment that they would ordinarily receive if there were not a shortage. A good example would be patients who have been unable to be treated with the many chemotherapy medicines that have been in short supply in the last few years (Gatesman and Smith 2011). Or there are patients for whom access to a very limited resource may always be a matter of luck or chance, as is often the case for those who are on transplant waiting lists. When these people lose, they potentially lose big, meaning they have not been able to be treated with something that could really help them. Furthermore, they lose by systemic design and not by happenstance (of course, they also will have had the bad luck to be sick or born with a disease for which there may be no covered treatment, but this may be distinguished from misfortune). The depth or amount of their loss should probably be calculated by what the consequences of the loss actually are. However, even if they lost something of such major value that it could threaten their lives—it is difficult to imagine anything more costly than that—and hence they qualify as the very archetype of a loser, they are not really losers in the sense that nothing could have been done to prevent one patient from obtaining the resource and another from not getting it. That is the nature of scarce-resource rationing. In many situations, it may even qualify as a horrible, catastrophic result, but if the loss is entailed by the unavoidable circumstances of the rationing scheme, then while it is perhaps tragic, it is nonetheless part and parcel of the system itself, and hence acceptable.

This conclusion is predicated on the assumption that the rationing scheme is fair and that all contestants who are similarly situated—in this case, medically—would be treated the same or would have a reasonably equal opportunity to receive the resource in question. The eligibility rules would be applied equally and in a disinterested and nonpartisan way to all. There would be no "special" people or VIPs who could either edge their way ahead of others to obtain a better chance of being considered for the resource, or, once there, have an edge over their competitors for other (morally irrelevant) reasons. In other words, the system would not be rigged in favor of one group over another. Even if the nature of the shortage of resources—be it organs, drugs, or money to buy other things—is draconian or exceedingly harsh, a just prioritization method and allocation algorithm would be sufficient for declaring anyone who lost out on something to have done so fair and square. They would have no reason to complain that they had been treated in an inconsiderate and inequitable manner: the fair rules were followed fairly and all patients were covered under the same rationing plan, so the result may have been due to bad luck but not foul play. Moreover, if the system had been set up with adequate input from those potentially affected by its decisions—that is, present and future patients—there would be little genuine cause to complain if someone did not receive a resource as a result of a fair application of the rules. This does not mean that these patients would not have suffered a loss, because they most assuredly would have. Of course, this is a utopian vision and bears little likeness to reality, especially in situations that breed desperation such as those involving critically ill patients and their families. As I described in chapters 2 and 3, existing systems of rationing, while striving for better justice in application, are still susceptible to gaming and manipulation to favor some over others. And a strong argument could perhaps be made that the patient who could conceivably have received a liver in Memphis had it not been for Steve Jobs moving there, or in Los Angeles had it not been for the intervention of the Japanese gangsters, had suffered an unjustifiable loss: they may not have lost fairly.

These are examples of people who have failed to receive something of real, possibly life-saving, value such as a heart, kidney, liver, or vital chemotherapy drug (Case #3). What about patients who have been denied something of marginal or no benefit (Case #1)? Certainly, patients who have not received a treatment that could not help them at all would have no claim to say they had been denied anything of any value whatsoever, so they could therefore not have suffered a loss. The state of affairs with interventions of marginal benefit is more complex, because if they have lost anything, they have not lost much. And if all similarly situated patients are also refused this therapy, say, as a result of a reasoned rationing process where it is decided that interventions that offer only marginal benefits (however these may ultimately be defined or determined; see chapter 4) would not be covered, then it is a justifiable loss. Of course, if the reason the line is drawn where it is was due to draconian stinginess in funding a healthcare rationing plan (for example) and the definition of marginal benefit is hence placed so that it really isn't so marginal at all, or if the plan applied mostly to people who had little choice in the matter (as in Oregon), then our conclusion might well be different.[16]

The main differences between our current healthcare system and that under a generalized and centralized approach to planned rationing would be that the latter would presumably be more regulated and the rules would more justly govern the allocation and distribution of resources for all who are covered by the plan. In a wealthy country like the United States, it is likely that there would be fewer losers under rationing than there are at present, simply because receipt of healthcare would in all likelihood not be left to the vagaries of the market, employment, and so on. Nonetheless, I would suggest that there would be a class of patients who currently lose, and most likely would continue to do so under rationing, and these losers would not do so by chance or bad luck, as portrayed in the third case I presented earlier in this chapter.

Many people are members of socially and medically marginalized groups on the basis of ethnicity, socioeconomic status, and other factors. These individuals suffer bias for morally arbitrary characteristics over which they have little to no control. These patients have traditionally had less access to both basic and advanced medical care. Examples include African Americans, poor people, and undocumented immigrants (Committee on Understanding Eliminating Racial Ethnic Disparities in Health Care 2003). It is widely recognized that many of these people suffer from the differential ability to obtain the same kinds of healthcare for themselves as others who are similarly ill. For instance, ethnic minority groups have significantly lower access to primary medical care than those who are members of more favored majority groups (Flores and Tomany-Korman 2008; Howard, Carson, Dajuanicia, and Kaufman 2009; Marshall, Urrutia-Rojas, Mas, and Coggin 2005; Cruz-Flores et al. 2011). Being able to gain access to the healthcare system can be equated with being eligible to participate in a contest for a scarce resource. A patient must be in the examining room if she is to be deemed potentially qualified to be a "contestant." In much the same way, potential participants in a game must first meet certain eligibility requirements and these must not discriminate against possible contestants for capricious and/or unjustifiable reasons. And, while there is little doubt that contests can be rigged so that unsuspecting participants can be duped into believing that they have a fair chance to win, they at least have been able to enter (of course, it may also be true that it is crueler to deceive people into thinking they are equal to others, all the while knowing that they are not).[17]

Getting into the doctor's office is necessary, but not sufficient. Even if the system was biased at the point of entry but became fair afterward, we could expect that all people from then on would be treated equitably. And, except for potential differences attributable to medical history or genetics, outcomes for a specified disease and treatment would be expected to be reasonably equivalent. Unfortunately, this is not case. For example, black patients have surgery less often for lung cancer and have fewer cardiac catheterizations for equivalently severe heart disease, when compared with similarly (clinically) situated white patients (Farjah et al. 2009; Gregory, LaVeist, and Simpson 2006). In the case of organ transplant, these factors play out in both eligibility for transplant and the short- and long-term success of the transplant (Goldfarb-Rumyantzev et al. 2006; Singh et al. 2010; Gruttadauria et al. 2011).

Though there are fewer published analyses looking at undocumented immigrants in the United States, the fact that they are often the subjects of such overwhelming nativist vitriol suggests that they, too, suffer as a medically marginalized group as much, if not more, than African Americans (Pitkin Derose, Bahney, Lurie, and Escarce 2009; Bustamante et al. 2012). Certainly, there have been many efforts, some even initially successful, to effectively bar them from any access to public resources such as education and medical care (with the notable exception of emergency care). Since many—if not most—of these people are ineligible for Medicaid or Medicare assistance, those who need chronic care are often left in desperate circumstances.[18]

It is not just people who are born the "wrong" race or the "wrong" ethnicity who may be the victims of biased allocation decisions, because there is also data that show that rural patients (still a significant part of the U.S. population) have a smaller chance of getting access to organ transplants than comparably sick urbanites (Axelrod et al. 2008). And homeless people both in the United States and Great Britain are clearly at risk for many health problems, at least some of which may be attributed to significant barriers to obtaining healthcare (Axelrod et al. 2008). Even women are commonly treated differently (and less well) than their male counterparts with similar medical conditions (Basu, Franzini, Krueger, and Lairson 2010; Brannstrom et al. 2011; Sondak, Swetter, and Berwick 2012).

Since getting into the system does not guarantee fair and equivalent treatment, it is reasonable to conclude that the medical establishment may be biased at multiple levels. One could thus view patients who suffer from this form of discrimination as individuals who, by virtue of birth and/or bad luck because of morally irrelevant features about themselves, are predisposed to be "losers" under "normal" conditions. When resources are even more constrained such as with formal rationing, when the emphasis on allocation is not necessarily need, but ability to benefit this designation would be more applicable. Therefore patients such as these could pay an extra penalty in addition to the misfortune of being sick, by having a lower chance to obtain needed healthcare that could help them. But, unlike others who lose by bad luck, these patients lose also because they never really had an even chance to compete. Hence, these people are unjustified losers. Since rationing could only provide more opportunities to disallow certain kinds of people from equal access to the types and quantities of healthcare resources available to others, it could only exacerbate the consequences of an already unfair social system. It is reasonable to presume that not only could there be more losers of this sort, but they could stand to lose more—that is, of course, unless structural and systemic features of the rationing plan were such that they could mitigate many of these currently extant biases.

Should There Be Compensation for "True" Losers?

As I mentioned earlier in this chapter, it is not uncommon for losers in some kinds of contests to receive a consolation prize, such as a second-place ribbon or a special T-shirt for having competed. While these awards are of little intrinsic value, they do recognize the achievements of the participants in some fashion. But healthcare is a fundamentally and categorically different enterprise, and the competition is for a prize that possesses a form of value perhaps unique in its capacity to (potentially) contribute substantively to an individual's well-being. While there is little question that people who compete in high-stakes games in which the winner earns both glory and riches would hold that their endeavors are of the utmost importance to them, their argument rings somewhat hollow when compared to the worth of a liver to a patient in danger of imminent death from organ failure. The former can frequently try her luck again and hope to do better the next time out, but the latter generally has just one chance. It thus seems that loss is experienced by both, but only suffered by one, so they are not comparable. Moreover, if the athlete loses because of cheating by the winner, she may protest and, if successful, be awarded the prize. Such redress is not available to the heart-failure patient who does not receive a heart.

Daniels (2008, 140) asks the question "What do we owe people when we cannot protect their health by restoring normal functioning—for example, people with certain disabilities?" By this he seems to be implying that we (society) owe something to people who, because of some deprivation via the "natural lottery" or by accidental acquisition (say, by involvement in an auto accident), are "losers" in some essential sense by not having as much health as (on average) other people have who do not possess any disability. The consequences of the outcomes of just or fair allocation decisions with inherently scarce resources (when they are made using criteria to maximize efficacy or outcome for example) can be tempered by telling people—both deciders and patients/families—that they will be cared for and won't suffer. In other spheres of life society occasionally tries to make up for losses to individuals or groups of similarly situated people. For instance, one could interpret affirmative action programs, or the official government payments to Japanese Americans who were interned during World War II, as attempts to compensate for past (and occasionally current) discrimination (Tatesihi and Yoshino 2000).

Short of totally reforming the structural and systemic inequities in the American healthcare system, ones that in all likelihood could prove to be resistant to change even under a planned, universal rationing scheme, should there be some form of tangible compensation or redress for people who lose in an unjustifiable manner? That answer may be trivially simple: of course. More germane to real life though is whether something like this is feasible, and I very much doubt it. I will just spend a short time analyzing the situation and will show the implausibility of creating a system to rectify, to individuals or groups, the inherent bias that helps create this class of losers.

Given that they lose through no fault of their own and the odds of winning are less for them than for other comparable patients who are not members of a minority group subject to prejudicial treatment, then I think a case could be made for owing them something as restitution for these existing institutional or societal biases.[19] As people who have been discounted in allocation decisions because of factors about themselves over which they may have had little control, they may be owed compensation as individuals. However, as members of groups that as a class may be treated in much the same way as discrete persons are, recompense for being "born losers" may be realized only as a reform of the system.[20] Ideally, the best form of making amends for their loss is to think of them as a class, and then to aim fixes at the framework as a whole to remove any systemic forms of prejudice that are the ultimate reasons they are inherently more likely to be losers rather than winners. This is not to say that single patients would not experience real harms when denied an intervention to which they should have had access, solely because of some identifiable feature whose presence (or absence) should be irrelevant to a medical decision involving care.

However, in the short term, and in the absence of the ability to remove endemic and ingrained discrimination from society, we could perhaps think of other, conceivably more tangible forms of loss compensation, incorporating approaches that have been tried in other public sectors— for example, higher education, employment, and the like—and that have included various forms of affirmative action. But this would require identifying who the potential losers are and adjudicating the credibility and validity of their claims. For many types of healthcare interventions or treatments, the end result of losing might very well be death or severe and permanent disability, so then it would fall to survivors to make the claim, a tangled mess that has bedeviled other forms of claims for past injustices (Kershnar 1999; Sher 2005).[21]

If some form of compensation were feasible, who should be charged with fulfilling the obligation of compensating these losers? This question is both pertinent and quite similar to those asked about situations when an individual or group asserts a claim about a violation or infringement of a presumed (human) right. The claim must be lodged against somebody or something and identifying the guilty entity with convincing evidence can often prove maddeningly frustrating (not to mention the difficulty of enforcing actions against those properly judged guilty). For problems due to societal or widespread prejudice, it would make sense that "society" would be the source of recompense ("society" might equate with the regional or federal government). As I suggested above, the best way to approach compensation for these kinds of losers might be to attempt to change the various sources of bias in the diverse aspects of the healthcare system and society in general. This requires trying to remove or diminish any preformed discrimination against populations of people so that the losses they may suffer in future rationing allocation decisions would be similar to others from more fortunate background circumstances. Alternatively, one might think that those who benefit from the allocation

decision—the winners—would be the ones best situated to provide recompense to the losers. But do winners in this sense really "win"? After
all, if they obtain something to which they would ordinarily be entitled
(in a just world where there would be enough stuff that is good so that
no one would have to do without a true benefit), they receive their just
deserts as persons.[22] But there are at least two arguments against this idea.
First, the size of the losers' group may far exceed that of the winners (such
as with organ transplantation: the numbers of those who die waiting or
who are even denied access to being listed are much greater than those
who actually receive transplants), so that it may impose a great burden
on the winners to be required to contribute to some sort of consolation
fund. Second, personal healthcare, in its very imperfect form in the United
States, is either the responsibility of the individual (commercial insurance
or no insurance) or the state (Medicaid, Medicare), and hence the provision of compensation to the losers should come from this traditional
source. And this would certainly be the case even under a form of organized, universal healthcare insurance incorporating even the mild form of
rationing I have argued might be acceptable to the American public.

The truth of the matter is that most healthcare rationing will not involve life-or-death decisions but more pedestrian, even mundane, interventions, similar to healthcare in the absence of explicit rationing. But
there will still be people who are—or who think they are—losers. The
stakes for these types of allocation decisions may be lower than for those
involving organ transplantation (for example), but those who win will be
happy and those who lose—for whatever reason—will be unhappy and
possibly angry, probably out of proportion to what they have lost. Such
is the case now, and there are no reasons to expect that things would be
different were open rationing in effect. In any case, the important point
is that a generous rationing system could ideally be more structurally fair
and offer more benefits to more patients than anything that exists today.
But no matter how just the features of allocation and distribution are,
they must be applied equitably. If that is not the case, then patients who
lose now for unjustifiable and morally indefensible reasons, will continue
to do so, but with the added insult of a veneer of impartiality.

Conclusion

Healthcare is of singular importance to people because of its potential to
further universal concerns in maintaining or improving health and thus
enabling people to pursue other important interests. This statement is

even more to the point because medicine in general has been able to make such significant strides in its ability to cure some diseases and ameliorate the symptoms of others. Indeed, the capacity of modern medicine to treat and palliate has led some to declare that it plays a unique moral role in society and should count as a "primary good" (although not the only one) (Daniels 2008, chap. 2). It is this last fact that determines that healthcare must compete with the other goods that a reasonable society should offer its people, including education, security, infrastructure, and so on. Where the lines are drawn and how the funds available are apportioned to support these various domains of public interest is a matter of heated debate. No matter how this is decided, there are limits to the absolute amount that can be spent on any one area, even if the potential need seems to be inexhaustible. Once that upper boundary is set, then rationing of one form or another must occur. And once that happens some people will, by design, not get what they might want or possibly require to substantively preserve or improve their health. If it is something that can truly be beneficial, that can really help them by relieving suffering, then it is difficult to view them as anything other than people who have lost something valuable. I have called these persons "losers" because they miss out on something that they might have received had conditions (in this case, financial conditions) been otherwise.[23]

But not all patients lose the same amount or in the same way. Some don't receive what they might want, but when that is something of little or no value (to anyone), it is difficult to characterize them in the same way as those who have truly not had access to an intervention of potentially great value, such as a drug that can cure a disease or palliate it well, or an organ for a transplant where the chance of success is good. Depending on the wealth of the healthcare system and how well it is funded, the absolute numbers of losers in this last category could be relatively few, but it is easy to imagine societies in which the resources are more constrained than others and in which the priorities are set such that many patients will have to do without interventions that could undoubtedly help them. Planners will have made decisions to privilege some needs over others, like childhood immunizations over heart transplants, or some groups over others, such as the young over the old. While this state of affairs may be unfortunate, even tragic, it is a fact about rationing, no matter how generously funded the plan may be.

However, there are steps that can be taken to make these painful outcomes more acceptable, including creating a rationing scheme that is intrinsically and procedurally fair. While not absolute, it is reasonable to believe that a just system of prioritization and allocation that is equipped with proper safeguards will warrant just decisions and outcomes, even if it is an example of imperfect procedural justice (Rawls 1999, 74–77). But life itself is inherently unfair and our societies do not go to extreme lengths to rectify all of the inequities of life brought on by both brute (bad) luck and the biases of others. Racial and ethnic prejudice, gender discrimination, and so on continue to be pervasive, regrettable, and seemingly ineradicable components of our lives, regardless of where we live. As much as we may try to formulate a rationing plan that diminishes the corrosive effects of bigotry, it will be imperfect. Even though the institution of the MELD score for liver transplants has lessened the overt racial inequities in the recipients of liver transplants, it has done little to remove the socioeconomic disparities that limit the access of many people of color to the system. It has also done little to eliminate the ability of some to use their wealth or influence to improve their chances of receiving an organ, which therefore entails lessening the prospects of others (see chapters 2 and 3).[24] Hence, the tragedy of a "normal" or "expected" justifiable loss is amplified by the addition of unethical and systemic problems in the underlying healthcare delivery structure, which no doubt reflects those extant in society. In some sense, the entire arrangement is rigged to ensure that the chance of losing is greater for some than others. As Kilner (1990, 181) notes, "The poor as a group are consistent losers. . . . Such predictable discrimination for reasons beyond the victims' control is most odious when peoples' lives are at stake."

But it is losers who also suffer the indignity of not having an equal chance of winning compared to their clinical equivalents that justify my claim that they may be owed some form of compensation or consideration for having suffered their loss. It is not the loss itself that grounds this assertion; more precisely, it is the way it came about and the reasons for it. It is the additional risk of losing (the increased odds, if you will) that warrants these patients' entitlement to redress. It is not that these same people are not subjected to bias and prejudice and the effects these have on their ability to obtain equal consideration for medical care in the health system we currently have in this country. Rather, it is that the implementation of a just rationing plan would only offer a veneer of legitimacy to the allocation of resources but do nothing to alleviate the injustice of existing inequities of access and treatment. I have suggested that these facts, both real and projected, would support the notion of restitution. However, any attempt to compensate people for a loss they have already experienced is imperfect and would fall far short of equaling the value of what they have lost. In the real world such individually or group-based reparations or compensation for even justified losses would hardly be feasible in the spirit of "ought implies can."

Nevertheless, the conditions of our current healthcare system support systematic biases that result in unjustifiable losers. It is to be expected that even a generous national rationing plan would by itself do little to rectify structural discrimination or personal prejudice on the part of the dispensers of healthcare resources. If anything, we could anticipate an exacerbation of the disadvantage experienced by certain populations of patients. Rather than devising compensation schemes, we would do far better to address the fundamental social causes that make for such losers. Short of that, perhaps the best way to minimize the effects of patients being "cheated" by the system, either by accident or by design, is to ensure that the appeals process is sufficiently robust to compensate for and rectify unjustified losses.

6

Limits to Fairness in a Democracy

"Politics is the art of the possible."[1]

"Ought implies can."[2]

In the late winter of 2003 a major medical error was discovered to have occurred at Duke University Medical Center in Durham, North Carolina. Mistakes, many grievous, are unfortunately made every day at hospitals, clinics, and doctors' offices throughout the United States; as reported by the Institute of Medicine in 2000, as many as 90,000 patients may die each year in the United States as a result of medical errors (Kohn, Corrigan, and Donaldson 2000). Many of these are not noticed or caught by anyone. Some result in major harm to patients and some of these may end up in court as the subject of malpractice lawsuits. This one was a whopper. Not only was it a terrible blunder that undoubtedly played a major role in a young girl's death, but due to a perfect storm of contributing factors, personalities, and unpredictable events, it wound up on newspaper front pages and TV evening news programs all across the country and beyond (especially in Latin America). This is the (abbreviated) story of Jesica Santillan. But it is much more than a sad account of sloppiness in managing complex medical systems. I want to present it because of what happened after the initial brouhaha settled down. It is the secondary plot—the aftermath of the medical error—that is important for my purposes and the topic I wish to discuss in this chapter.

Jesica (she was universally referred to by her first name in almost all of the media accounts) was born in 1985 in Mexico.[3] A sickly and fragile child from birth, she was diagnosed with a restrictive cardiomyopathy around the age of five years (this occurred in Texas, where her family had taken her for help). In simple terms, this meant that her heart was unable to pump the amount of blood needed to supply her body; as a consequence, her tissues were starved for oxygen. It was unclear why she had this condition, but generally it is both progressive and fatal in children and adults and curable only with a heart transplant. The earlier the transplant can be done after diagnosis the better, since the lungs can also be affected in a secondary way, and if treatment is delayed for too long it may be necessary to transplant both heart and lungs (Colan 2006, 442–443). Because of a relative who lived in a North Carolina town not too far from Duke (where they were told there were doctors who could help Jesica), the family made their way to this country using the services of a smuggler (a so-called mule) in 1999, four years before her eventual transplant. They did not apply for a visa to seek medical services for Jesica and were therefore in the United States illegally. The Duke pediatric cardiologists quickly confirmed the diagnosis and recommended a transplant, but because of the enormous cost, this treatment was unavailable to her at the time. With the assistance of friends and a local American sponsor, fundraising began in earnest. Within a couple of years they had made significant headway and it was determined that it would be acceptable to list her for a transplant. This was all perfectly appropriate and aboveboard because UNOS permits up to 5 percent of all transplants to be allocated to patients who are not citizens or permanent residents of the United States, and currently there is no rule that comments on the legality of their immigration status.[4]

As expected, Jesica's medical condition deteriorated with time. Indeed, she followed the natural history of relatively untreated (and untreatable) restrictive cardiomyopathy: both her heart and her lungs were beginning to fail, and do so irreversibly. If she were to live she would need one of the rarest and most unlikely of transplants, a combination of heart and lungs. As she became progressively sicker, her priority status—the urgency with which her clinical situation mandated some form of treatment—was elevated until she was listed as "Status 1A." These are the patients with the highest and most critical need for an organ. On February 7, 2003, she received the heart and lungs she and her family and their supporters had been hoping and praying for. Naturally, no operation of this type is ever risk-free and she would have anticipated a potentially rocky postoperative course, but no one could have predicted what actually happened. Shortly after the surgery was completed, the Duke doctors made an awful discovery: a major error had been made and Jesica had received a heart of the wrong blood type. Her surgeons had inadvertently accepted organs they should not have. The mistake had permeated the system and was not caught until it was too late. In addition to taking prompt emergency medical and surgical steps in an attempt to mitigate the potential terrible consequences of the accident, Jesica's surgeon immediately told her family what had happened and promised to do everything he could to save her life. He also apologized profusely and, in some reports, was said to have broken down in tears during his mea culpa.

Jesica's medical condition continued to deteriorate, despite all the efforts of her medical team. Her transplanted heart started to fail and a decision was made to list her for another transplant in a last-ditch attempt to give her a chance. By this time the local, national, and even international news media had gotten hold of the story (it was apparently leaked to the press by the North Carolina man who had assumed the role of the family's guide through the complexities of the medical system). Via an interpreter (because the Santillans did not speak English) an urgent plea was made by her parents (especially her mother) for another heart for their daughter. On February 20 (almost two weeks after the initial surgery) she received her second double-organ transplant. During this period she suffered catastrophic brain damage and was declared dead by whole-brain criteria on February 22, after which she was removed from artificial life support.

As documented so well by Morgan and colleagues, the initial public story of Jesica's travails was one of sympathy for her plight and that of her family (Morgan, Harrison, Chewning, and Habib 2006; see timeline on pp. 22–23). It wasn't until eight days after her initial surgery that the media started reporting that she was an illegal immigrant and describing how the family arranged to enter the country. After that, it seemed as if it was a competition between two emerging tropes: one that she was a victim of "big medicine" and the other about her immigration status. The latter focused on the fact that she was "illegal," a standing that gave her no right to take organs from clearly more deserving U.S. citizens. This theme was amplified by the knowledge that she had received a second transplant, thus provoking an argument that by so doing, *two Americans* died for lack of a heart (and possibly even more, since she also received two sets of lungs).

Even though some may think that the current bitter climate on immigration reform and the standing of undocumented immigrants is harsh and shrill and that this is a relatively recent development, the Santillan case demonstrates that this fight has been going on for quite some time. In many ways this was a perfect setup for adding fuel to the nativist sentiment that has been a mainstay in the United States almost since its founding. But here, the social indictment of Jesica and her family—and most important for my argument, the indictment of the transplant allocation system, for permitting someone like Jesica to receive a scarce resource that some think should be reserved for others they consider more like themselves instead of lavished on unworthy "others"—reveal that there may be limits to what can be done with a communally held asset, like solid organs. It demonstrates, I believe, a lesson to be learned for any attempt at a more broad-based and universal healthcare rationing system.

In chapter 3 I described the features of fairness that should comprise any decent and just rationing system so as to make it palatable to the largest number of people who would be affected by its benefits and burdens. Critical to this process was establishing a procedure by which reasonable discussion between rational people could establish the rules by which the five central principles of Fairness of any policy could be followed. To reiterate, these included the core values of *transparency*, meaning that any debate about various methods of rationing, as well as how they would be accomplished, would be open to inspection by all; *relevance*, which governs the kinds of rules that could be acceptable: they would have to be judged as relevant to the situation to which they were applied; *fairness*, which states that similar situations would be treated similarly without special preferences (no VIPs or their opposites); the ability to lodge an *appeal* or to protest a misapplication of the rules or mishandling by the "system" or by people who work in it; and finally, *enforcement*, or the built-in power to ensure that the rules are implemented in the way they are designed to be implemented. Importantly, implementing such a plan on a national, "universal" basis would require endorsement by as large a majority percentage of the population as possible. It could not simply be arbitrarily imposed by one group on another (no matter how benign their intentions, as in Oregon, for example). This suggests that some compromises with the ideal approach would undoubtedly have to be made and incorporated into the plan to win support from as many people as feasible.

Of course, this process describes an ideal system, one to which we might aspire but that might be exceedingly difficult to accomplish under real-life circumstances. As the story about Jesica Santillan demonstrated, we live in a society that continues to express prejudice against a variety of people for morally irrelevant traits that they happen to possess. How likely is it that the design and implementation of a public rationing plan can be deaf or immune to these beliefs, as unjustifiable as they may be from an ethical point of view? It is perhaps to be expected that in a country composed of diverse voices with unequal and unevenly distributed sources of power and financial strength, as well as vestiges of latent and occasionally blatant prejudice, there will be a tension between those arguing for liberal equality and justice, and those striving to maintain a social status quo. In this chapter I want to discuss what a democratic polity could reasonably be expected to accept that could place limits upon any conception of a theoretical ideal of fairness (and thus not what they *should* accept). I should state at the outset that it is not my intention to defend this point of view, only to argue that it must be considered in any discourse about implementing a comprehensive, universal rationing plan. In so doing I wish to examine the risk imposed to two of the core principles that would undoubtedly come under assault in any dialog about the actual implications of taking them seriously: fairness and appeals.

The Challenge of Fairness

Before I launch into an in-depth discussion of this complicated topic, I want to provide two more examples to illustrate the complexity of this problem. These show that the challenge of inclusivity in rationing does not simply concern undocumented immigrants. This story was reported in the spring of 2011 from upstate New York:

> Convicted rapist Kenneth Pike, of Auburn, N.Y., is expected to undergo a life-saving heart transplant that could cost up to $800,000—a price that will be paid courtesy of New York state taxpayers. The expense has outraged many crime victim advocates and community members, who say they cannot understand how the justice system can provide big-tag services for convicted felons arguably at the expense of innocent patients. "From a moral standpoint I think everyone should have a chance at life," said Carol Speach, a media sales professional in Auburn. "But realistically, I think no he shouldn't. I know innocent people with health problems who have medical bills coming out of their ears and can't afford it." The question has been the talk of the small suburban New York town: Should taxpayers shell out for convicted criminals to receive services that some payers could probably never afford themselves?[5]

And this story from the *Sacramento Bee* from 2002:

> A California inmate has become the first person to receive an organ transplant while in state prison, adding fuel to the debate over the costs of providing medical care to an expanding, and aging, prison population. In an operation performed without fanfare at the Stanford Medical Center three weeks ago, a 31-year-old two-time felon was given a new heart. The taxpayer-financed operation and subsequent aftercare, which prison officials estimate could carry a total price tag of $1 million, is certain to raise questions as to whether there are limits to the kinds of treatment ailing inmates must be given. "We don't have a policy per se," said Russ Heimerich, a spokesman for the California Department of Corrections. "We have a requirement, based in law and in losing many, many lawsuits, to provide

medically necessary care to inmates. The courts have told us that inmates have a constitutional right to healthcare. You and I don't, but inmates do. . . . We have to do whatever is medically necessary to save an inmate's life." The inmate, whose name is being withheld by the department for reasons of medical confidentiality, is serving a 14-year sentence for a 1996 robbery in Los Angeles. Prison officials say he will not be eligible for parole until late 2008 because this is his second felony conviction. After a longtime heart problem caused by a viral infection became critical, he was transferred to the Stanford Medical Center from the prison system's medical institution at Vacaville. He received a new heart from an unidentified donor Jan. 3, and has been returned to Vacaville. A spokeswoman for the medical center said the cost of the procedure was $150,000 to $200,000. But that does not include security costs, aftercare or post-transplant medication that can run as much as $21,000 per year. Department of Corrections officials have estimated that total costs could reach $1 million before the inmate is released. After his release, he will have to seek private insurance or qualify for government-run medical coverage such as Medi-Cal.[6]

It is perhaps not surprising that these stories (and a number of others like them) provoked widespread outrage when the news media got hold of them and they became well known by the public. In much the same way that the saga of Jesica Santillan was transformed from a heartrending tale of a girl who made her way to a "mecca" of modern medical care to receive a life-saving heart transplant into one of an illegal immigrant—a criminal—taking a communal and scarce resource from more deserving Americans, the accounts of prisoners—even those convicted of violent, heinous crimes—being as eligible to receive a scarce resource as law-abiding citizens, stimulate an emotionally wrenching sense of moral outrage, of a grave injustice being done. It seems to be irrelevant that UNOS states that it is perfectly acceptable for undocumented immigrants or citizens of other countries to receive transplants in the United States,[7] or that since 1976 it has been the law that incarcerated prisoners must receive standard-of-care healthcare:[8] public opinion seems to differ, and often is quite strident.

And in these stories lies a cautionary and important problem for any plan of universal healthcare rationing. A "tyranny of the majority" may place limits on what can be accomplished with public resources and how comprehensively and widely the net of distributive justice may be cast and implemented. So we must consider how the undercurrents of deeply held prejudices against the non–native born, many ethnic minorities, and all sorts of people who have departed from what is commonly thought of as mainstream, acceptable behavior can place boundaries on who can receive the anticipated benefits of what healthcare reform and universal, generous and planned rationing can bestow.

In a 1996 essay titled "Should a Criminal Receive a Heart Transplant?," Schneiderman and Jecker (1996) suggested a dichotomy of justice. Under the general rubric of justice—with particular reference to its application for healthcare—they distinguished between a foundational ethic of medicine (medical justice), in which doctors are sworn to provide the same (appropriate) kind and level of care to all patients irrespective of any other factors, and a second and parallel kind they called societal justice, by which they referred to the restrictions placed on the egalitarian ideal of the former. In the latter, certain prejudices or preferences (this may be a kinder or more benign way of stating it) may be expressed as the boundary of tolerability, as in the ability to permit felons to be eligible for organ transplants. This clearly departs from the usual conception of the ideals of justice that we uphold, at least in argument and the abstract, as a goal toward which we should strive. And clearly there can be a conflict between what morality dictates and the reality of what societal justice may demand and therefore what may be publicly acceptable or permissible.

Most of the time we think about the limits of what a health insurance plan might offer as a matter of money, a purely financial consideration. And for the most part this is undoubtedly correct. This means, as in Oregon (see chapters 2 and 3), the total number or kinds of healthcare services made available to poor and low-income people were determined almost entirely by how much money was to be allocated to pay for the plan during each two-year budget period. Of course, this was dependent not only on tax receipts but on critical decisions of the legislature to devote *x* amount of the total budget to the OHP rather than to some other need in the state, such as infrastructure. As recounted by Fox and Leichter (1991), the willingness of the legislature to be reasonably generous was due in large part to the persuasiveness of Senate President John Kitzhaber (himself a physician). But, as they also relate, the magnanimity of the legislators was neither unbounded nor continuous and the plan suffered from downturns in the economy as well as pressing needs for funds elsewhere. Finally, and not discussed very much at all, was the willingness of the state's citizens to be taxed to pay for the OHP. While the tales of Coby Howard, Donna Arneson, and others clearly demonstrated that purse strings and heartstrings can be tugged by similar forces, the news story about Horacio Alberto Reyes-Camarena is another case entirely, as reported by ABC News' Brian Robinson in May 2012:

Thanks to the state of Oregon, a law-abiding citizen in need of a kidney transplant may have to die so that death-row prisoner Horacio Alberto Reyes-Camarena can live. Reyes-Camarena, 47, has been on Oregon's death row since 1996, when he was convicted of repeatedly stabbing 32- and 18-year-old sisters he met in a farm-labor camp. The older woman survived 17 stab wounds to testify against him. Every year, as Reyes-Camarena appeals his conviction, Oregon—which is struggling through budget cuts and having a tough time providing a basic education for its children and healthcare for its poorer citizens—pays a reported $121,000 a year to keep Reyes-Camarena on dialysis. Last month, his prison doctor determined he was a good candidate for a kidney transplant. With the state funding his medical care, Reyes-Camarena could be placed on a transplant waiting list ahead of others who did not commit any crimes and become the state's first death-row inmate to receive an organ transplant. That has outraged crime victim advocates, who cannot understand how the justice system can "reward" convicted murderers at the expense of innocent patients.[9]

I suspect that the citizens of Oregon would react with outrage (as indeed they did) when contemplating having their tax dollars go to fund something like this, rather than something else. Tax receipts, like kidneys, are not limitless and choices must be made on how to spend them, and in a democracy we need to give strong deference to the will of the people. Even if the people can be in error, especially with opinions about moral rights and wrongs, their "will" cannot be lightly dismissed as irrelevant. This does not mean that we must always bow to the wishes of the majority, especially when they reveal grossly immoral preferences. But there may be times when absolute moral purity will be unreachable; the goal then should be to pursue other means to persuade the majority to change their views so that they are more consonant with ethical standards. As Fleck (2009) has suggested, we may have to settle for an approach that is "just enough" (although it is not entirely clear where the minimal benchmark of this standard should lie).

Of course, we have accomplished national public policy changes that have been unpopular at the time even though they have been right, such as advances in civil rights (including racial/ethnic, gender, and now gay rights, including marriage equality in an increasing number of states). Some might also cite various Supreme Court decisions expanding other rights and individual dignity (*Roe v. Wade* in 1973 and *Estelle v. Gamble* in 1976 are examples). As most people know, the former recognized (or established according to some) a right to electively terminate pregnancies prior to the ex utero viability of the fetus, and was founded on a constitutional right to personal privacy. The latter found that incarcerated prisoners cannot be denied access to a reasonable (or the prevailing) standard of healthcare, because to do so would in essence comprise a form of secondary, additional punishment.[10] But one of the often-stated accusations against *Roe v. Wade* is that it "created" a right where none existed, and that something as socially disruptive as legalizing the practice of elective pregnancy termination should be the result of democratic deliberation and hence legislation or voter referenda. The idea is that this is a more representative form of action, which presumably reflects the majority will of the people, and would be more accepted in the general population.[11] There is clearly a tension between judges making (or interpreting) law for everyone else and then endorsement (or rejection) of what they say is the law by a majority of the people.

The second court decision granted prisoners a "right" to medical diagnosis and treatment paid for by the local, state, or federal government (depending on which entity had jurisdiction or control of the facility housing the inmate). Ironically (and some would argue inexplicably and indefensibly, if not incoherently), prisoners would have access to free or subsidized healthcare they would not have had if they had not been locked up. On the "outside" they would have been on their own, and even if they had wanted to see a doctor or go to a clinic, they might not have had the financial means to do so, like millions of other Americans without health insurance. Thus, people who had violated the law, flouting the mores of civil society, could get something for "free," a good that others might not be able to obtain for themselves despite the fact that they were law-abiding citizens. (The similarities to the reactions to the Santillan case are both striking and not surprising.) Many people view this as a deep injustice and think that the solution would be to deny felons such access. And while this may be viewed as an affront to common morality, or a waste of taxpayer dollars, it reaches a boiling point when it is not simply money that is at issue, but a critically scarce, life-saving resource such as a liver or heart.

So we may conclude that mandating equality of access to prisoners in healthcare and rationing has both a legal and moral justification even if it is controversial. But as with the abortion debate, which remains deeply divisive in the United States, the ability to implement the law's requirements with respect to organ transplantation in actual practice turns out to be quite difficult. And it is not simply the pedestrian public that often harbors these opinions. As recently demonstrated in a survey of liver transplant professionals, providing this life-saving treatment to some—but not all—felons, was felt to be absolutely contraindicated (Secunda et al. 2012; Griffin and Prieto 2008). Of great interest was the fact that a distinction was drawn between felons serving a life sentence and those in jail for lesser offenses, with the latter being more acceptable as potential recipients. Of course, a major problem with attempting to differentiate between criminals who have been convicted of crimes of varying gravity is that it once again gets us entangled with a cutoff problem: How heinous a crime is too heinous? Should only those convicted of first-degree murder be eliminated from consideration? What about prisoners in states that have "three strikes and you're out" laws, by which some people who have been convicted of, say, three nonviolent property offenses such as burglary can be sent away for life? Should they be placed in the same (im)moral category as violent offenders (Chen 2008; Tonry 2009)? Or what about people who are imprisoned (including for murder) who have then been freed after their innocence has been discovered, sometimes many years after their convictions? Finally, we might reflect on the societal acceptance of transplanting "white-collar" criminals (such as Bernard Madoff), who may have effectively been sentenced to life. The point is that attempting to parse where the line, or cutoff, should be drawn is no less difficult for this continuous, complex variable that it is for age or marginally beneficial treatments. It seems as if the only way to succeed at this task would be to place the line at either zero (eliminate prisoners and undocumented immigrants from consideration) or include them within the "umbrella of care." Either way, we must cope with the apparent conflict between moral ideals of justice and those less-than-exemplary attitudes held by many people whose approval (or at least acquiescence) would be required to implement any sort of reasonable rationing plan that affects everyone.

Finally, I wish to say a few words about one of the cardinal aspects of fairness—that is, the need to treat similar people similarly when they are clinically alike. Adhering to the dictates of this principle demands a very high standard, particularly within organizations that treat a complicated mixture of people. While it is true that my colleagues and I created (and implemented) a policy for the allocation of drugs during a scarcity that forbids treating some people as deserving of special consideration, thus permitting them greater access to a rare medication than others who could also benefit from it, it has yet to be put to a true test of its strength and durability (Rosoff et al. 2012). Furthermore, I fear that in the absence of a more far-reaching set of rules embraced by all institutions, it will be very challenging to maintain the standard set by the policy. However, if such an egalitarian approach faces these kinds of challenges within a single institution, it would not be difficult to imagine the problems if one attempted to impose this method more broadly. More important perhaps, creating a policy like this, even when accomplished with comprehensive support and input from community representatives, offers a cautionary lesson of both hope and warning. It was done and is working within a "closed" and focused environment, but it may be a different matter altogether if it were applied more extensively and opened up to broad public scrutiny and criticism. It is unlikely that its essential fairness would be viewed either kindly or reverentially by all and thus remain unscathed.

The same problems plague the discriminatory views voiced by many against undocumented immigrants. From what services of a civil society should they be excluded? Should it be all healthcare, or just some parts of it, such as organ transplantation where there is an absolute scarcity of resources (as opposed to money)? Should Jesica Santillan, a child dying of heart disease, be denied a transplant simply because her parents brought her to this country in search of a cure to save her life? In many ways, attempting to dissect varying degrees of illegality or culpability is no different than trying to decide what kinds of prisoners are less bad—less evil if you will than others.

When I have discussed these cases with both bioethics and clinical colleagues, we generally begin with the worst case, such as a confessed murderer and rapist. No one would want to save his life with a transplant, especially when one could offer the organ to a law-abiding patient. Indeed, many would just as soon deny him any kind of healthcare. But as we move toward more "tolerable" offenses, finally ending up with the innocent person who was unjustly convicted or the man who robbed a convenience store to pay for food for his family or the desperately needed medical procedure for his daughter, people clearly start equivocating. Moreover, if anyone in the group has or has had a relative or friend who has been in prison, they also tend to be more tolerant or flexible.[12] There seems to be a direct relationship between the gravity or assumed evil of a person's actions and the public's willingness to exclude him from the benefits society may offer (such as healthcare). Social condemnation, or what people believe to be one's just desert, increases as their perceived departure from societal normal increases. But the degree to which this view governs the way we give people access to resources may be correlated with how scarce those resources are and whether the allocation to an individual felt to be less deserving would have a perceptible impact on another who was understood to be more so.

In some ways, the views expressed toward those felt to be less blameworthy than others are similar to the views commonly heard about transplantation in people whose medical conditions are believed to be a result of lifestyle choices. For example, should smokers be eligible for heart transplantation or alcoholics for livers (Kotlyar, Burke, Campbell, and Weinrieb 2008; Kroeker et al. 2008; Neuberger 2007; Neuberger et al. 2008; Secunda et al. 2012; Volk et al. 2011; Wilmot and Ratcliffe 2002)? Or, should smokers with chronic obstructive pulmonary disease be eligible for a lung transplant (Tong et al. 2010, 2013)? So, in reality, socially marginalized groups of all kinds may be excluded from many of the benefits available to others who are not identified as members of these groups, but the kinds of prejudicial views voiced against them are clearly more blurred for what might be labeled as borderline cases. How seriously should we take these often-discriminatory views when designing a healthcare rationing system?

So far I have been discussing the acceptability of allocating critically and finitely scarce resources like organs when the potential recipients are considered to belong to a group that is out of the mainstream. They have this status because of some attribute they possess or have acquired, such as criminal behavior, so they're thought to have forfeited their "right" to be considered a candidate for allocation. Are similar concerns voiced about the distribution of more flexible and fungible resources, like money? It is clearly a major leap to move from livers to dollars where we have much more discretion in how much we apportion the latter for healthcare, but the contours of the concern are very similar. For example, it seems to me that unease about giving an organ to an undocumented immigrant or a prisoner is based on a two-pronged argument. First, these individuals have broken the law in one form or another and thus have violated the rules of civil society. Therefore, they should not derive the benefits that society has to bestow on its members beyond some minimal standard of housing, sustenance, basic medical care, and so on. This is their just desert. Second, the entire (cadaveric) transplant system is based on the voluntary donation of organs on the death of a patient. Presumably full disclosure about potential recipients might have a corrosive effect on the willingness of individuals prior to death to donate (such as on advance directives like driver's licenses) or their families on their behalf postmortem, if they knew that a murderer or illegal immigrant could receive these organs instead of a "law-abiding American citizen." It is not too far a stretch to suppose that taxpayers might have similar concerns about the uses to which their hard-earned dollars might be directed. This could include any kind of healthcare for marginalized people, from relatively inexpensive (and highly cost-effective) interventions like primary care and prenatal care, to vaccines for childhood illnesses, all the way to hemodialysis and cardiac surgery.[13] One can get an inkling of how this might play out by observing the acrimonious rhetoric in the debate over providing in-state tuition for undocumented adolescents applying to state colleges and universities.[14] In this situation, it surely is a case of anger over spending public money on people who are believed to not deserve it.

Can we legitimately say that things like organs, scarce drugs, ventilators, and ICU beds during an influenza pandemic—that is, absolutely scarce resources—are somehow different and their allocation constitutes an emergency that can justify abandoning or neglecting our ordinary sense of inclusiveness and hence limit accessibility to the "worthiest" members of society? If the answer is yes, we of course must provide reasons why we should do so, as well as deciding who should be worthy enough to qualify for coverage. If there is no crisis (or perceived crisis present or looming), I suspect that most people don't think about giving convicted felons and undocumented immigrants healthcare, be it emergency or high-level, high-tech care like radiation therapy or chemotherapy for cancer, heart bypass surgery, or even hemodialysis for renal failure. This doesn't mean that they are indifferent, but these issues are not brought to their attention. Most people who might be angry are probably more concerned about other issues of more immediate relevance to their lives. I realize that this is somewhat cynical, but it may be a case of "out of sight, out of mind," because we tend not to devote a great deal of attention to issues that exist below the radar. But the minute something like organs for crooks hits the news, it seems to awaken many of our baser impulses and prejudices, occasionally yielding a backlash that can have terrible consequences not just for felons and undocumented immigrants, but for many others as well.

There were concerns, and I think legitimate ones, that critically scarce resources during the anticipated influenza pandemic in 2009 would initially be available to all but that the allocation system would later encounter problems. As the needs increased and the amount of life-saving interventions and supplies dwindled in comparison, we feared that emotions like xenophobic nativism would take over and the undocumented would feel the full brunt of exclusionary policies. Indeed, there was a fear among some that this type of bias could be an expression of a majoritarian belief that certain populations had no claim on scarce resources. Those most marginalized would include the undocumented and prisoners, but one could readily imagine other groups also fitting these criteria. Indeed, the danger would be to expand those on the list to exclude once we got a taste of its acceptability and its apparent instrumental utility for those fortunate enough not to be precluded from care. In a way, this is a slippery-slope argument, and its force is clearly due to our realization that something like this could actually occur (Rosoff and Decamp 2011).

There are assuredly other domains in which society and its medical representatives make little or no distinction between different kinds of people for the purposes of trying to save their lives. Indeed, this is a paradigm of medical justice. This is unquestionably true in the emergency department, where trauma surgeons and others do not differentiate between victims and perpetrators when treating those injured by violence. They obey the rule of sickest first, although occasionally this may be modified to eliminate counterproductive attempts to save the lives of those deemed irreparably lost, in order to redirect resources to others with better survival chances. And, while it is certainly controversial in the abstract, there is little dispute among military medical ethics experts that on the battlefield and under standard battle triage methods, the duty of the physician and her team is to save the sickest or the one most likely to survive first, irrespective of the uniform the patient is wearing, or even if the patient is not wearing a uniform at all (i.e., is a civilian).[15] Admittedly this can be a contentious approach when physicians are faced with overwhelming numbers of casualties that vastly exceed their capacity to care for them. However, in the heat of battle and with the often-extreme patriotic fervor stirred up during an armed conflict—especially one that enjoys broad public support—it may be extremely difficult to uphold these moral commitments. One can easily imagine the popular outcry that would accompany media stories of a grieving family whose son or daughter was lost in the casualty triage station "because" an enemy soldier's life was saved instead. The fact that the captured and wounded enemy soldier was in the custody of "our" side and hence a prisoner of war would, I suspect, make as little difference as the fact that Jesica Santillan was a very poor, desperately ill child whose control over her destiny was limited or nonexistent. While some might argue that these are the occasions during which our deeply held moral sentiments and values are best put to the test, it may be difficult to adhere to these ideals in a pluralistic society that depends on some measure of common or mass support for national efforts to be successful.[16]

Distribution of Public Resources

Some might contend that the issue of "ownership" of healthcare resources, be they livers or dollars, is integrally important to any decision on how they might be controlled and who gets to oversee their distribution. For example, the organ transplant organization system in the United States is publicly managed and funded by the federal government. Potential donors (actually their families or their estates) are not paid for their "donation" (if they were, it would not be a donation, but a salable and potentially marketable commodity; indeed, the sale of organs is illegal in this country and most others). Thus, people decide to give their organs (or not) for a variety of reasons, but none of them have to do with the possibility of financial remuneration (Alden and Cheung 2000; Baughn,

Auerbach, and Siminoff 2010; Boulware et al. 2002; Bratton, Chavin, and Baliga 2011; Davidson and Devney 1991; Gill and Lowes 2008; Iltis, Rie, and Wall 2009; Institute of Medicine, Committee on Increasing Rates of Organ Donation 2006; Rodrigue, Cornell, and Howard 2006a,b; Siminoff, Mercer, Graham, and Burant 2007; Siminoff, Burant, and Youngner 2004; Siminoff, Burant, and Ibrahim 2006; Vernale and Packard 1990). As it happens, marketing campaigns to attempt to increase the number of available organs often concentrate on the "gift of life." And while the gift is presumably given to an individual, most of the time cadaveric organs are transplanted into recipients who remain anonymous (at least initially) to the family of the deceased. Representatives of the local organ procurement organization (OPO) are usually charged with obtaining consent from the family if prior authorization has not been given by the donor, such as on a driver's license or other valid advance directive, and if the family does not try to override this antemortem decision. The organ is then retrieved and placed into a general system in which it is offered to doctors and hospitals that could use it most effectively. The important point is that it is a public system. Therefore, in a sense, the organ "belongs" to the public and is a communal resource, available to any patient who meets the agreed-on medical and psychosocial criteria for transplantation.

Generally speaking, ownership confers the ability to dispose of the property as the owner sees fit, within certain limits, depending on what kind of property it is. We place restrictions on how such transfers can take place and under what conditions. For example, you can't just sell your house to anyone you like: the title has to be free and clear of certain kinds of liens, there are types of prejudicial sales that one is not free to engage in (such as refusing to sell to people you don't like because of their ethnicity), and so on. And some things are more commoditized than others. Even though we tend to regard our organs as a sort of personal property, we prohibit people from selling their kidneys, even though the transaction may be purported to be free of coercion and one into which all parties enter freely and openly (well, perhaps not openly due to the illegality of these transactions). One cannot sell one's freedom and enter into a status of involuntary servitude or slavery. But goods owned collectively may be a different sort of property. I am not speaking of things like joint ownership of a piece of land, for instance, but of a public space (a park), or a building (the local library or town hall), or general funds. Presumably the public, either via voting through referenda on the ballot, or via their elected representatives, exercise their power of "ownership" to dispose of funds (tax dollars) the way they wish, under some limits. Without getting into an involved discussion of political philosophy, I want to explore what might be the boundaries of the preferences the public can legitimately express about how their tax dollars are used for social spending purposes (such as healthcare). Can a majority permissibly (legally or morally) exclude certain people or groups from consideration for resources like health insurance or certain kinds of coverage?

Much of this discussion also hinges on how we view these marginalized groups: as full or less-than-full members of society. If the former, then they are owed the same rights and privileges and pieces of the pie (theoretically speaking) as others; if the latter, then less so up to and including complete exclusion. Even if we have a moral and/or spiritual or even theoretical dedication to the ideals of egalitarian inclusiveness, we live in the real world where such sentiments may be more honored in the breach than reality. How to reconcile the need for legitimacy of a policy and the limits of what may be publicly and politically acceptable and tenable is a major challenge. At the same time we may live in an intolerant society in which the tyranny of the majority may yield outcomes that are less than perfect.

Actions often speak louder than words and the very fact that incarcerated felons and undocumented immigrants, poor African Americans (as well as perhaps the rural and older poor), and so on, exist at the borders of society and have diminished access to the general benefits available to others simply because of who and what they are, demonstrates that their marginalization is, in one sense, deliberate. Our society chooses to treat these people in this manner, and whether it is a result of an active, calculated process of institutionalized, legal racism, ageism, or nativism or simply a kind of "out of sight, out of mind" disregard of the plight of these people, the end result is the same. Now I am not arguing that American society would intentionally and consciously vote to exclude poor American citizens from access to a universal healthcare system. Indeed, while the popularity and merits of the Patient Protection and Affordable Care Act of 2010 can be debated, it is a legislative attempt by the country to expand the umbrella of healthcare to more people, especially those who either choose to not buy health insurance, or those who can't afford to. And even the partial and spotty expansion of state Medicaid programs under the law should help attain this goal.[17] But the states already exclude undocumented immigrants from Medicaid (except for emergency treatment), and the inability of such patients to obtain dialysis for kidney failure (a program funded by federal Medicare) has wreaked financial havoc among a number of private and public health systems.[18] Furthermore, the new healthcare reform law will do nothing for illegal immigrants (Galarneau 2011).

While imprisoned people—who comprise an alarmingly high percentage of the U.S. population and an even greater proportion in some communities—are entitled to the standard of care in medical treatment due to a series of Supreme Court decisions dating back to 1976 (*Estelle et al. v. Gamble*, 1976), few would argue that many prisoners receive anything close to what is available outside the jail walls. On the other hand, as illustrated by the outrage accompanying the stories I related earlier about felons being eligible for transplants, it is both tragic and held by many to be a disgrace that those who have flouted the norms of society, often violently, can receive a good for free that must be purchased by the unimprisoned and often forgone for financial reasons. This belief that people get something they don't deserve, either because they are here in this country illegally and didn't "earn" it or because they have thumbed their nose at civil society by committing crimes, energizes the prejudice against these (and other) groups. It also fosters resentment about the allocation of healthcare resources to them, whether these resources are concrete, noninterchangeable things like organs or more fungible stuff like tax dollars. While I would argue that these feelings should not be translated into policy, they cannot be ignored and methods to account for them would help garner support for a more inclusive and generous healthcare system.

Finally, a word needs to be said about the risks of a slippery slope. Under this conception, if we agree to permit the exclusion of some obvious groups that are unpopular—even hated—by large numbers of people, and certainly so when one envisions them getting "something for nothing," there could be a danger that if this step were taken, it would be much easier to both define and eliminate from healthcare coverage other groups on the margins of society. For example, one could imagine that these might comprise the homeless, the long-term chronically unemployed, or individuals with severe cognitive dysfunction (either acquired as in dementia or after a traumatic brain injury or hypoxia, or congenital); the list goes on.[19] Indeed, anyone who could conceivably be construed to be worth less than others or to contribute less than their fair share or who is in any way on the receiving end of group bias or hatred, could become a target for refining a healthcare system to make it cheaper (fewer people covered) or just more exclusive, reserved for "true" or "real" Americans who are taxpayers.[20] While slippery-slope arguments almost always suffer from simplicity, they have a real attraction (perhaps because of this feature) and can gain traction in some cases (Burgess 1993; Govier 1982). In the situation under discussion, our history in the United States as well as elsewhere would tend to support the concern about the risks of taking a big step and permitting institutionalized, legal discrimination against large swaths of the population. Indeed, in the case of exclusion from healthcare, the danger stems from starting with big groups (prisoners and illegal immigrants, which comprise many millions of people) and then moving to smaller and perhaps less visible ones, rather than the reverse. Either way, I believe that the peril is real and can serve as a caution as we proceed.

Ultimately, the question is about how public prejudices against one or more groups in the United States can adversely influence the ability to adopt comprehensive rationing. I have argued that since we find the allocation of truly and finitely scarce resources such as organs or drugs acceptable, even when the result of not receiving them may be grievous harm to individuals, then we should find a generous and fair rationing system to be immensely more tolerable since the number of people who suffer from not receiving something will be negligible. Nevertheless, the creation of a fair system in a democracy requires us to listen to the concerns of the public, who will ultimately be responsible for paying for a system that affects them in a very deep and integral way. Moreover, if we endorse the central concept that the system must be fair in a manner described in chapter 3, it therefore must be supported in large part by a majority of the populace to garner legitimacy. Will the American people tolerate generosity toward groups that are on the margins of society or significant minorities? This is an empirical question that must be addressed. I suspect that the tolerance of the American people might be more reasonable than the individuals they elect as their representatives in Congress. But we will have to see.

The Limits on Appeals

In this section, I want to briefly discuss the potential problems with the principle of permitting appeals for poor treatment due to misapplication of the rules. The issues and challenges I wish to examine here are related to, but differ from, those I presented in the previous chapter. Here, I am not arguing that the public will not permit the fair exercise of appeals power; indeed, the availability of such a process contributes to maintaining justice in the application of the rules. Rather, I want to present some potential obstacles to implementing a workable method of adjudicating disputes that bear a connection to the issues I presented earlier with respect to democratically imposed limitations on fairness. As an example, we can imagine a situation where a patient's family believes that their relative has been denied, say, intensive care including mechanical ventilation, pressor medications to maintain blood pressure, hemodialysis, and so on, and wishes to contest this decision. Let us assume that the reason given for the denial of these interventions is that in the expert opinion of the doctors, the interventions would offer no more than a marginal benefit to this patient, and therefore they would not be covered by the health insurance system. The family believes that this opinion is incorrect. What avenues should be available to them? What should a fair appeals process demand? Or, more specifically, what kinds of appeals should be sanctioned?

Under current conditions, patients initiate appeals, more properly labeled lawsuits, whenever they feel they have been mistreated by the healthcare system. Grievances can be based on real harms perceived to have been caused by doctors, nurses, or ancillary personnel, but even minor complaints have been known to lead to legal action, as demonstrated by the significant number of "frivolous" suits that continue to be quite common (Hochberg et al. 2011; Golann 2011). The risk of being sued can prompt physicians to adopt a defensive posture, ordering more tests than clinically indicated, which can perversely lead to even more potential injuries (Bishop, Federman, and Keyhani 2010; Schifrin and Cohen 2012). Of course, not all complaints result in a suit and many are settled at the local level by some form of arbitration. More complicated are disputes with larger organizations such as big insurance companies when patients (and often their physicians acting on their behalf) go to battle to obtain something the patients have been denied that they believe they are entitled to. Frustration with a system that often appears uncaring or deaf to complaints can lead to legal action. Sometimes this prompts physicians to lie for their patients (as I discussed in chapter 3). Hence, it would appear as if there are a number of routes available to angry or aggrieved patients, any one of which may be taken to attempt to satisfy a claim of mistreatment. This is not surprising considering our present-day mixture of private and public insurance programs, the large number of uninsured, and a completely separate group of patients who obtain much of their healthcare in the Veterans Administration system. What could be expected, and more important, what could practically work if we created a comprehensive, universal health system with rationing?

No matter how generous the benefits, there will continue to be people who believe that they have been treated poorly by the system. I could imagine three general classes of complaints.[21] The first would be rela-tively straightforward. The allegations would involve a misapplication of presumptively fair rules. For example, a patient may object to a judgment that states that the system will not pay for a certain kind of operation he wants on the grounds that it is primarily cosmetic and a decision has been made a priori not to cover these sorts of procedures. The reasoning is that the type of cosmesis in question is not essential to most people's welfare (say, a rhinoplasty, as opposed to reconstructive surgery after trauma to the face). The complainant could attempt to either persuade the system to recognize him as qualitatively different from other nose-job patients, or try to get the entire exclusion overturned; either way, he is arguing against a legitimate exercise of a fair rule.

The second category of complaints would involve objections to the rules themselves. These could take the form of stating that the process to create the allocation method was incorrect or fundamentally flawed in such a way as to make any resulting decisions or allocations of resources incorrect. This accusation would have both moral and presumably le-gal force if, and only if, it could be conclusively demonstrated that the process by which the system was constructed was inherently incorrect. For example, if we accept that the five principles as I described them in chapter 2 (and reiterated above) were themselves somehow defective and using them as a guide would inevitably result in a product that was unavoidably unfair—either to everyone, or perhaps to a class or group of people—in a way that could not be justified, then such a claim could be legitimate. However, if the rules were created using an open and demo-cratic process that was guided in good faith by these principles, then it is reasonable to conclude that there would a better-than-average chance (perhaps much greater than this) that the resulting rules were themselves fair. Therefore, if the patient was the one I described at the beginning of this section, and it were judged that intensive care would have minimal ability to improve the person's condition, and if it had been previously de-cided that all patients in similar clinical situations would be treated with compassionate palliative care, then there would be little cause for protest.

However, the third cause for complaint is more complex. In this situa-tion, the grievance would be based on the belief that the rules themselves are corrupt solely with respect to some people and not others. For ex-ample, basing this view on the previous section, we could imagine a state of affairs in which democratic deliberation in setting up the healthcare system resulted in one in which it had been decided a priori to exclude undocumented immigrants or some other identified group, say, people over the age of seventy, since this is the group identified by Callahan (2009) as one that might reasonably be denied access to many kinds of technologically advanced healthcare services. Let us further suggest that it is my father/mother/brother who has just turned seventy years old and he/she gets very sick with pneumonia and respiratory failure or has a heart attack and develops intractable left-sided heart failure. Ordinarily—that is, for younger patients—the standard might be mechanical ventilation in the ICU for the former until (or if) she gets better or perhaps the implantation of a portable left ventricular assist device in the latter, which could help her live for several more years to see her grandchildren get married. However, with the age cutoff having been accepted as reasonable within the constraints of rationing, these therapeutic options are unavailable and such patients die. Is this fair? Is it (or can it be) acceptable?

The answer is that it could be, assuming that older people—meaning those over the age of seventy, as Callahan proposes—agreed with younger people that this was an appropriate form of limiting medical interventions in the interest of saving money or reallocating it to more fruitful uses. However, if the decision-making process was more like that in Oregon, where most decisions were made by people unaffected by the outcome, then we might come to the opposite conclusion, and the individuals complaining about the fairness of the system might have a legitimate point. Under these circumstances, it would be reasonable to say that the rules themselves were suspect if not corrupt. Moreover, it is almost inconceivable that other large groups would agree to be classified as second-class (or even no-class) recipients of health insurance. However, the danger for some extremely marginalized populations (prisoners, illegal immigrants, etc.) is that they won't even be consulted; they will have to rely on other parties to serve as their advocates.

In our current healthcare system, undocumented immigrants generally do not have access to legal methods of obtaining healthcare, since it is illegal to employ them, so any form of private or public health insurance would be only obtainable by fraud. Of course, there is nothing to prevent them from purchasing medical services on an à la carte basis, or availing themselves of acute care in emergency departments (which are generally reimbursed by Medicaid). We could reasonably say that this system is mean-spirited and plausibly even immoral. Perhaps it is no more unfair than the many other inequities that already exist in our healthcare system. But what if this form of discrimination persisted under a comprehensive (and generous) systemic reform with rationing, in which most of the present unfairness and inequalities were minimized if not eliminated by making health insurance or coverage available to everyone else in an extensive benefit package? This would mean that the resulting system was prejudicial by design, not happenstance. Could the sincere application of the five principles as the guiding doctrines for formulating the rules for rationing and the delivery of healthcare actually yield this result? Probably not, since it is impossible to imagine how treating clinically similar patients similarly could produce this outcome. But this may be a case where there is an absolute limitation on fairness that is ultimately determined by the willingness of the public to endorse a system utterly dependent on public acceptance.

Can There Be Solutions?

I want to emphasize that I am not stating what should be the case but what may be the case. This is a discussion about practicality: the definite limits on what could be accomplished should we engage in a serious discussion about implementing a truly broad healthcare reform with universal coverage and generalized planned rationing to deliver high-quality care and control costs. No matter how generous and expansive the coverage and benefit package, an honest and open debate about who should be offered what could have negative consequences. But would these consequences be so terrible as to justify abandoning the entire project? Should the incorporation of morally indefensible provisos—for example, provisos excluding some people from coverage because of the group to which they belong—prevent the implementation of a system that could vastly improve the lives of the remainder?

The main issue for the application of fairness and justice and creation of a comprehensive system of healthcare rationing is distributive justice. And clearly this is ultimately dependent on who is considered deserving of justice. Should it be everyone, everywhere? Or is this an ideal that must be contingent on what can be accomplished within the constraints of a diverse and (reasonably) democratic polity? In the actual, real world in which we would be attempting to implement a form of universal, comprehensive, and centralized healthcare rationing, it must be decided to whom it would apply. Would it be like Oregon, where the health plan only covered the poor and near-poor? Or would we aim toward something more thorough that embraced as much of the population as feasible? Short of some form of executive fiat or judicial ruling that dictated that the benefits of justice and fairness applied to everyone who lived in the United States, considerations of what might be politically feasible should be examined and taken seriously. And the practical and moral implications of excluding some portions of the population for who or what they are must come under careful scrutiny before being adopted.

If the only feasible plan that could be reasonably accepted by the majority of the public was one that involved grievous violations of justice by excluding say, a bit fewer than 4 percent of the total U.S. population from consideration for any healthcare coverage,[22] would this be so intolerable that it would be worth relinquishing the entire project (which, of course, would bestow massive benefits on the vast majority of Americans, not to mention having the potential to constrain healthcare costs)? While I do not have any data to support my conjecture, I would hazard a guess that this would be considerably more bearable than eliminating anyone over the age of seventy from access to potentially life-saving medical interventions. That being said, we do need to consider the extent to which we can permit the tyranny of the majority to set the rules. To quote Rawls (1999, 172, 395–396):

Yet since the political process is at best one of imperfect procedural justice, he [the citizen] must ascertain when the enactments of the majority are to be complied with and when they can be rejected as no longer binding. In short, he must be able to determine the grounds and limits of political duty and obligation. Of course, it cannot be denied that prevailing social attitudes tie the statesman's hands. The convictions and passions of the majority may make liberty impossible to maintain. But bowing to these practical necessities is a different thing from accepting the justification that if these feelings are strong enough and outweigh in intensity any feelings that might replace them, they should carry the decision.

In this chapter I have discussed the potential obstacles that might hamper the imposition of any universal healthcare plan (with or without explicit rationing) that would include equal coverage for marginalized people or groups, such as undocumented (illegal) immigrants and convicted and incarcerated felons. For any process that requires the passive acquiescence, if not active consent, of those affected by it, it might be very difficult to unilaterally impose a plan that could be interpreted as taking something away from the majority to give to a despised or less-than-equal minority population. This is especially true if rationing is involved, as it undoubtedly would have to be. Even if the rationing plan were generous to a fault, as I suspect it would have to be in this country, some things would necessarily be denied to some people, and even if they are interventions that no reasonable person could unequivocally declare to be of significant benefit, I have little doubt that there would be an immediate suspicion that the resources saved would be diverted to use for less-than-worthy groups. Since one of the main goals of a universal rationing scheme would be to save money (as well as to deliver more equitable care to everyone), there could be ample but erroneous support for this view. The fact that it would seem to make sense could also undermine public backing for the plan.

Of course, one could counter this contention by using the example of the Oregon Health Plan, in which a number of actually effective treatments were denied to significant numbers of patients due to budgetary constraints (although one could argue that the overall utility of the non-covered condition-treatment pairs was not that great and certainly was much less than the utility gained by being able to insure more patients). But, as I have suggested previously, one of the major ethical flaws of the OHP was that the rules were by and large made by people not directly affected (i.e., covered) by the plan. Although it is true that public input was sought and was incorporated (where thought to be appropriate) into modifications of the plan, this does not negate the fact that the recipients had little power to effect changes. And most important, people who wanted health insurance via the OHP had to accept it as it was or not be insured at all: they had no choice. In the larger context of a universal national healthcare insurance plan, this would not necessarily be the case, because presumably almost everyone would be covered (although whether that would indeed be true is the topic of this chapter).[23] And they—or their elected or appointed representatives—would be delegated to make decisions on what the eventual plan looked like. As Schneiderman and Jecker have asked, would the majority of average U.S. citizens placed in a hypothetical Rawlsian "original position" choose to extend healthcare coverage to illegal aliens (I choose this descriptor deliberately) or to convicted and imprisoned criminals?[24] I would be surprised if they did.

While it may be true that overuse has diminished the deep practical wisdom of the two aphorisms with which I headed this chapter, they have bearing nonetheless on the implementation of any workable healthcare rationing in the United States. If it can be agreed that this could (or would) be a significant problem, we should decide two things. First, what kind of a problem is it and for whom? Second, can anything be done about it? I will address these in order (also because the latter issue is much more complex).

If we as a democratic nation decide, after serious deliberation, that we cannot offer anything other than, say, emergency or some sort of bare minimum of healthcare to the marginalized groups I have discussed as plausible targets of discriminatory animus (and it is likely others will crop up), who would be affected by this choice? Obviously, the first to feel the weight of this judgment would be the members of the excluded groups. They would be the ones who would presumably die earlier than they otherwise might, suffer unnecessarily, and so on. But there could also be unintended side effects. I have no doubt that those who would vote to exclude prisoners and the foreign born would do so because of a belief that these people don't deserve our largesse. But extending the healthcare umbrella to cover everyone could also serve a less morally uplifting and noble purpose as well, namely one of instrumental self-interest (be it enlightened or not). For instance, in communities that have large numbers of the undocumented, especially children, not vaccinating the young could cause a loss of herd immunity, leading to an increased risk of individuals from the favored groups getting sick from diseases we thought were almost eradicated, such as mumps and polio.[25] Another example is from the height of the HIV epidemic, where there was resistance to providing condoms to male prison inmates due to some sort of (misguided) notion of prudery. As was noted at the time, spreading HIV in prisons could endanger members of the community outside the jailhouse walls because significant numbers of inmates are released each year and those who acquired their infection while incarcerated would then be able to spread the disease to others.[26] Finally, it is well known that uninsured patients cost the system (i.e., everyone else, the taxpayers, etc.) considerably more than had they been insured up front (Bradley et al. 2012; Cunningham 2010). So the prudent, perhaps selfish approach would be to immunize as many kids as possible and restrain one's moral outrage in order to supply the condoms, if not providing reasonable levels of healthcare to all.[27]

A possible solution to the second question is much more complicated and may actually be untenable (at least in a morally acceptable way). Schneiderman and Jecker clearly accepted the limits on what can be done in a democratic society that relies on some level of public acceptance for universal programs to function. In their example, they discussed a heart transplant for an imprisoned felon, but they raised the hypotheticals of this man being in prison for life, or being convicted of a violent crime, and so on, to raise the ante, so to speak. And certainly in a system where resources are as constrained as they are in organ transplant, and where the source of the organs is wholly dependent upon the voluntary donations of individuals and families, it seems unrealistic, if not absurd, to suggest that we could expect any other type of conclusion. That is unless, of course, we wish to compel organ retrieval from all eligible dead (or soon-to-be-dead) people, a prospect that seems highly improbable in the United States. But in a well-funded universal healthcare system, even with rationing, it is very plausible that resource constraints would be relatively minimal for most people, unlike organ transplant. So, while I definitely understand their reasoning, there are counterexamples.

The struggle for civil rights for disenfranchised African Americans is a notable one. When *Brown v. Board of Education* was decided in 1954 by the U.S. Supreme Court, it was by no means the majority view in this country that African Americans either deserved equal legal rights to whites or that they were in fact intellectually or socially equivalent. Even when the landmark civil rights legislation of the 1960s was passed by Congress—arguably a much more democratic method of instituting civil social change—sentiments were similarly lagging behind. But due to a convergence of strong and persuasive political rhetoric (much of it from the voice of President Lyndon Johnson), the public gradually fell in line and supported the laws and their intent (Rodriguez and Weingast 2002–2003; Goldzwig 2003). Indeed, the most recent reauthorization of the Voting Rights Act passed both houses of Congress with overwhelming majorities.[28] And, of course, the election of Barack Obama, a black person, to the presidency in 2008 and his reelection in 2012 speak to the ever-increasing acceptance of racial equality in the United States.

In this same vein, some might point to the growing public affirmation of marriage equity (i.e., "gay marriage") and the advancing legislative and judicial approval of this remaining form of overt and legal discrimination. Against this is the well-known argument made by opponents of elective termination of pregnancy that its legality was based on a court ruling rather than the will of the people, notwithstanding a long history of polling data demonstrating the public's support for the right of women to control (most of) their reproductive choices. And while these examples may reflect the increasing moral maturity of our society, it should not be forgotten that much of the outcry over Shana Alexander's 1962 *Life* article about the deliberations of Swedish Hospital's "Admissions and Policies Committee" (see chapter 3) was due to the characteristics of patients and their lives used in determining who would have access to the life-saving dialysis. Readers in large numbers objected to using social worthiness as a criterion for life or death. So perhaps there is even more reason to hope that regrettable decisions may not occur.

These examples provide evidence endorsing the proposition that it may be possible to create policies that are the "right thing to do" and that public opinion, if not initially favorable, can be brought around. I would also argue that extending general healthcare to all is not only morally sound but fiscally wise. While it may be reasonable to further discuss the restricted allocation of scarce resources—like livers and hearts—based on societal pressures, in a wealthy country like the United States, we should be able to find room for compassion and inclusion without too much effort or sacrifice. So I end this chapter by endorsing a view of hopeful—but (very) cautious—optimism, perhaps betting that the "better angels of our nature" will win out over those who express a much darker and less inclusive outlook.

7

Summing Up

It has been my task in this book to construct an argument to convince readers that large-scale healthcare rationing of a certain kind is potentially feasible in the United States. To do so, I have suggested that the already existing general acceptance of the organ transplant system (for example), in which the stakes of not receiving a scarce good are dramatic and irreversible, leads one to believe that an approach incorporating many of the elements that contribute to its social success (distinct from its medical success) could be assimilated into a much more universal rationing program. Many other authors have already pointed out the United States already engages in significant healthcare rationing, either by overt planning (such as Medicare's DRGs or diagnosis-related groups) or, more commonly, by the subtle methods of restricting access by financial wherewithal. We (actually, insurance companies and federal agencies such as the Centers for Medicare and Medicaid Services) accomplish the latter by limiting the choices people have based on how much money they have, where they live, where they work, and so on. These other writers have almost exclusively concentrated on financial rationing. While hardly ignoring the crucial role that money plays in rationing, I have chosen to focus on the mechanics and ethics of how rationing could plausibly be instituted to accomplish the dual goals of offering decent healthcare to as many people as feasible and to do so economically and fairly.

Of all the countries that belong to the club of wealthy industrialized, technologically advanced, "first-world" nations, the United States stands alone for not having created and implemented a thoughtful, reasonable, and comprehensive healthcare system to enable its residents—citizens and others alike—to obtain a sensible and practical array of effective health services. While most countries with a universal health insurance program finance it primarily with public monies, others have adopted a mixed public-private approach that accomplishes similar goals (Schoen et al.

2010). Unique among its peers, the United States possesses a crazy-quilt patchwork of private, semiprivate, and public insurance, and shamefully for many millions of its citizens, no insurance at all. The supposed justification for this hodgepodge is that it celebrates both the libertarian ethos on which this country was founded and the primacy of the marketplace. It has prospered in part because those who have vested interests in maintaining the status quo have spread rumors and stoked fear of the dreaded "socialized medicine" and "death panels," helping to doom attempts to accomplish real reform. Even a cursory analysis of what we have reveals how preposterous this notion is: while we can claim the dubious distinction of having the most expensive healthcare in the world on a per capita basis, we unfortunately do not get good value for the many billions spent. As amply demonstrated in a detailed report from the Institute of Medicine, the United States is at the bottom or dead last among industrialized nations in health outcomes. Even more damning, perhaps, is our standing with respect to some relatively poor countries, including our arch political nemesis, Cuba.[1]

Equally important, it is estimated that by the year 2020 the U.S. healthcare budget will comprise 20 percent of the entire GDP, up from a mere 18 percent or so in 2011 (Keehan et al. 2011; Berwick and Hackbarth 2012). As most (perhaps all) commentators suggest, this continued growth is unsustainable unless we perversely wish to subvert all other priorities and needs for federal money to feed the apparently insatiable maw of medicine (Orszag 2011; Sutherland, Fisher, and Skinner 2009; Berwick and Hackbarth 2012; Riggs, Hobbs, Hobbs, and Riggs 2011). Moreover, while it may be true that America has the "best medicine in the world," it only applies to those who can afford it, a steadily shrinking portion of the citizenry. And even though the Affordable Care Act (ACA) should extend health insurance to many of the currently uninsured, there will remain an unconscionable number of people without insurance, including the eleven to twelve million undocumented immigrants currently living in the country, as well as those people who have the bad luck to live in states that have chosen not to participate in the ACA-sponsored Medicaid expansion to incorporate many of the uninsured. So, while the ACA represents a major step forward, and contains many provisions that may slow the escalation in overall healthcare spending (although this is by no means guaranteed), it is hardly the panacea its most enthusiastic boosters claim it will be.

There are two substantive reasons to undertake a comprehensive reform of healthcare in the United States. The first is practical, in that if we do not do something to interrupt the steady increase in healthcare costs we will bankrupt ourselves. What this means is that if we continue with our present chaotic and relatively unregulated pastiche of approaches to cobbling together insurance for those who possess it we cannot but inevitably come to financial disaster. The second is a moral reason. Not only is our present situation incredibly expensive, but it ignores the fact that millions and millions of people must make do with either substandard or no healthcare at all. This is indefensible. I think there's little doubt that we have the capability and means to provide comprehensive and decent healthcare for all who live in this country. To fail to do so is morally unjustifiable. To not act to change the status quo for the better permits a continuation of a situation in which a lack of respect for the dignity of the individual seems paramount. For if we have the capacity to relieve suffering in our fellow human beings but refuse to, what does this deficiency of concern say about our sense of social morality? Of course, rationing of any type in isolation would not fix the problems with U.S. healthcare. It must be combined with other steps to make its application and implementation both effective and tolerable.

Thus, for reasons both moral and of practical political necessity, I have repeatedly stated that any conceivable national health system that placed limits on the availability of some treatments (i.e., rationing) must be generous enough to make the transition from what exists for most people an improvement over what they currently have and relatively painless and indiscernible to the remaining minority. But the question of how both of these moves would lead to a constraining of the exploding healthcare budget (even if the rate of increase has slowed during the recent recession) or, more hopefully, a decrease in the overall national healthcare budget to bring it more in line with what is spent in other technologically advanced, industrialized nations is a big one. Furthermore, if one is going to reform healthcare in such a radical way, one might as well attempt to relieve the moral and public health shortcomings of the disjointed conglomeration we currently employ, by ensuring a decent level of healthcare for all. Importantly, it remains to be adequately explained how one could vastly expand the number of people covered by comprehensive health insurance (which would include virtually everyone) and control or cut costs at the same time; superficially it would appear to be an impossible task.

As I write this, almost 50 million Americans lack health insurance of any kind, 47 million receive Medicaid, and about 49 million have Medicare coverage.[2] This cumulative figure comprises almost half of the entire U.S. population. Presumably the remainder has some form of private insurance (including Veterans Administration healthcare). This compound mixture of payers—commercial, government, and private—has produced a multilayered system of interlaced providers and patients of almost unimaginable complexity that is the most expensive and one of the least efficient in the world. For years people have been clamoring for a change, if for no other reason than to control spiraling healthcare costs that threaten to bankrupt the country and certainly limit our ability to allocate funds for other, equally deserving, needs. I would think that most people who are able to assess this situation both impartially and compassionately, would judge it to be intolerable from a practical or instrumental standpoint as well as a moral one. In addition, for a moment thinking hypothetically, these same people might say that it doesn't necessarily have to remain this way. There is a solution(s). Other countries have developed approaches that are capable of delivering high-quality healthcare (certainly higher quality on a population basis than America) at a fraction of the cost. Why not here?

Most careful and critical analysts believe that some form of healthcare rationing is the inevitable and logical answer to the current and undoubtedly worsening crisis. It is probably the only realistic approach to both cost control and an equitable distribution of the wealth that we would undoubtedly think appropriate to spend on healthcare, assuming it is coupled with some form of universal health insurance for all Americans.[3] It is the only plausible way to accomplish the dual goals of financial restraint and providing all with what they need (and should want).[4] Integral to my approach is how to make the American people understand that rationing does not have to be a bad thing, because it need not entail shortages or shortchanging people from what they believe they are entitled to (even if they can't obtain it now).

The Reign of (Rationing) Terror

During the writing of this book, I was asked to do an ethics consultation on a man in his fifties who had end-stage liver disease (let's call him Mr. Doe). Out of sheer desperation his daughter called me to see if there was anything I might be able to do to help her father. It turns out he was extremely sick and had been evaluated for a liver transplant. He was felt to be a good medical-surgical candidate. However, he lacked the comprehensive insurance that could pay the doctors' bills and cover the extremely expensive medications that he would need for the rest of his life. His daughter implored me to go to the hospital administration to plead their case and let her father be placed on the list for a liver (of course, this was no guarantee that he would receive a transplant before he died of his disease, but being listed was an absolute prerequisite to proceed). Unfortunately, there was nothing I could do. A sad fact of organ transplantation is that there are not enough organs for all who could potentially benefit from receiving them, and recipients have to be able to pay the high costs of the operation and its aftermath. This patient could have been rejected for a variety of others reasons having nothing to do with his disease, including not having reliable transportation to get to the clinic, living in an inadequate home that might predispose him to infectious complications when he was immunosuppressed postoperatively (to prevent graft rejection), and having few friends or family to help take care of him after the transplant. None of these is any more tragic than not having enough money, except for the fact that they generally happen together: poor and underinsured (and uninsured) people tend to have more psychosocial problems than people with more financial resources.

Nevertheless, something the patient's daughter said stuck with me: they could bear not getting a liver if he were only given the chance; losing without ever getting in line was the most galling, coupled with the fact that he was barred from consideration for reasons that had nothing to do with his medical and social ability to benefit from and support the transplant. It was solely due to his lack of sufficient money. She was making the point I have tried to argue throughout this book. She accepted the fact of rationing, and the real possibility that if her dad were placed on the list he could die without receiving a liver. That was simply a matter of fact, the state of affairs necessitated by an absolute resource scarcity. What she couldn't tolerate was being denied an opportunity to be considered because of money. This suggests that it may not be that rationing per se is what bothers people, but what is rationed and why. The hard sell is that we need to ration healthcare, because we need to ration money. In effect, we are saying to people that the reason they are not getting X is that we don't have enough money to pay for it, not that it doesn't work, or some other reason. Perhaps for the same rationale that Ms. Doe and her father were angry about their situation—that the denial of a transplant was purely for financial reasons—the American people can't get their heads around the idea that money is the issue, and not a shortage of some "real" resource, which they could understand, in much the same way they understand—and *accept*—that there are not enough livers for everyone. Perhaps we simply need to reframe the argument.

Of course, some might criticize this point as being naive in the extreme. It might be said that potential organ transplant recipients (or people vying for a ventilator during a flu pandemic or a needed drug during a scarcity) have no choice in the matter; they must submit to the system if they wish to take advantage of what it has to offer, the possibility of a cure. It implies that the choice of participating in the transplant system or supporting it with donations of organs is, in reality, a form of Hobson's choice wherein there is the appearance of an option when there truly isn't one. I think this is an incorrect analysis. I pointed out in chapter 2 that a fundamental and integral component of the organ transplant system is its essential fairness (albeit within the constraints of a medical and surgical process that demands a certain level of personal compliance, psychological strength, social support, and financial wherewithal). True, there are occasional examples of blatant gaming of the system, both by patients and their doctors, as I related in chapter 3, but it is a rather interesting feature of this rationing method how rare those stories actually are. Furthermore, there is a basic dedication to improving the fairness of the system, as I illustrated by the examples of the changes wrought by imposing liver and lung numerical scoring systems to minimize the effects of physicians manipulating the priority listing structure (Moylan et al. 2008; Liu, Zamora, Dhillon, and Weill 2010; Merlo et al. 2009). There would be no reason to engage in this kind of activity if fairness were a secondary concern and there truly was an attitude of "take it or leave it." Given the severe shortage of organs, there would be little doubt that more than sufficient numbers of patients would be willing to participate, even in a grossly biased allocation program; consequently, there is no reason for the system to be fair except that people want it to be fair for both ethical and practical reasons. It is fair because its organizers and users think it must be fair. Furthermore, fairness may also contribute to the altruistic desire of people to become donors (although this may be somewhat debatable, as the discussion in chapter 6 suggests). Hence, people who "lose" out on an organ are sad, and their families mourn their loss, but it is rare to hear of an accusation of prejudice or callous disregard or injustice. I think that it is likely that the inherent fairness of the system engenders both trust and consent—hallmarks of legitimacy—and creates an atmosphere wherein people readily accept the fact of rationing. I believe there is a lesson to be learned from this and to be applied more widely.

Healthcare rationing: scary, yes; a four-letter word that should only be whispered under one's breath or even banned from public discourse, no. What is infinitely scarier is what could happen to the whole edifice of American healthcare if rationing is not instituted. It has often been said applying the label "rationing" to a situation in which allocation decisions must be made in the setting of resource limitations is frightening

(Baily 1984). In point of fact, in contemplating the title for this book I was repeatedly advised by colleagues not to use this "dirty word" in the title—or for that matter, anywhere in the book—for fear of frightening off potential readers who would not venture on to the meat of the argument because of the negative emotions induced by the mere mention of health-care rationing. I was counseled to employ euphemisms such as "prioriti-zation," "scarce-resource distribution," and the like. "Rationing" is bad, they said, allocation is good, or at least more palatable than rationing. I believed otherwise, which is why I have not shied away from using this word throughout this book. Indeed, I have structured my argument on the premise that rationing of healthcare in general does not have to be scary.

Unfortunately, the face of rationing for many people is this: as former Alaska Governor and Republican vice presidential candidate Sarah Palin wrote on her Facebook page in 2009 (referring to the then-proposed leg-islation that would eventually become the Affordable Care Act, otherwise known as "Obamacare"):

The Democrats promise that a government healthcare system will reduce the cost of healthcare, but as the economist Thomas Sowell has pointed out, government healthcare will not reduce the cost; it will simply refuse to pay the cost. And who will suffer the most when they ration care? The sick, the elderly, and the disabled, of course. The America I know and love is not one in which my parents or my baby with Down Syndrome will have to stand in front of Obama's "death panel" so his bureaucrats can decide, based on a subjective judgment of their "level of productivity in society," whether they are worthy of healthcare. Such a system is downright evil.[5]

Because of this kind of fear mongering, formal rationing is viewed by many as a primary constituent of government-run, "socialized" medicine, itself an assault on the libertarian spirit that the United States prides itself for fostering and promoting, and a massive expansion of government in-trusion into the autonomous lives of individual Americans who should be free to pursue their dreams—including whatever healthcare they want or can afford—unencumbered by the restraints associated with what would necessarily be a major overhaul of how we deliver medicine. It is part and parcel of a system that will eliminate free choice—in doctors, hospitals, pills, you name it—and turn off the ventilators of older patients just to save money. Moreover, it will necessitate the formation of panels or tri-bunals of all-powerful Oz-like arbiters who will decide who *deserves* to live and who does not, a sort of modern day version of Swedish Hospital's Admissions and Policies Committee that had the ultimate control over who could gain access to the few existing dialysis machines (chapter 3).

As I have argued throughout this book, it is inconceivable to me that, should we somehow be successful in enacting a plan that encompassed reasonable rationing as a first principle, it would not be both broad-based and extremely generous. Indeed, one plausible concern might be that it could be too generous and thus be self-defeating, its munificence reflecting the necessary political compromises entailed by any democratic legislative endeavor. However, if we also employed sensible cutoffs as I suggested in chapter 4 (as well as the savings to be expected from decreasing the massive administrative overhead associated with private insurance, etc.), we could expect to have sufficient funds to bestow a very liberal, if not lavish, benefit package on almost everyone. We would save considerable amounts of money as well, mainly because what we would be replacing is so grossly inefficient, bloated with administration and laden with perverse financial incentives. This would not eliminate the ability of people who were so inclined to purchase even more healthcare if they chose to. And Palin would not have to fear that children with Down syndrome or her elderly parents would be arbitrarily excluded from access to healthcare because of who they were or for what illness or disability they may have. Indeed, any comprehensive healthcare plan that is morally justifiable in the way I have suggested (chapter 3) would be known more for its inclusiveness that for who it excluded.[6] And this really doesn't seem so frightening a prospect after all.

Nevertheless, it would be both naive and foolish to disregard the antipathy—if not hostility and downright fear—that many Americans have for any kind of overt rationing. As Oberlander and White have observed, Americans like the *idea* of controlling costs and reining in out-of-control spending on healthcare; what they don't like is someone *telling* them openly they can't have something (i.e., rationing):

There is also good evidence that many Americans oppose reform if it means reduced access to medical care. The public is eager for cost controls that limit their rising medical bills, not for restrictions on the availability of services. ... Cost-control approaches that emphasize the need to ration and reduce consumption of medical care are politically vulnerable. Reformers can insist that they want to limit only inappropriate care in line with evidence-based medicine. The intent, in other words, is to rationalize medical care rather than to ration it. Opponents, however, will still deride any government policies to substantially change medical practice or reduce medical services as a "one-size-fits-all" bureaucratic nightmare that threatens the doctor-patient relationship. (Oberlander and White 2009, 1288)

This pessimistic outlook suggests that we must avoid evoking or stimulating the "scarcity principle" discussed in chapter 1, or any public, open discussion of rationing; it is much better to do it quietly, almost secretly, so no one notices. Indeed, the introduction of the DRG system two decades ago was virtually ignored by the public (although not by hospital executives and doctors), even though it represented an extremely plain and undisguised attempt to control costs by limiting hospital reimbursement and thus restricting (rationing) inpatient stays. Patients didn't pay attention because it wasn't called rationing and they went home when their doctors told them to, assuming it was because it was safe and they were better, not due to the influence of cost-control measures.

Furthermore, as I have indicated a number of times throughout this book, the forces arrayed against any comprehensive healthcare reform that includes overt rationing, no matter how fair and generous, would be formidable. If we ignore for the moment those factions who would reflexively object to any apparent loss in their personal financial fiefdoms and perquisites that could occur with such reform, such as pharmaceutical companies, insurance executives, and medical device makers, there are also those people who legitimately and on principle oppose any move to increase what they might interpret as a greater influence of government over peoples' lives. And certainly a healthcare reorganization of the scope I am suggesting would fit the bill. While we could argue about the level of intrusiveness, it would unquestionably represent an expansion of a government-controlled and centralized program that could affect a number of different aspects of daily life, much as Medicare does now (but more so). It would be a specious argument to say that it would not be "socialized" medicine, as indeed it would be. For those who would be unalterably opposed to the very concept of a program labeled as such, there may be no gainsaying them. But I suspect that most of these individuals readily accept the strictures and benefits of Medicare for themselves and their loved ones, and it is not too far a stretch to suggest that there are more similarities than differences between what we currently enjoy in these programs and what I propose.

Importantly, I have presented several real-life and existing systems that ration medical care that have been quite acceptable (sometimes reluctantly, I admit, but only because of the onerous consequences of failing to receive something that can help, not because of unfairness) to those most affected by them. In the case of organ transplantation, the allocation of extremely limited numbers of livers and hearts entails that most people who could benefit from a transplant won't get one. And, except in the case of kidney transplants (and sometimes with cardiac failure as well, with the newer, more portable and functional LVADs), those who fail to receive an organ die. While the experience of rationing scarce drugs and ventilators for pandemic influenza is much more limited, what history we have also supports the view that when we understand that we have no choice but to ration, and if it is seen as being done fairly and openly, it can be accepted or even celebrated. Hence, it seems plausible to suggest that if we could convincingly argue that funding must be limited in much the same way as livers are, we could create a tolerable healthcare system rationing plan, but with the beneficial caveat that no one would suffer a significant loss because of the plan. Indeed, the United States has experience with something like this in its not-too-distant past.

Rationing during Wartime

In April 1941, some eight months before the Japanese launched their attack on the U.S. naval base at Pearl Harbor, the Roosevelt administration created the Office of Price Administration and Civilian Supply (OPACS) to control inflation and regulate the supply of various consumer goods in the economy, especially commodities. At the time, and somewhat later in retrospect, this government agency was viewed by many as yet another New Deal organization to combat continuing economic problems from the still-present Depression (and by some as representing more government intrusion into their lives). While OPACS was established well before the first bombs fell in Hawaii and was ostensibly aimed toward controlling potential threats to the fiscal health of the nation, it was clear to government officials—career civil servants and Roosevelt administration political appointees alike—that it was only a matter of time before America was brought into the war then raging in both Asia and Europe. As we would hope our government officials should be, they wanted to be prepared for what they considered the likely, if not inevitable, course of events. Their predictions were correct, and they were prepared (Galbraith 1943; O'Leary 1945; Rockoff 1981).

Indeed, within weeks after the attack, the Emergency Price Control Act of (January) 1942 was introduced in Congress and then passed with a large majority. It bestowed a more formal legislative imprimatur on these efforts, but the bureaucratic mechanism and structure had already been put in place and only awaited official legislative authority and funding to begin the task in earnest. The act constituted the Office of Price Administration (OPA), into which OPACS was enveloped. The goals remained the same: to regulate the supply of goods and products, and to some extent demand, such that wartime shortages would not lead to rampant inflation, hoarding, and scarcities. For some items, such as various metals deemed vital to the production of war matériel, the process conserved articles and diverted their customary consumer use to war manufacturing.

The result for the duration of the war and somewhat beyond was the rationing of a wide variety of goods, especially foods. Importantly, one of the main objectives was to make distribution of scarce commodities fair so that both rich and poor could claim equal access to items in short supply. And since controls were exerted at the production or wholesale and retail levels, the chances of a black market were much less. This is not to say that cheating did not occur, but for a country the geographic size of the United States, with a population of about 132 million,[7] and a complex economy, it is perhaps surprising that the system worked as well as it did and with as little overt fraud and under-the-table activity as was documented (Mills and Rockoff 1987; Bentley 1998; Witkowski 1998; but see below).

Moreover, it is noteworthy that the powers that be decided that the wealth of the country could support a general lifestyle that did not involve draconian sacrifice in material comforts, unlike those suffered by the British and other combatant countries nearer to the front lines. Indeed, a significant component of the thinking that went into the discussion about how to allocate goods to achieve the dual goals of supporting the material demands of the war effort and persuading a perhaps skeptical public to endorse—even embrace—what was explicit rationing, was purposefully constructing it so that the shortages that did occur were tolerable and could be viewed as the kind of sacrifice it would be natural for citizens to make and endure during wartime. Thus, because the country could afford it—*even though it didn't have to*—the crafters of this policy sufficiently understood the mindset of Americans to comprehend that sacrifice would be infinitely more palatable if it wasn't too harsh.[8]

So it is noteworthy that this system was by and large both acceptable to and accepted by the overwhelming majority of Americans. It was viewed as fair and evenhanded, even though it was a massive government program run by government bureaucrats working via a government agency (Bartels 1983; Jacobs 1997; Leff 1991; Bentley 1998, chap. 1). Of course, this was undoubtedly helped by the fact that rationing and price controls gradually started easing toward the end of the war and were mostly ended by 1946. So some might say that this was a time-limited programmatic response to a national emergency, with every reason to believe that it would not last very long, with the amount of personal pain of doing without access to unlimited and unregulated quantities of stuff also being limited. But no one knew how long the war would last in 1942, and yet the rationing plan was still viewed as reasonably just and most of all, tolerable.

John Kenneth Galbraith, one of the economists who worked at OPACS and then OPA during the war and was a principal architect of its policies, has remarked:

We were saved partly by the fact that the supply of civilian goods, while it did not keep pace with demand, increased beyond any pre-war calculation. *Never in the long history of human combat have so many talked so much about sacrifice with so little deprivation as in the United States in World War II.* In 1938, the last year of peace in the world, $140 billion worth of goods and services were available for personal consumption. In 1940, the last year of peace in the United States, $156 billion worth were so available at comparable prices. After four years of what were called wartime sacrifices, $173 billion worth were to be had in 1944 and were had. More goods still were available for the next year. Munitions, manpower and other military needs in World War II were supplied out of the increase in production with this further increase for civilian use. An unsuspected and mighty resource of the Republic was the idle plant and idle men of the depression by whose re-employment the war was sustained. *A war that required a pro rata cutback in civilian consumption would be a new and disenchanting experience for Americans.* (Galbraith 1981, 172; my emphasis)

Several significant insights can be gleaned from Galbraith's pithy observations. First, because of the immense wealth and productivity of the United States, even with our entry into a world war (on two fronts) and with the economy being wholly diverted to wartime production, we were able to make rationing not unduly harsh for virtually all Americans. Second, rationing was viewed as reasonably fair: rich people received the same number of ration coupons per capita as poor people. And, third, Galbraith's final point about the possible "disenchanting experience" for Americans if they were forced by circumstances to undergo a major decrease in their access to consumer goods (i.e., foodstuffs, clothes, etc.) serves to show us that the palatability of rationing and the support for the program was dependent upon the degree of suffering imposed on the quotidian lives of the public. He had the insight that Americans' toleration for ongoing—especially government-imposed—deprivation is shallow (even when tempered by wartime patriotism). One can only wonder how this country would have fared if we had been faced with the true shortages of food and other consumer goods as were the British.

These remarks may have great bearing on how to think about constructing a healthcare rationing system that is, at a minimum, tolerable (and, it is to be hoped, much more so). Hence, it may not be a categorical truth that Americans are unable to accept some kinds of restraints on their unfettered liberty entailed by rationing. But I wish to emphasize Galbraith's last point as extremely significant, because he believed much of the success of the wartime rationing was due to the fact that material suffering was minimal. The wealth of the United States is such that a similar lack of hardship should also be attainable with any kind of reasonable healthcare rationing plan. It could be feasible to craft a comprehensive system that incorporated sensible rationing that reins in healthcare costs (and their growth) by curtailing access to only the least medically effective interventions (as well as eliminating most administrative overhead and other waste), while simultaneously offering almost everything else within reason.

Some might question the accuracy of my analogy between the rationing of commodities during World War II and my postulated rationing of healthcare. During the war, we were presumably fighting for the survival of the nation (or so it was portrayed); we were attacked and the country was as united as it perhaps could be behind the war effort.[9] Healthcare rationing has no identified "enemy" equivalent to Japan and Germany, or so the argument assumes. But I might suggest that there is such an adversary, and one that presents perhaps almost as much of an existential threat to our future welfare (if not more) as the Axis powers ever did. After all, except for America's entry into the war with the Japanese bombing of Pearl Harbor, the continental United States was barely threatened (I am not counting the German submarine attacks off the East Coast in 1941–1943 or the Japanese attacks on the Aleutian Islands). The danger to our present and future economy by runaway healthcare inflation is perhaps just as much a menace, and conceivably more, than that posed in the war. Indeed, a successful (and truthful) public relations campaign could potentially represent the "enemies" of comprehensive healthcare reform—insurance companies, the medical product industries, even some physicians and hospitals, to mention but a few—as "evil," just as U.S. government propaganda so successfully portrayed the Japanese and Germans (Dower 1986; Koppes 1987).

Another point of disanalogy might concern the fact that there was no gaming of the rationing system during the war, meaning the rich were prohibited by law from obtaining more than their allotted share. The latter may be true, but it is false to say that there were no violations; indeed, there was a robust black market in many commodities (Clinard 1946). One well-known study suggests that "in Britain controls produced less evasion, less black marketeering, and less open defiance than in the United States, at least during the years of actual conflict" (Mills and Rockoff 1987, 197); indeed, dodging of the rationing system was actually quite widespread in the United States (Rockoff 1981a; Clinard 1952). This does not mean that the system was not successful or not actually embraced and endorsed by the vast majority of Americans. Rather, any imposition of controls that induce scarcity can be expected to induce some forms of gaming. The trick is to make the decisions about how to allocate the available goods, whether they be gasoline and automobile tires or livers, as inclusive and as fair as possible. And where deficiencies or "holes" in the system are discovered when put into practice, plug them to the extent possible. Of course, unlike gasoline and tires, the possession and control of transplant organs is considerably more limited and centralized, but the point still holds. Finally, as pointed out by Galbraith, wartime rationing was not draconian at all, and that fact—in addition to the patriotic jingoism that accompanied its imposition and undoubtedly played a part in its acceptance—contributed in a major way to its tolerability. The same could be true for rationed healthcare.

By drawing this analogy between the rationing of commodities in the United States in the Second World War and the potential for healthcare rationing in the present day, I do not mean to imply that this correspondence is a strong one. Rather, I simply wish to point out that we have carried out rationing before against seemingly overwhelming odds and that we do formal rationing now (organs and pandemic flu, etc.). I think there is no categorical reason to believe that it could not be accomplished again, at least inasmuch as the American public could be persuaded to accept it under certain conditions. Whether it is politically feasible is another question, which I will address shortly.

(Some) Requirements of Tolerable Rationing

It is very simple to state that we need a universal healthcare plan that incorporates rationing as a central component in its approach to control costs and ensure that all receive adequate benefits. The moral and economic arguments in favor of this solution are strong. But that is the easy part. Convincing people that rationing is not anathema and is not to be feared is a challenge, and admittedly perhaps an insurmountable one. On the other hand, I have pointed out that not only do we have a historical record of accepting consumer-goods rationing during wartime, but also of healthcare rationing as a standard of care in the absence of crisis. In chapter 2 I discussed the allocation of organs in the widely regarded and tolerated, centrally controlled (but regionally administered) transplant system, the proposed (and partially executed) rationing of vaccine and intensive-care beds and their affiliated high-technology (and limited availability) equipment needs during an influenza pandemic, the prioritization and distribution of life-saving drugs during acute shortages, and finally, the healthcare rationing plan devised and implemented in the state of Oregon in the early 1990s. All have their flaws as well as their strengths. To a greater or lesser extent, all have been successful. And, most important, within certain limits and caveats, they have all been accepted by both the general public and those most directly affected by their decisions.

Of course, except for the Oregon Health Plan, one could argue that none of these situations permitted a choice. If we want to take advantage of transplant technology and all it can offer to some people (i.e., those fortunate enough to receive a liver or heart or kidney), then we must accept the fact that are insufficient numbers of organs for those who could potentially benefit from them. Despite that, we have no shortage of people willingly lining up to be on the transplant list, hoping they will be the lucky one to get a transplant, but knowing the odds are heavily stacked again them, and that there is no "consolation prize." The same is true for other existing rationing plans (once again, excepting Oregon). Even so, these forms of rationing are accepted, even lauded as exemplary attempts to make do with the resources we have available.

But I have also argued that there are characteristics of a rationing scheme that could make it considerably more palatable, in addition to the fact that any realistic method that would stand even a ghost of a chance of being enacted in the United States would have to ensure that its beneficiaries receive an extremely generous range of services. Indeed, I suspect that, like some commodities during World War II, the amount of scarcity might not be visible or noticeable by many (perhaps most) people. Of course, oral histories of rationing during the war are replete with stories of having to make do with less of this or that, supplementing one's diet with vegetables grown in the multitude of Victory Gardens, running out of ration coupons for butter or eggs or meat before the month was out, and so on (Bentley 1998). But few, if any, people went hungry. And, as Galbraith pointed out in the quote above, toward the end of the war, restrictions were loosened on most consumables such that rationing was no longer required in much of the economy. Any reasonable reapportionment of the vast sums we spend on healthcare per capita could, with proper allocation, stewardship, and economies of scale, offer extremely generous benefit packages that would probably represent a minimal-to-absent burden on the vast majority of Americans. And certainly for those millions who have no insurance or are underinsured, such a plan could prove to be an unparalleled boon. If this claim is true (or close enough to be true), rationing per se would not be a mechanism to control the fair and equitable distribution of scarce resources, simply a more efficient way.

Nevertheless, more detail is required to flesh out what I mean by "generous." After all, generosity implies expensive. If the services offered are too lavish, then the goals of rationing—egalitarian distributive justice for the greatest number who could benefit and, equally important, saving money and controlling costs—would be pointless, because we would simply be shifting expenses and the financial burden from one pot to another. Moreover, if we did this correctly—both medically and morally—and extended healthcare benefits to everyone (perhaps excepting the groups I described in chapter 6 and that I will address again below)—we could actually end up spending even more than we do now. Thus, this generosity would also have to be as inclusive as feasible. A further benefit of this approach, which might help alleviate some of the expenses incurred by both generosity and inclusiveness, would be the reduced costs and enhanced health of those individuals who were previously uninsured or underinsured (Bradley et al. 2012; Hall, Hwang, and Jones 2011). Therefore, generosity must be tempered or balanced with other cuts and efficiencies that would, in sum, result in net savings. Where might those savings come from? (I should note that the following is by no means meant to be a comprehensive listing of all the changes that might be required to reform healthcare in the United States. Rather, it is merely a series of suggestions, most of which are not new and have been suggested by many others.)

I have suggested—without saying so directly—that the American public might settle for a collection of services that either gave them more or less what they had been accustomed to or greatly enhanced what they had never had, presumably to lessen the "shock" of moving to a new system. In essence, the largesse of such a plan would serve as a sort of inducement, if you will (not that it couldn't be easily defended on other grounds) to entice people to accept something that is called rationing, which necessarily implies shortages and doing without. By demonstrating that what would be missing would be either invisible (the bureaucracy contributing to administrative overhead) or negligible (ineffective therapies, marginally beneficial therapies), coupled with all of the resources that would still be or newly available, this approach could go a long way toward diminishing skepticism and suspicion. And this must be coupled with a major campaign to sell the public on the advantages of reform, if for no other reason than to counteract the firestorm of negative advertising that will undoubtedly accompany any attempt at comprehensive change. And, of course, generosity by itself, without corresponding savings elsewhere in the system—as I have discussed several times—is a recipe for breaking the bank. If we simply gave everyone lavish Medicare benefits without looking to cut someplace (i.e., no rationing), then it would be a fruitless enterprise.

I have already proposed (as have others) that eliminating access to marginally beneficial care, especially at the end of life, could result in significant cost reductions. As has been repeatedly noted, healthcare expenditures in the last six months of life in the United States account for a notable percentage of both public and private medical expenses (Gawande 2013; Morden et al. 2012; Riley and Lubitz 2010; Unroe et al. 2011). It is reasonable to conclude that these interventions do little to extend life, and do much to make people miserable (it is noteworthy that almost half of hospice referrals occur within the last two weeks of life and 35 percent less than seven days before death).[10] Of course we would have to put a great deal of public thought and debate into what criteria to use for defining marginally beneficial treatment (as much as that can be done), and this confronts the cutoff problem, but a not unreasonable first approximation might be to limit access to those interventions with less than 1 percent chance of success, as originally suggested by Schneiderman and colleagues (Schneiderman, Jecker, and Jonsen 1990; Schneiderman 2011a,b,c). Limiting access to costly treatments that have little chance of efficacy (and at the same time often precluding access to more beneficial palliative and hospice care), especially those that take place in hospital intensive-care units, could result in significant savings without a corresponding escalation in harm. Taking this step might also help to check the exploding growth in the number of ICU beds in the United States, and hence their use (Halpern and Pastores 2010; Barnato et al. 2010; Kohn et al. 2011). An obvious companion to the regulation of marginally beneficial care would be to target the enormous waste in the current healthcare system in the United States, ranging from the gross inefficiencies of private insurance to the high use of ineffective or unproven treatments to the overuse of many others (Tilburt and Cassel 2013; Rao and Levin 2012). But in order to eliminate these practices, both better data and enforcement of clinical guideline applications would be required. This step would demand more and superior clinical research—especially comparative-effectiveness analyses—to supply the information needed to help physicians help their patients and keep costs under control. Similarly, it might be wise to empower the FDA to increase the level of evidence it needs to approve drugs and devices. (For example, it may be prudent to insist that new and very expensive anticancer drugs offer more than a median of several months of extra life, and actually contribute substantively to improvements in quality or length of life.) But this step would clearly only be one component of a comprehensive "remake" of American healthcare. What other measures might complement these sorts of restrictions on access to medicines and procedures, for example?

It has frequently been mentioned that the levels of administrative overhead that permeate the management and operations of healthcare (especially in the private sector) are astoundingly high and correspondingly expensive, especially when compared to public systems, such as Medicare (Berwick and Hackbarth 2012; Casalino et al. 2009; Sullivan 2013; Fineberg 2012; Young and Olsen 2010, especially chap. 4). Other sources of waste include the liberty with which doctors prescribe and use unproven treatments, including off-label uses of medication with little (if any) evidence to support their utilization (as an example) (Rosoff and Coleman 2011). Simply eliminating private insurance (except as a supplement for those who might wish to purchase it) as a major source of healthcare financing in this country and switching to a Medicare-like primary provider could save huge sums by cutting out administrative waste. (There would be no more highly paid CEOs of for-profit insurance companies, minimizing the number of people in doctors' offices and hospitals needed to process claims and deal with the myriad of different insurers, etc.)

Any restructuring of the healthcare system must of course involve doctors. Most important, it would have to address the way that many (if not most) doctors and the institutions where they practice are paid for what they do. It is not novel to note that the fee-for-service reimbursement system that pervades both publicly and privately financed healthcare offers perverse incentives to do more stuff. Another way to state this is to view American healthcare as a business that sells stuff (both services and things such as devices) and thus commoditizes medicine. Doctors and hospitals and clinics are agents or brokers in this business and hence suffer an enormous conflict between serving their own interests and those of their patients (Schroeder and Frist 2013; Laugesen and Glied 2011; Spiro, Lee, and Emanuel 2012). Of course, combining this proposal with restrictions on the freedom of doctors to prescribe what they want to whomever they want would threaten the treasured and almost sacrosanct principle of physician autonomy (Emanuel and Pearson 2012). The opposition of doctors to these kinds of restrictions is nothing new, because it was this threat that motivated the implacable opposition of the American Medical Association to national health insurance and to mount its major campaign to defeat the creation of Medicare in the early 1960s (Marmor 2000b, chap. 3, 38–41). It is unlikely that this suggestion would be any more acceptable to most nonsalaried physicians than to their forebears fifty years ago, especially specialists who are exceptionally well paid such as cardiothoracic, orthopedic, and neurologic surgeons, cardiologists, and medical oncologists (Tilburt et al. 2013).

What steps could be taken to sweeten the bitter pill and perhaps make it (somewhat) more palatable? First, physician salary levels could be less disparate, but still generous, and could compensate those in the primary-care "trenches" considerably better than they are today. While it is certainly true that the aforementioned specialties are exceedingly highly paid, they are a minority of the total and while they would feel some pain individually, it would be difficult to publicly complain about one's poverty when one is making a substantial salary that puts one well within the upper 5 percent of income levels in the country (Vaughn, DeVrieze, Reed, and Schulman 2010).

Second, one could relieve the debt burden on newly graduated medical students that is often carried for years into their professional lives and plays a role in the choice of specialty, greatly diminishing the attractiveness of relatively low-paid areas such as general pediatrics, internal medicine, and family practice (Grayson, Newton, and Thompson 2012; Youngclaus, Koehler, Kotlikoff, and Wiecha 2013). This could occur via substantial subsidies to both public and private medical schools to minimize out-of-pocket costs for students (the funds could come from the savings to be realized elsewhere in the system).[11] Students could receive incentives, such as greater subsidies or lower tuition costs to motivate them to pursue primary-care careers or careers in other underserved areas.

Finally, physicians have complained for years about the financial (and other) burdens imposed by the medical malpractice system in the United States. There is also evidence that this system imposes significant unnecessary costs on healthcare (Mello, Chandra, Gawande, and Studdert 2010). There are a variety of proposals that could accomplish tort reform in a manner that is fair to both physicians and patients and would presumably save money along the way. These proposals would diminish the impetus to practice defensive medicine and decrease the costs of malpractice insurance, a major financial load for private-practice doctors and institutions (Brody and Hermer 2011; Kachalia and Mello 2011). While there are no doubt a number of other measures that could be contemplated that would mitigate the negative effects of lowering the salaries of many doctors and switching from a fee-for-service reimbursement model to one of capitated payments and salaried physicians, I offer these only as a beginning and to make the point that compromises must be considered to enhance the attractiveness of comprehensive reform.

One further problem that needs to be addressed in any broad health-care reform (incorporating rationing) is the danger of moral hazard, or the principle that the presence of insurance (in this case health insurance) promotes greater use of medical care because the insurance protects the insured from experiencing the full effects—or cost—of the intervention (Stone 2011). Hence, people with good insurance use more medical resources than those without it even if they have a comparable level of illness (or health). So, a good tends to promote a bad. Indeed, Stone goes on to summarize how some people use the moral hazard to argue against providing more insurance, since doing so will only promote poor behavior and overutilization:

Nevertheless, proponents of moral hazard use this theory about how insurance affects individual behavior to prove—or rather justify—a political viewpoint about public policy. The moral hazard argument makes a normative leap from individual behavior to policy prescription: because health insurance induces people to use more medical care than they need or can afford, health insurance leads to a waste of social resources. With scarce resources gone to waste, society as a whole is worse off with insurance than without it. Therefore, we should not expand insurance and we should put limits on the insurance that already exists. The lesson for public policy is that society is better off with less insurance. (Stone 2011, 889)

How can this trap be avoided if everyone has insurance and it is generous, meaning that all people could need is provided as part of the benefit package? What is to keep people from abusing the system, by accident or design? As Stone also points out in her paper, there are a number of errors in the assumptions the theory of moral hazard makes, not least of which is that there is a gatekeeper of sorts at the entryway to the healthcare system, a doctor or nurse or some other triage-and-assessment individual. If, as was suggested earlier in this chapter, the financial and legal incentives to order more tests and do more interventions and treatments were removed, doctors could rely more on their professional, unbiased judgment for their recommendations and the threat of moral hazard would be greatly diminished. Furthermore, if certain kinds of interventions were removed from the "menu" because of their ineffectiveness or their very low likelihood of success (marginally beneficial treatments), this would tend to further erode the significant power of the moral hazard. Where it would continue to have influence might be in the accessory private insurance market utilized by those who wished to avail themselves of coverage for all of the services—perhaps unnecessary or even frivolous, such as elective cosmetic surgery—not covered by the basic benefit package.

Acceptability of Rationing

What features of rationing plans—both past and present—have made them acceptable to the members of the public affected by them? I believe we can divide them into two broad categories. First is what I have just discussed, namely the lavishness with which the program would be funded. It would be natural to think that people will not mind changing to something that gives them more of what they want (compared to what they have now) or no less, so long as the transition itself is relatively seamless. It is no doubt true that even under the most generous of rationing schemes some people might not have access to what they want (although not necessarily what they need). I illustrated this in chapter 4 with the example of marginally beneficial treatments. Now the fact is that most patients and their families don't know something is marginally beneficial until it is offered to them, it doesn't work, and then we try to take it away. But if we established up front that (for example) prolonged intensive care would not be available for patients with advanced, incurable cancer (or heart disease, or liver failure for patients who aren't transplant candidates, or those with progressive, severe dementia, etc.), because such interventions don't help people (indeed, they often lead to unnecessary and prolonged suffering), the protests could be less effective. This is especially true when these fruitless interventions are compared with all of the other, clearly helpful things we would be able to do, and for whom.[12]

Another obstacle or challenge might be resistance to how to fund such an expansive plan. With the current mixture of private and public insurance and the tremendous variety in the kinds and amounts of benefits provided by the former depending on the policies offered by employers (usually), there is enormous variability in the services available to patients. While Medicare generally provides a basic benefit package, there is state-to-state heterogeneity in what Medicaid will fund, so these kinds of regional and insurance-plan disparities are widespread throughout the healthcare system as it exists today. With a universal healthcare plan that covers everyone (with perhaps the caveats that I discussed in chapter 6), it can be assumed that a high level of consistency of benefits would result. Of course, if we continue to have a secondary market of private insurance to provide services not covered under the basic (and I submit, generous) package, some people will still have more than others, but they would be in the minority, in the same way that those who buy cosmetic surgery today are vastly outnumbered by those who do not. This state of affairs does not introduce instability now and it is unlikely to do so in the future if the basic group of covered services is generous enough to garner endorsement by the majority of the public. Presumably, the funding mechanism could be similar to the mechanism used to pay for Medicare, either as a supplement to taxes or some other mechanism. However, no matter which funding method is utilized, it might be impossible to avoid the belief in some people that they were paying for something for someone else who "had not earned it" or its corollary, "getting something for nothing." The libertarian hostility to distributive justice could present a major stumbling block, but perhaps no more so than for any other expansive social welfare program. And, if cloaked in the patriotic mantle I suggested would be vital for marketing the program and obtaining the affirmation of the populace, it could potentially counter if not overcome the resistance posed by this form of opposition. Moreover, we already provide Medicare and Medicaid to poor people whose financial contributions are far less than what they receive.

Importantly, if everyone has the same form of insurance, it would be difficult for one group to claim they were denied something some other group received within the system, and, of course, this is an essential element of fair treatment. Following the proposals of Daniels and Sabin, I have suggested that several attributes of any kind of goods rationing—meaning the prioritization and allocation of items that are (relatively) scarce and are considered valuable by everyone or almost everyone—would make the system tolerable. These include first and foremost the concept of fairness. I have described this as not simply the understanding that similar situations will be treated similarly, but as embracing the idea that there are no "special" people deserving of increased access or improved prospects for receiving the scarce resources simply because of who they are. Of course this could be viewed from two different perspectives. Most of the time we might think of "special" people as those designated as "very important people" or VIPs. Because of their social status, their wealth, their personal and societal connections, or even their unique knowledge of, or access to, inside information due to their situation in life, they are designated as meriting exclusive entrée to, or treatment from, the system. This could include jumping to the head of the line or simply receiving extra consideration when it came time to decide who should receive what.

The circumstances surrounding possession of exclusive information is a special case that warrants separate mention. Ordinarily, when we think of VIPs in a healthcare setting, it brings to mind relatives of physicians or hospital administrators, highly placed staff, wealthy donors or potential donors, politicians, and so on. But there are others who might be able to acquire information about the good to be rationed—for example, a scarce drug or an influenza vaccine or even a shorter waiting list for an organ transplant—that they come to have by virtue of some social situation. This could include knowing people who have access to confidential facts who then let them in on the secret, or even simply knowing what everyone else knows but having the ability to take advantage of it better than others (such as having easy access to transportation). While there was no evidence that his Croesus-like personal wealth enabled him to buy a liver, as it is suspected the Japanese Yakuza gangster brothers did, Steve Jobs was able to find out about the shorter waiting times in Memphis and both take time off from work and fly there to obtain his transplant (chapter 3), a prime instance of the asymmetry of information benefiting one person over others. One could argue that saving his life was just as important as saving another's who did not have the advantages that he did, but that is missing the point, which is that fairness includes equality at both the front and back ends of the "transaction." Jobs should not have had an improved opportunity to save his life versus another patient's simply because of his situation or status.[13] Examples such as this breed cynicism and erode trust in the overall fairness of an allocation or rationing system, and thus undermine its general legitimacy. The moral character of a system may be better exemplified by how it treats its least powerful members, rather than its most influential. Hence, any attempt to impose a comprehensive healthcare rationing plan—no matter how generous it may be—must adhere to the principle that both rich and poor alike are treated with similar dignity and access. As with the commodity ration books of World War II, all are equal, the main difference being that the wealthy were not *legally* permitted to purchase more food, but it seems reasonable that they could buy more private healthcare if they chose to.

Without question, there will always be people who seek to exploit flaws or loopholes in what is essentially a fair system. More often than not, these will be wealthy individuals who possess the resources to capitalize on shortcomings in the allocation procedures. The purpose of vigilance, constant reviews, scrutiny, and policing of how the system actually works is to ensure—to the extent possible—that "gamers" are as few in number as achievable, and to understand these failures in order to minimize the chances of further cheating. If these sorts of guidelines are followed, it can be presumed that the system can only become more fair with time, and experience with the transplant system has suggested that this claim is true.

This leads me to consider whether special attention should be paid to the least well off—broadly construed—when we devise a fair rationing scheme. Many would think that this is a primary constituent of distributive justice or fairness in allocating resources. Regarding this point, I call to mind Rawls's "difference principle," which he devised as a mechanism for fairly distributing resources in a manner that tolerates disparities between individual recipients (Rawls 1999, 65–70). In this approach, distribution schemes should be devised such that inequities would be permitted if they did not harm those at the bottom or the least well off. In a healthcare rationing scheme that is based on a generous benefit plan, but that still permits those who have the wherewithal to purchase extras if they so choose (but in which this freedom does not harm or detract from what is offered to everyone else), it would seem as if Rawls's proposal could be accomplished. Naturally this would have to be predicated on the adequate provision of resources in the insurance scheme that enabled people whose health outcomes are worse for social reasons (and not simply because of limited access to healthcare) to overcome some of these obstacles.

Of course, paying specific attention to the least-advantaged patients and their families, especially in an overt, perhaps programmatic manner, could raise the hackles of those who feel that "giving" resources to the poor is unearned welfare that others should not be forced to support through taxes (for example) unless they wish to do so. This evokes the old libertarian lament about compelling people to be charitable rather than leaving it to their altruistic impulses, which may or may not result in sufficient help being available to those who need it the most. For those who hew to this view, the "welfare state" is anathema. But while they may rant about being forced to contribute their hard-earned dollars to Social Security, Medicare, and other social programs for the impoverished, they still do so, possibly because these programs are now entrenched in the public's consciousness. The creation of a large, new government-controlled social welfare program encompassing healthcare, which truly does affect everyone at one time or another, might be enough to drive them absolutely nuts. The answer to that—as it was with the creation of Medicare—is to counter the arguments and vitriol, not to back down.

The other hallmark of an ethically justifiable plan that is fair includes openness or transparency such that there are no secret clauses or rules or small print that are invisible or opaque to public scrutiny, especially by those who are most affected by the plan. Another important principle is what has been called relevance, or the idea that the rules and features of the plan would have to be judged as both reasonable and appropriate for the situations for which they have been devised. There must also be a venue and mechanism by which persons can appeal decisions by which they believe they have been treated unjustly. Finally, there must be a procedure in place by which the rules can be enforced. The scheme may be grand and seemingly just, but without the ability to ensure that those who deliver services and who allocate resources do so by the rules, then the appearance of justice is simply that, a sham or a veneer covering up a corrupt system.

Taken together, under reasonably ideal but certainly attainable circumstances, such an approach could achieve a real system of procedural justice, doubtless impure, but capable of delivering a far more equitable and even-handed kind of healthcare to the citizens of the country that can possibly exist now. Generosity and fairness: What is not to like?

Of course, this may simply be a fantasy. No one could plausibly argue that the United States of today could enact laws creating a total revamping of the country's healthcare system. Given the fractious and dysfunctional political scene—one that seems irretrievably ensnared in the vice-like grip of moneyed interest groups, disease-advocacy organizations, and others speaking for factions that stand to gain or lose enormous sums based upon the outcome of various pieces of legislation—any effort to remake American healthcare would make the fight over the Affordable Care Act seem like a minor tiff. However, let us assume for a moment that patriotic altruism, or at least enlightened self-interest, could hold sway and a serious discussion about the fiscal implications of continuing as we are, as well as about the moral failure exemplified by our disjointed and grossly inequitable approach to healthcare, took place. Let us further imagine that it was decided that all people in the United States should have, as a matter of right, access to decent healthcare—and because we are a rich country, it would be considerably more than a basic minimum.[14] Even though we could most likely afford to offer generous benefits to all U.S. residents, would we want to?

In chapter 6, I suggested that there very well may be limits to what a democratic society could (not *should*) endorse in terms of comprehensive coverage in what would actually be a not-so-universal health insurance plan, rationing or not. Even if we could get past the various special interests who would try to derail such an approach at every point along the way, it seems both politically and socially inconceivable that U.S. voters would permit lavish benefits to be bestowed on those they may deem unworthy. Now, who the unworthy happen to be at a given moment in time has been a shifting and evolving target over the last two hundred years, so this perhaps offers a glimmer of hope in that yesterday's outcasts may be today's most upstanding members of society. Thus, it may be possible to argue for more inclusivity on this basis.

However, there are some "others" whose "otherness" has withstood the test of time. Included in this somewhat exclusive group are incarcerated felons and undocumented immigrants. The latter have consistently been the victims of an ironic nativism in this country composed of immigrant groups; whether it is the Irish of the late nineteenth century, Eastern Europeans in the early twentieth century, Asians in the 1920s, etc., etc., the common theme has been ethnically identified groups from someplace else (Reimers 1998). While it could be hoped that appeals to the foreign ancestry of most citizens may be able to somewhat mitigate this animosity, this kind of argument has not been notably successful to date. Hence, I remain pessimistic that those individuals who are considered outside of the protections of the law, and thus our moral and legal concern—like the undocumented—could share in the benefits available to everyone else living in this country under a sensible and magnanimous healthcare rationing system. Even an appeal to the prudent financial self-interest of voters (i.e., it costs more *not* to offer any basic healthcare compared to the provision of emergency services only) may not be successful. There are just too many emotions and politics involved.

Despite repeated rulings of the Supreme Court that incarcerated prisoners must receive the prevailing standard of medical care (which in a system of universal, generous rationed care, could be expected to be a fairly high standard), it is realistically implausible that this could conquer the antipathy—if not downright hostility—that many have toward this population group (*Estelle et al. v. Gamble* 1976; Kahn 2003; McKneally and Sade 2003; Morgan et al. 2008). The only counters to this view may be two observations. First, because of our penchant for locking people up, the United States has the highest incarceration rate of any developed country.[15] Hence, there are huge numbers of people who have left the criminal justice system entirely, are not in jail but still under some form of court supervision, or are related to someone who is or was a convict. It is possible to imagine that these people are not completely indifferent to the welfare of prisoners; since they are numerous, their views could count. Of course, they tend to be overrepresented by people whose political voice has never been very loud (the less well off), but that could be potentially overcome by their numbers. Second, most of the time the public aversion to providing "free" stuff to prisoners bubbles to the surface only when it is publicized—for example, via a news story of a felon who is listed for a heart transplant. This is actually a somewhat weird (if not perverse) example of the "rule of rescue" that I described in chapter 3. In the same way that we rush to express our concern over the identified life that is endangered and whom we believe we can save if only we immediately devote excess resources to saving the person at risk—be it Coby Howard, who wanted a bone marrow transplant but lacked the money, or the Chilean miners who were trapped in a mine—we express our disgust and outrage about the system of providing prisoners with healthcare even if it means scarce resources, only when the person becomes identified. Otherwise, it stays in the background. So, if the healthcare plan with rationing encompasses prisoners but does nothing to diminish resources available to law-abiding citizens (unlike organ transplants), it may be more palatable.[16]

Nevertheless, it is reasonable to consider whether practical, realistic compromises such as these would be a worthwhile trade-off to enable comprehensive healthcare reform with the sort of rationing I foresee to be enacted. Could we accept a system that continued to exclude undocumented immigrants as we do today, not because it is the wise or prudent thing to do, but because it is the only way to buy the endorsement of people who simply could not stomach the idea of criminals getting these potentially lavish benefits? I previously alluded to the libertarian aversion to people getting handouts (not to charity, though, which stems from an individual's wish to give; forced giving is anathema). While it plausible that we could overcome this general antipathy to gain endorsement of a general program, I remain pessimistic that a system that was inclusive for all could survive the inevitable assault that would occur should such marginalized groups be included in its coverage. It is a fight that merits fighting, but it might be foolish to sacrifice the entire effort for the sake of pure justice. As the epigraphs in chapter 6 state, politics is the art of the possible, and what we should do must be tempered by what we *can* do. What needs to be carefully considered is not whether this amount of legislated injustice is a bitter pill, but whether it is a poison pill.

Final Thoughts

Throughout this book I have strived to present both a moral and a practical argument in defense of my thesis that rationing is both the right thing to do and a reasonable solution to the seemingly insurmountable challenges that bedevil us with financing and delivering healthcare in the United States. I have consistently suggested that rationing done correctly, by which I mean fairly (as defined in chapters 2 and 3) and generously (as I have proposed could be the most feasible and plausible way to make it palatable to the American public), would be something that could be sellable—even attractive (I am perhaps going out on a limb here)—to a skeptical population. I have shown that we already tolerate overt rationing with considerably more serious consequences for those who fail to receive what could save their lives. I fully realize the political difficulties—perhaps impossibilities—in defending large-scale healthcare rationing in the United States of the kind that I have been discussing. However, if at least some of the challenges and difficulties of doing so are because there are psychological and philosophical objections to rationing itself, then I think I have presented a reasonable justification to overcome them.

In many ways I am making a psychological argument. Others have demonstrated the economic or fiscal case for universal care and systematic rationing. But what I have wanted to accomplish was to present a case for rationing to overcome the emotional obstacles that prevent even initiating a conversation, much less a debate on the merits of this method of allocating resources and distributing the benefits and burdens of restricted funding for healthcare. By showing that we already ration in planned, open, systematic, and acceptable ways that pretty much everyone knows about and seems to think are acceptable, we could begin to think that rationing may not be anathema—the four-letter word—contrary to what so many believe. Furthermore, by explaining the details of current systems that employ rationing, I have distinguished them from the hidden, adventitious, and often arbitrary methods that are so often found in current practice. Hopefully, we would not further entrench these approaches, in which so often what is available to patients is defined by how much money they have, the small-print terms of their insurance policy, and where they work. This is not to say that money and socioeconomic factors do not play a major role in access to organs for transplant, because they most certainly do: a poor person or one with minimal social support or one with marginal insurance benefits will be shut out of the liver or heart or cadaveric kidney transplant programs just as assuredly as someone who cannot meet the stringent medical criteria. These are problems we have yet to work out, and it is doubtful that even a munificent and comprehensive healthcare rationing program would do much to solve them. However, it could go far to mitigate the negative consequences of the current system.

We must also not neglect the not inconsiderable "sales" job that such a major effort would require. As I have mentioned on numerous occasions throughout this book, the individuals and groups who could line up as opposing such a major overhaul of healthcare in this country would be legion. Their complaints and accusations, as vicious and vitriolic as they often may be, should not be ignored or written off for the kernel of truth they contain. A thoughtful analysis of the possible reasons for the furor raised by the initial inclusion of language in the Affordable Care Act to reimburse physicians for discussing end-of-life care planning with Medicare patients has theorized that the legislative language in the bill may have helped spawn much of the hyperbolic rhetoric that followed. Piemonte and Hermer suggest that the inclusion of text mandating a list of topics that should be discussed, raised the specter of government decrees, just the sort of authoritarian "Big Brother" kind of fiat feared by libertarian-leaning Americans (Piemonte and Hermer 2013; Smith and Bodurtha 2013). Better that the directives from the government be more open-ended or perhaps in the form of suggestions rather than edicts to calm edgy nerves for a undoubtedly controversial policy. This may be a useful lesson to keep in mind as we contemplate the sort of radical reform required by both financial necessity and moral urgency.

Several types of people or groups could be expected to be most scared of rationing as an integral part of comprehensive healthcare reform per se. First and foremost—because they are the ones who have the most to lose financially—would be people and organizations that currently profit from the status quo. These individuals and corporations also tend to have deep pockets and history suggests that they would reach deep into their pockets to mount a spirited—and probably vicious—attack against any form of change that might diminish their influence and financial stake in healthcare as it exists today. Examples might be highly paid insurance executives and hospital administrators, drug and device manufacturers whose bottom line may suffer if drugs and medical technology were prescribed more in accordance with the evidence that supports their use, and doctors who get paid more when they do more.

Second would be people vulnerable to manipulation by the first group. They will be (and have been) the targets of the disinformation and smear campaigns mounted by those protecting a valuable fiefdom to which they believe they are entitled by right. The objects of the advertising are all the individuals whose financial and social hold on life and its benefits may often be shaky, and who are easy prey for those who wish to take advantage of their insecurity. They are also inevitable targets for those who would portray rationing as "death panels" and attempt to undermine their perhaps tenuous peace of mind by fearmongering. The specter of all they might lose rather than all they might gain by generous and comprehensive healthcare redesign (with sensible rationing) is bound to induce alarm and evoke the "scarcity principle" (chapter 1), the combination of which may doom any attempt at major reform.

Those who champion the adoption of a more fair and effective system must be aware of these lurking dangers and be prepared to combat them. Advocates for both the Clinton-era healthcare reforms and the Affordable Care Act have been surprised by the firestorm and less effective than their opponents in this fight. They shouldn't be again. Indeed, taking a proactive approach might be well advised. For example, they could take advantage of many of the common irrational-thinking errors described by Kahneman and Tversky (and others) and employ (or exploit) them for the task of convincing the groups who need to be convinced of the merits of healthcare reform and rationing and to counter the arguments and misinformation of their antagonists (Kahneman 2011; Tversky and Kahneman 1973, 1981). Whichever tactics are utilized, the significant point is that supporters of reform should not be taken unawares and must be prepared for the battle that would undoubtedly ensue. They must also recognize that fighting an emotional and dirty rhetorical battle with rational argument is destined to fail.

Finally, we must also be prepared to contend with those who do not resort to propaganda, lies, and vitriol, but who have principled and philosophical objections to a centralized, government-run healthcare system that would restrict the availability of some services and hence limit free choice. These individuals certainly do exist but their voices are often drowned out by the shouters and screamers from both sides who dominate the conversation. Nevertheless, their views must be heeded and dealt with seriously. These opponents might argue that a market solution with even fewer controls than what currently exist would result in more freedom, flexibility, choice, and cost savings than any form of socialized medicine with rationing. It is to be hoped that the advocates of such a view would be willing to engage in an honest and open debate on the merits of these opposing concepts of how American healthcare should function; if so, this could only foster a better understanding of what is at stake and the advantages and disadvantages of the contrasting standpoints. However, my fear is that such a high-minded discussion might be lost in the war of the words and ads that could dominate the battle.

If we are smart, and perhaps a bit lucky, we will ration smart. If we realize before it's a major crisis (if it isn't already) or too late (if it isn't already) that we have to ration healthcare as a major public policy for the welfare of the people of the United States and the good of the government, we will do so wisely. If we are fortunate, we will look to how we have allocated livers, hearts, and cadaveric kidneys for how we might begin to craft a fair and equitable system. But unlike organ transplants, we have more than enough money to buy beneficial medical treatment and preventive care for everyone who needs it: no one need die waiting for a heart bypass or a pacemaker or a hip replacement or antibiotics or (effective) chemotherapy. No one should be denied therapy for cancer or diabetes or ICU care for premature babies or substance addiction if there is a reasonable opportunity for benefit. But people will not be allowed to have anything they might want, especially quack treatments, drugs that don't work (it doesn't matter if they are cheap or breathtakingly expensive), and endless time waiting for miracles to occur. People will have to play their part and accept the fact that we can't fix everything, that we don't have a bottomless pit of money to wait for miraculous cures, and that everyone dies eventually.

Like food, rubber, and metal in World War II, and like organs today, money is not limitless, even though we seem to act as if it were. More important, the dollars we can afford to devote to healthcare do have some definable upper boundary beyond which we will most definitely say "enough," especially when it becomes obvious that we can or will no longer go into debt to finance all that we wish to buy. And even though the money available for healthcare probably won't run out, it will increasingly hamper our ability to pay for anything else. What would we wish to sacrifice to maintain what at best is a seriously dysfunctional and seriously inequitable, if not morally and medically disgraceful, system? The longer we continue to feed the maw of this voracious and never satisfied beast,[17] the less competitive we will be in the global marketplace, and existing social and health inequities will only get worse.

We need to have what I hope would be a reasoned and legitimate debate about the role of government in our society, although all too often it degenerates into an impassioned and irrational fight between groups whose interests are intimately and integrally tied up in the outcome. If we believe that a reasonable benefit, indeed a right, of citizenship (and perhaps simply of residency) is to possess the capacity to take advantage of the opportunities that society and our economy have to offer, then the best healthcare, broadly construed, is a singular key to attaining that ideal. We have already accepted that maintaining and guaranteeing public and environmental health are legitimate functions of government because these features of our lives affect us all. It is then not too much of a stretch to include healthcare in that mix, for we are all similarly vulnerable to the adverse effects of poor health and the damage it can do, not only to individual well-being but to the flourishing of society. It is especially tragic when we leave lives behind that are so situated because of a lack of healthcare when it is so well within our grasp to remedy these circumstances.

Is there a fundamental, elemental difference between livers and dollars? In one sense, of course there is. With dollars, we can buy almost anything (except more livers)—that is, they are fungible. We get to decide not only how many there are (within some sort of upper limit without specifying exactly what that limit is), but what we get to spend them on: we have a choice. With livers, there is a finite supply that is real and immune from any true effort to manipulate their numbers. If we continue to rely on livers that come from dead people for transplantation, there is an absolute upper limit of the number available. Furthermore, you can't really bargain with livers or exchange them for something else; a liver is only good for a liver transplant. While few people may *act* as if there is no limit to the number of dollars out there that can be used to purchase all sorts of healthcare, no matter how exotic or unnecessary or ineffective it might be, I suspect that most of us know that there is a limit to how much we can spend on medicine. The easy part may be figuring what that limit is; the hard part will then be to decide what to spend our healthcare budget on.

And it is indeed the absolute limit to the number of dollars we can commit to healthcare that justifies rationing, in exactly the same way the absolute limit on livers (or kidneys, hearts, ventilators, etc.) justifies rationing in those clinical situations. If we didn't care about paying for anything else other than healthcare, we very well might not need rationing, but we do. We want to have schools, roads, a military, and all the other social goods that communally raised and pooled funds pay for. Of course, this statement doesn't say anything about how the money should be divided up between these various needs, but the recognition that the pie is of finite size is an important initial goal. What remains is to determine how important healthcare is among all the other objectives that are also clamoring for their piece of the pie.

Sacrifice of a certain sort would almost certainly be necessary, but as I have suggested, the kinds and amounts of sacrifice could be relatively small for those who should count the most: patients. There is no question that pain would be felt by the health insurance industry, which would undergo a vast contraction under this proposal. Those who make their living trying to figure out how to administer the vast array of health plans and game the system to keep hospitals and clinics and practices afloat and financially viable will suffer, because the necessity for their services will be reduced to a minimum. Industries that produce devices and expensive technologies could see their market share decreased as the demand for their stuff diminishes; presumably, the creative and successful entrepreneurial types in their midst will find new things to invent and new markets to explore. Doctors (at least some of them) could also suffer, because the highest paid among them would see a decline in their earning power as the commoditizing of medicine was altered; at the same time, however, perhaps those physicians engaged in primary care would see salary increases, the overall student debt could be dramatically lowered, and true tort reform could see malpractice rates and the costs of defensive medicine plummet. No fundamental reorganization of such a significant segment of the nation's economy and a vital component of peoples' lives could be accomplished without individual groups believing they are receiving the brunt of the sacrifice. However, it would again be an important component of promoting such a vast change to emphasize the benefits and not the (transient) burdens. It would also be instructive to look for historical precedents; as Fox and Markel point out, "antagonism to reform in the months, even years, after it is enacted is often fierce and vitriolic: but it has a half-life" (Fox and Markel 2010, 1749).

Nevertheless, it should be acknowledged that not all opposition to comprehensive healthcare reform and/or rationing is cynical and self-serving. There are clearly some people and groups who have strong philosophical objections to the imposition of a major government-controlled program funded by taxpayers that necessarily limits choice. I have referred to some (not all) of these arguments as "libertarian." There are also those who object on principle to the idea of extending healthcare benefits to those they deem "unworthy" or "undeserving," such as the poor, undocumented immigrants, and perhaps prisoners and other social outcasts. If that is so, then they should represent their case openly and honestly in free debate on the merits of their views. While idealistic, it is considerably more justifiable and noble than employing shadowy front groups to scare vulnerable and impressionable people rather than honest and frank discussion.

One final memorable clinical encounter may be instructive. A number of years ago I cared for a young man who had metastatic bone cancer. He had been living with it for some time and it had started progressing, probably for the final time. I thought that he could benefit from what

I described to him as a "minor surgical procedure," and it was, at least compared to other kinds of operations such as, say, open-heart surgery. But he said something to me that I will never forget, and it has influenced the way I think about patients and what doctors and nurses do for them and to them. He told me, "Doc, it may be minor to you, but it's happening to me, so it's major." And indeed it was. Of course, this is also true for the kinds of rationing or allocation decisions we may make, either because we want to, or because we must (like organs and scarce drugs). It is relatively straightforward and simple to sit in a conference room and discuss who should be on the list, who should get what and why, and how to follow the rules correctly. It is quite another matter when sitting across from a sick person and her family, someone who is desperately looking to you for hope that you can make her better. Most important, that you will be her advocate and fight for everything she needs to get well. The inevitable tension and conflict between what someone wants, what someone needs and what is available, along with the professional role of the doctor as safeguard of both "the system" and the patient's best interests, threaten to be overwhelming and potentially unsolvable. Conserving resources for an unidentified someone else, when confronted with a real, live sick person whose welfare you are pledged to advance, is a very difficult position for both the doctor and the patient. But, as we have seen, patients can accept not getting something that could save their lives, if the system is set up in a certain way. But it is less easy to accept—if at all—if the reason for rejection is not seen as fair or as frivolous (e.g., due to a lack of money).

Indeed, it may be valuable to recall that in his State of the Union Address in 1949 President Harry Truman presented his proposals for a comprehensive group of social programs to ensure that Americans would be able to have the kinds of flourishing lives so many of their fellow citizens had recently died to protect. In his "Fair Deal," he offered programs to guarantee that all Americans would have health insurance, be fully employed and paid a decent wage, and that racial and religious discrimination would be outlawed[18] Not surprisingly, perhaps, the Congress that was elected in 1948 (along with Truman) did not warm to many of his legislative aspirations, notably (for my purposes) universal health insurance. Nevertheless, Truman was keenly aware of the significance and importance of the word "fair" in any proposition to the American people (if not Congress). The passage of some sixty-five years has done nothing to lessen the noteworthiness of fairness, both in word—and, most powerfully—in deed.

So where do we go from here? It is inevitable that the system will break if it continues to grow in cost the way it has. I remain pessimistic that the

Affordable Care Act will restrain expenditure growth significantly over the next ten or so years. Furthermore, the compromises that were made to ensure its congressional passage, combined with the 2012 Supreme Court case that ruled the Medicaid expansion mandate unconstitutional, mean that we will continue to have unconscionable numbers of people without health insurance (almost all of whom are poor or near-poor). If that is true, then something has to give. Indeed, as repugnant as healthcare rationing is portrayed to be for most Americans, it may pale in comparison to their hatred of more taxes, which will undoubtedly be called for to finance the ever-expanding entitlement programs of Medicare and Medicaid to which they also seem so attached. Otherwise these entitlements will have to be reduced, perhaps dramatically, and in a manner that could pale in comparison to the relatively minor restrictions I have suggested would be sensible, justifiable, and possibly achievable. I would not like to think of reasonable and generous rationing as the lesser of two evils, but that may be another way to "sell" it to a suspicious public that is often held psychologically captive by special interests, who may be hurt by rationing and who control enormous budgets for advertising and lobbying of legislators eager for campaign contributions.

As I stated at the end of chapter 1, I fully realize the practical political and social challenges that await anyone with the audacity to attempt real comprehensive healthcare reform in the United States, especially of the type I have discussed in this book. Some might suggest that we should take incremental, perhaps hesitant steps, so as to not upset the powerful interests that remain heavily invested, both philosophically and especially financially, in the status quo. Certainly, even a cursory review of the brutal and (some might say) ruthless, take-no-prisoners fights over the doomed Clinton health reform proposals and the recent (and ongoing) Affordable Care Act clearly demonstrates the obstacles that would undoubtedly be arrayed against this kind of reform. Nevertheless, some legislators, pundits, public intellectuals, talk-show hosts, and the like may retain some remnant of dedication to the collective good of the nation. If so, then it is difficult to imagine how some could honorably and honestly defend a view that the present state of affairs is a good one and that it is acceptable for so many Americans to go without decent healthcare or the security that good health insurance provides, because it is specious to argue that the millions who live this way do so out of choice rather than necessity. If true, we might then hope for a principled debate on the merits of various approaches to delivering healthcare in the United States.

I have presented a variety of strategies, based on existing systems, that could make an end result palatable to its eventual users (all of us), but it could be plausibly (and cynically) maintained that the American public has perhaps the least powerful voice in what would happen, and that they can be—and are—easily swayed by sophisticated and none-too-subtle advertising campaigns often appealing to their most basic fears. Leaving the status quo behind and moving into an unknown and untried future tends to frighten most of us if we let it, and we can be confident that the vested healthcare industry, as well as others who might wish to exploit such an opportunity for their own selfish concerns, will be lined up waiting for the fight. The certainty of this looming struggle could discourage many, but it shouldn't deter the attempt. Some might even maintain that it is a sisyphean fight, doomed to failure. But the stakes are much too high to adopt that stance. Decent, comprehensive healthcare and the benefits it bestows on people is an unarguable good—good for them and good for the nation. When the means are available to accomplish it, it seems immoral not to make the effort to try.

Notes

Chapter 1

1. Congressional Budget Office, *The Long-Term Outlook for Health Care Spending*, http://www.cbo.gov/publication/41646.

2. http://www.unos.org.

3. News-savvy readers will recall a recent case of a child with cystic fibrosis (a congenital, autosomal recessive inherited disease that often destroys lung function) whose desperate parents sought help from the courts to change the allocation system for donor lungs so that their daughter could be eligible to receive (small) adult lungs rather than waiting for a child's organs; this would improve her chances for a transplant (see http://www.slate.com/articles/health_and_science/medical_examiner/2013/06/sarah_murnaghan_s_lung_transplant_organ_donors_should_be_compensated.html and http://www.usatoday.com/story/news/nation/2013/06/07/lung-transplant-girl-ethics/2397701). Of course the parents were primarily interested in saving their daughter's life, but they were criticizing the system's *fairness*, not the sad fact that there are not enough organs for everyone who could benefit from a transplant (see chapter 2).

4. http://www.donatelifeohio.org/debbie-rice-father-died-waiting-for-a-heart-transplant.html.

5. http://www.ashp.org/DrugShortages/Current.

6. Of course many people might argue that the defense budget is relatively immune to cost-cutting and hence seems a rather poor example of rationing, but it is one nonetheless, if only because a finite budget is passed that is not open-ended.

7. Of course, projections and forecasts are created to estimate the amount of money that will be needed, but these are only approximations. The actual budget and the sources of funding for Medicare and its different components are quite complicated. As explained by the Congressional Budget Office:

The various parts of the program are financed in different ways. Part A benefits [inpatient hospital costs] are financed primarily by a payroll tax (2.9 percent of all taxable earnings), the revenues from which are credited to the HI [Hospital Insurance] trust fund. Beginning in 2013, an additional 0.9 percent tax on earnings over $200,000 ($250,000 for married couples) is also being credited to the trust fund. For Part B, [physician professional charges] premiums paid by beneficiaries cover just over one-quarter of outlays, and the government's general funds cover the rest. Federal payments to private insurance plans under Part C are financed by a blend of funds from Parts A and B. Enrollees' premiums under Part D [prescription drug benefit] are set to cover about one-quarter of the cost of the basic prescription drug benefit, although many low-income enrollees pay no premiums; general funds from the Treasury cover most of the remaining cost. Altogether, in calendar year 2012, receipts from the payroll tax were equal to about 36 percent of gross federal spending on Medicare, beneficiaries' premiums were equal to about 12 percent, and general funds allocated to the program's trust funds amounted to about 37 percent; the trust funds are also credited with money from other sources. (http://www.cbo.gov/publication/44587)

8. See Cohen 2012 for a recent, concise discussion of this.

9. *Oxford English Dictionary* (online edition), http://www.oed.com/view/Entry/158517?redirectedFrom=rationing#eid.

10. *Estimates for the Insurance Coverage Provisions of the Affordable Care Act Updated for the Recent Supreme Court Decision*, report 43472, Congressional Budget Office, July 24, 2012, http://www.cbo.gov/publication/43472.

11. This state could be referred to as the so-called third phase of modern medicine, as labeled by Callahan, the first two phases being those marked by major gains in population health by relatively inexpensive public health measures such as good sanitation, clean water, vaccines, and antibiotics. Phases 1 and 2 were characterized by measures that could benefit pretty much everyone, while Phase 3 is distinguished by more individualized medicine in which technological and scientific advances benefit fewer and fewer people at great cost per treatment (see Callahan 1990, chap. 5).

12. Bob Cesca, "Keep Your Goddam Government Hands Off My Medicare!," *Huffington Post*, August 5, 2009, http://www.huffingtonpost.com/bob-cesca/get-your-goddamn-governme_b_252326.html.

13. See Goldsteen, Goldsteen, Swan, and Clemeña 2001 for a discussion of the effectiveness of the "Harry and Louise" ads and Bergan and Risner 2012 for the efficacy of more recent advertising to influence the debate on the Affordable Care Act.

14. I am grateful to Peter Ubel for pointing out this inconsistency.

15. Although it also should bar unfettered access to interventions that would provide minimal-to-no benefit, as defined medically. Amazingly, though, that restriction is also controversial, as I will discuss in chapters 2, 4, and 5.

16. The former means that the test result is positive, but the thing it was designed to detect was actually not there (the test was wrong). The latter means that the test was positive because it really did detect the thing it was supposed to detect. In a good diagnostic test, there is a very low false positive rate. Conversely, one also wants a low false negative rate, meaning that the test didn't miss anything that was actually there.

17. I discuss this a bit further on with respect to mammography.

18. This also raises the problem of unintended consequences. For example, it is well known that members of certain ethnic groups, on average, use many more resources at the end of life than others (see Blackhall et al. 1999; Braun, Beyth, Ford, and McCullough 2008; Fairrow, McCallum, and Messinger-Rapport 2004; Hanchate et al. 2009; Moseley et al. 2004). Any attempt to restrict access to high-tech ICU care in the end-of-life setting, even when most physicians might neutrally judge at least some of it as "futile" or not benefiting the patient, might have disproportionate effects on African Americans, a result which could harm trust in the medical system, which itself could lead to avoidance of doctors and healthcare in general.

19. This data is for 2008, the most recent year for which complete financial information is available. The data was obtained from the United States Renal Data System (http://www.usrds.org/reference.htm).

20. The point that requires emphasis here is that the patients with metastatic cancer and other grave conditions, who most certainly could qualify for dialysis as it's currently set up in the United States and often are actually receiving dialysis, would not be eligible for kidney transplants. Thus, dialysis is *not* serving as a bridge to transplant (theoretically, a "cure" for end-stage renal disease) but is an end in itself.

21. As I discuss in detail in chapters 2 and 3, one way we should not allocate resources is on the basis of morally irrelevant facts (especially social) about people that make some lives more "worthy" than others. This was one of the controversial issues raised by a very early description of the allocation of scarce resources—in fact, kidney dialysis machines—in the 1960s (see Alexander 1962, 102–125).

22. For instance, bevacizumab (Avastin®) prolongs progression-free survival by a few months in advanced breast cancer, but not overall survival (Robert et al. 2011). This means that women treated with this extremely expensive drug did not live any longer than those not treated with it, but their tumors seemed to take longer to come back (when they did return, they came back very quickly). Data like this is contributing to the FDA's review of this drug's approval for use in breast cancer.

23. I will be the first to acknowledge that we somehow think about money as fungible and qualitatively different than substantive material things, like kidneys, livers, or drugs. We can print money but we can't make livers (although we can make artificial kidney machines, so maybe they are somewhat analogous to dollars). Of course, the reality is that money doesn't materialize out of nowhere and isn't fundamentally different from other healthcare resources. This is a psychological distinction, to which more attention is due.

24. A few of the more notable ones include Fleck 2009, Ubel 2001, as well as Aaron, Schwartz, and Cox 2005.

25. There are a number of excellent reviews and analyses of the Oregon experiment, including Fox and Leichter 1991, Hadorn 1991, Kitzhaber 1993, and Oberlander 2007.

26. For example, see Fleck 2009, chap. 3. He points out that the "invisibility" part violates the demands of any just system to be publicly accountable, which derives much of its force from the arguments of Rawls 1999.

27. For example, see Emanuel and Wertheimer 2006 as well as Hurst and Danis 2007.

28. While this story serves as an example of what people fear about rationing and what it could personally mean for them and others, it is also an illustration of the potential limits of decisions that could be made to restrict access to scarce resources. I discuss this in detail in chapter 6.

29. For instance, several years ago it became apparent that African Americans were receiving fewer liver transplants than white Americans when controlled for geographic region (and thus availability of organs, donor rates, etc.) and degree of illness. This state of affairs suggested that there might be a disparity in access, similar to other situations of access to technologically advanced healthcare, such as sophisticated cardiac procedures (e.g., see Farmer et al. 2009; Shippee, Ferraro, and Thorpe 2011). To try to rectify this discrepancy, researchers looked at the influence of the MELD (Model for End-Stage Liver Disease) scoring system before and after it was initiated as a significant component of eligibility for transplant. Essentially, this disease-severity evaluation tool reduced the amount of subjective input by liver transplant doctors on who to refer and list for transplant. By lessening the discretionary power of the doctor, any overt or covert prejudice was minimized, leading to a virtual elimination of ethnic or racial disparities in the recipients of liver transplantation (Moylan et al. 2008).

30. However, we do decide whether to pay for transplants and the doctors, nurses, social workers, operating room technicians, laboratory technologists, hospitals, drugs, or surgical supplies. We have made a conscious determination to make sufficient funds available to support this life-saving activity (unlike the original Oregon Health Plan). Other funding decisions would be similar, although it should be acknowledged that saying yes is often easier and simpler that saying no, even if one has good reason for the latter and has to borrow money to support the former. (See chapter 3 for the breast cancer stem cell rescue/transplant story. I also discuss the "fungibility" problem in greater detail in that chapter and chapters 4 and 7.)

31. For example, the interminable debates in the 2010–2011 sessions of Congress to cut Medicaid and Medicare funding as well as limiting the funds for the long-term unemployed, but resisting attempts to raise taxes on the wealthy.

32. A PET (positron emission tomography) scan is a very expensive but increasingly available form of radiologic nuclear (i.e., low-radioactivity) imaging technology that can be valuable in detecting certain types of tumors, especially lymphomas (cancer of the lymph glands). In its latest iterations, it is frequently coupled with a CAT scanner (computerized axial tomography) to give extremely precise anatomical localizations of the "PET-avid" mass detected. Like most medical technology, it can be extraordinarily beneficial when used appropriately.

33. While some may think that this observation could be interpreted as an argument in favor of forceful imposition of rationing as a way of generating wide-

spread acceptance, this is not my intention. It is almost inconceivable that that scheme could be successful in the United States except when applied to a population that is relatively powerless to protest, like the poor people in Oregon.

34. There can also be a significant "framing effect" in how a scarcity story is portrayed to a target audience. For example, the proposal in 2010 for Medicare to pay physicians to have discussions with their older patients about end-of-life planning—something that surveys say happens infrequently but that seniors overwhelmingly wish to talk about (McCarthy et al. 2008; Morrison and Meier 2004; Keating et al. 2010)—was graphically depicted by opponents as doctors trying to knock off older people at the behest of the government, which would fund this activity (Tinetti 2012). Thus, an eminently benign, even admirable project that would be encouraged by modest compensation (that was then lacking) was demonized by groups with ulterior motives and political goals. Or consider how the suggestion of the U.S. Preventive Services Task Force to scale back the widespread use of mammography screening for women between forty and forty-nine years of age (irrespective of breast cancer risk status) was characterized as an attempt to take away a diagnostic tool responsible for saving the lives of millions, and its absence would absolutely lead to the deaths of goodness knows how many others. (See U.S. Preventive Services Task Force Recommendation Statement 2009; Squiers et al. 2011; http://www.huffingtonpost.com/2011/12/19/mammogram-advice-us-preventive-services-task-force_n_1156228.html.) While the data is somewhat controversial, screening rates for this young, low-risk population did not appreciably decrease after publication of the Task Force recommendation, suggesting the efficacy of the pro-mammography campaign (Pace, He, and Keating 2013; Block, Jarlenski, Wu, and Bennett 2013).

35. The last year for which complete data is available is 2007. In that year, 36 percent of deaths occurred in hospitals, 21.7 percent in nursing facilities, and 7 percent in the "hospital outpatient or emergency department," for a total of 64.7 percent in healthcare facilities (data from National Center for Health Statistics, *Health, United States, 2010: With Special Feature on Death and Dying*, 85, figure 33 (Hyattsville, MD: National Center for Health Statistics, 2011)).

36. For example, see Kilner 1990 and Ubel 2001.

Chapter 2

1. And even under the best of circumstances, influenza vaccine is far from 100 percent effective, especially in the most vulnerable populations of the very young and old.

2. This influenza virus is yet another that has its origins in the wild and domestic bird populations. Infections of humans presumably occurs via direct transmission from frequent and close contacts with infected animals, most often domestic poultry held in the close confines of a small family home. Further reassortment of the genes in the virus—specifically, recombination with a coexisting human influenza virus—can confer easy interperson transmissibility if the virus picks up genes responsible for human infectivity. The new virus would then have the virulence of

the avian flu (usually very high, meaning it kills a high percentage of those who are infected), along with the rapid infectivity of the usual seasonal flu and the lack of preexisting immunity in people because of the novelty of the recombined virus. These factors are what epidemiologists and infectious disease experts most fear.

3. ECMO has found a role in a variety of clinical settings in children and adults as a "bridge" to either recovery or heart transplantation.

4. Without getting too technical, there are two general forms of ECMO that depend on the type of hookup to the patient. The arterial-venous kind is the most complex and is used when the heart and lungs are not working well; venous-venous is a less complicated type mostly used in patients waiting for a lung transplant. The former needs one nurse per patient and requires a full-time ECMO technician to supervise and operate the machine and its assorted tubing, lines, and other components. In contrast, so-called V-V ECMO can have a technician operate two machines (and thus two patients) at once.

5. Of course, if the rate of H1N1 infections had then multiplied (as may experts feared) rather than tapering off, this approach would have offered only a very temporary solution.

6. In chapter 5, I describe patients who receive critical resources as "winners" and those who do not as "losers." One might be inclined to think of drugs as not in the same category as ventilators or livers, and very often they are not. However, a large percentage of the medications that have been in short supply have been chemotherapy agents for which there are rarely alternatives and that can often be life saving.

7. §299I of the Social Security Amendments of 1972, Pub. L. No. 92–603, 86 Stat. 1329, 1463–64.

8. This review is a very nice history of both clinical and scientific developments, as well as a concise story describing the politics that led to the creation of the ESRD program.

9. Because the program has grown almost exponentially (and has at the same time become a very big business for nephrologists and commercial providers of dialysis equipment, care, and associated supplies), the original budget estimates have exploded. Data from 2009 show ESRD expenditures at about $25 billion with about a 10–11 percent increase per year (the latest data is for 2009. (See http://www.usrds.org/2011/view/v2_11.asp, figures 11.4 and 11.5).

10. National Medical Care was created in 1968 by physicians at the then Peter Bent Brigham Hospital in Boston (now the Brigham and Women's Hospital), a major teaching affiliate of the Harvard Medical School. Today two of the biggest for-profit dialysis companies are DaVita and Fresenius. Fresenius merged with and took over National Medical Care in 1996. The former's webpage informs us that "DaVita Inc., a FORTUNE 500® company, is a leading provider of kidney care in the United States, delivering dialysis services to patients with chronic kidney failure and end stage renal disease. DaVita strives to improve patients' quality of life by innovating clinical care, and by offering integrated treatment plans, personalized care teams and convenient health-management services. As of June 30, 2012, DaVita operated or provided administrative services at 1,884 outpa-

tient dialysis centers located in the United States, serving approximately 149,000 patients. The company also operated 19 outpatient dialysis centers located in four countries outside the United States" (http://www.davita.com/about). Fresenius is even bigger, with 2011 net revenue of $12.8 billion and net income of more than $1 billion: "Fresenius Medical Care is the world's largest integrated provider of products and services for individuals undergoing dialysis because of chronic kidney failure, a condition that affects more than 2.1 million individuals worldwide. Through its network of 3,123 dialysis clinics in North America, Europe, Latin America, Asia-Pacific and Africa, Fresenius Medical Care provides dialysis treatment to 256,456 patients around the globe. Fresenius Medical Care is also the world's leading provider of dialysis products such as hemodialysis machines, dialyzers and related disposable products. Fresenius Medical Care is listed on the Frankfurt Stock Exchange (FME, FME3) and the New York Stock Exchange (FMS, FMS/P)" (http://www.fmc-ag.com/59.htm).

11. This is not necessarily true for kidneys, because there is always the alternative of receiving dialysis instead of a new organ, or more recently, for hearts, since the advent of small, portable left ventricular assist devices (LVADs) has enabled many patients who are either not eligible for transplantation for one reason or another, or who are waiting for one and don't receive one because of the shortage, to leave tolerable lives. There are currently no clinically available artificial livers or lungs.

12. Importantly, this means that we do not "harvest" organs from individuals who might be said to be "almost dead" or permanently unconscious (such as in a persistent vegetative state like Terri Schiavo) or comatose (people who have lost upper-brain or cortical function).

13. This is a well-discussed and controversial topic, with vocal advocates arguing for opposite points of view. I find Debra Satz's discussion against organ markets to be one of the most persuasive (see Satz 2010, chap. 9). While Michael J. Sandel's book is aimed at more general audiences than that of Satz, he also makes a somewhat similar although less comprehensive and detailed case (and unfortunately, less convincing to my mind) (Sandel 2012, especially chap. 4).

14. In Israel, people who have indicated their willingness to serve as organ donors (should the occasion arise) receive priority themselves in the allocation algorithm should they ever require an organ transplant. The goal is to increase the number of people amenable to (postmortem) donation. Not surprisingly, this approach has not been without controversy. The law was originally proposed in 2006, enacted in 2008, and finally activated in 2010. (See Lavee, Ashkenazi, Gurman, and Steinberg 2010; Guttman, Ashkenazi, Gesser-Edelsburg, and Seidmann 2011; Quigley, Wright, and Ravitsky 2012.)

15. The OPTN Charter reads: "This Charter governs the structure and operation of the Organ Procurement and Transplantation Network (OPTN). By accepting membership in the OPTN, each Member agrees to comply with all applicable provisions of the National Organ Transplant Act, as amended, 42 U.S.C. 273 et seq.; OPTN Final Rule, 42 CFR Part 121; this Charter; the OPTN Bylaws; and OPTN policies as in effect from time to time. The OPTN will conduct ongoing and periodic reviews and evaluations of each Member OPO and Transplant Hospital for compliance with the OPTN Final Rule and OPTN policies. All OPTN Members

are subject to review and evaluation for compliance with OPTN policies. All such compliance monitoring is performed using processes and protocols developed by the OPTN Contractor in accordance with the contract with the Department of Health and Human Services (HHS), Health Resources and Services Administration (HRSA), to operate the OPTN (OPTN Contract)" (see http://optn.transplant .hrsa.gov/policiesAndBylaws/charterAndBylaws.asp). An OPO is a local-regional "organ procurement organization." These groups perform the actual "grunt work" of obtaining consent, arranging harvesting of the donor organ(s), and other tasks. See http://www.carolinadonorservices.org for a representative example. As they state on their website, "Carolina Donor Services is the federally designated organ procurement organization serving 7 million people in 78 counties of North Carolina and Danville, Virginia. Our service area includes 107 hospitals and four transplant centers that perform heart, lung, liver, kidney, pancreas, and intestine transplants. Our mission is straightforward: Carolina Donor Services maximizes the passing of the heroic gift of life from one human being to another through organ and tissue donation. Our team of dedicated professionals work diligently to increase the awareness of the need for organ and tissue donors and to deliver the most sensitive approach to organ and tissue donation. We perform public and professional education, as well as coordinate the entire organ and tissue donation process."

16. Interestingly, as I discuss in greater detail in the next chapter, this evaluation does not include an assessment of the potential recipient's "social worth," or his or her past, present, or future contribution(s) to society. Objections to the use of these factors about people with reference to dialysis eligibility contributed to the furor over Shana Alexander's 1962 article in *Life* describing the procedures of the Seattle "God Committee" as they considered who should have access to the very few early dialysis machines they possessed (Alexander 1962). In theory, this means that prospective transplant candidates are considered for their medical characteristics, assuming they meet other criteria such as financial and social circumstances that would suggest they could pay for the process and be a good "steward" of the organ. Again, in theory, this implies that a Nobel Prize winner would have the same chance as a day laborer without a high school diploma, all clinical things being otherwise equal. In truth, however, the former would be much more likely to receive a transplant simply because it is more probable that he or she would meet the necessary psychosocial and economic criteria.

17. Although, if technology ever advances to the point that we have artificial organs to replace those that fail, we will be in the same boat we find ourselves in with dialysis. We will have to decide whether the only criterion for giving an artificial heart or liver to a patient should be the ability to pay—either via insurance or, as with dialysis, at government (i.e., taxpayers') expense—or whether we should determine that perhaps some individual benefit is too little to justify the expense. In this sense, then, the cost rather than the machine (organ) would be the communal resource that must be spent wisely and judiciously. We already have a little taste of this with two very expensive cardiac support devices. The first is the LVAD, referred to earlier. It is being used as both a temporary "bridge" to transplant, essentially keeping very ill patients alive until (or if) a donor heart becomes

available, as well as "destination" therapy instead of transplant (since there are not enough transplantable hearts) (Birks 2010; Flint, Matlock, Lindenfeld, and Allen 2012). But they are very expensive (Rogers et al. 2012). The latter indication suggests that more and more people will be living with these devices and money will not necessarily be an object so long as Medicare continues to pay for them. Similarly, implantable cardiac defibrillators are being used with ever-greater frequency, and Medicare pays for them at $25,000 for the instrument itself (in 2010: www.cms.gov/.../CMS_1414_P_ APCsDevicesSubjecttoNoCostFullCredit-PartialCreditAdj.pdf), and the associated fees, including professional fees from physicians, add thousands more. Once again, scrutiny as to how much benefit is sufficient to warrant using these devices is mostly absent.

18. The lung transplant program at my institution, now one of the largest in the entire country, requires that patients live within thirty miles of the hospital for up to one year after surgery. This is obviously prohibitive for many (maybe most) people. There are some notable exceptions to this dismal and shameful state of affairs. For example, the Veterans Administration health system will pay for transplantation for conditions judged to be service-related. And kidney transplantation is subsidized by the ESRD Program of Medicare, along with antirejection immunosuppressive medication for up to three years postoperatively (of course, one must take these drugs for the rest of one's life, so it is unclear what patients are supposed to do after the three years are up). (See Swaminathan, Mor, Mehrotra, and Trivedi 2012; Kovacs, Perkins, Nuschke, and Carroll 2012; Hynes et al. 2012.) It is also worthwhile pointing out that even comprehensive national health insurance would only reduce some disparities. Since people from lower socioeconomic strata tend to have more psychosocial challenges than their more advantaged, clinically similar peers (such as poorer housing, more mental health issues including substance abuse, etc.), the best health insurance in the world would be unable to eliminate these residual barriers to equality of transplant access.

19. I discuss this topic in greater detail in chapter 5, when I discuss the status of a group that I have labeled "losers"—that is, those who don't receive some resource that they might have in the absence of rationing.

20. For example, the development and introduction of the Model for End-Stage Liver Disease (MELD) and its counterpart for children, the Pediatric End-Stage Liver Disease model (PELD), over the last ten years have successfully reduced—if not eliminated—physician championing of their own patients' needs over other physicians' patients. This score, based on easily verifiable (and audited) lab test results that are reasonably immune to jiggering by overly enthusiastic and passionate doctors, has been highly effective in improving both equity and efficacy in allocation (Moylan et al. 2008). However, it is possible that at least some of this improvement may have been bought at a cost (i.e., in terms of outcomes: years of life saved as well as quality), since it means that the absolutely sickest patients ascend to the top of the priority list, even though they may be the riskiest to transplant (Bonney et al. 2009; Weismüller et al. 2011). One group has proposed a modification of the MELD score to take this anomalous feature of cadaveric liver transplant into account (Dutkowski et al. 2011). More recently, a somewhat analogous approach has also been taken for lung transplantation (Egan et al.

2006; Merlo et al. 2009), but as with the MELD score, the sickest lung transplant candidates may fare the worst (Liu, Zamora, Dhillon, and Weill 2010). Hence, just as there are patients who are not sick enough to be eligible for high-priority listing for an organ, there may also be people who are too sick to receive one. In an attempt to bring similar rigor and impartiality to the lung transplantation field, a "lung allocation score" or LAS has been developed and is in its early days of implementation and evaluation (Orens and Garrity 2009; Liu et al. 2010; Smits et al. 2011; Russo et al. 2011).

21. I have received numerous requests for the policy from institutions throughout the United States. It was published as an electronic-only appendix in Rosoff et al 2012.

22. I discuss a variant of this sort of tourism in the next chapter. It should be noted that this form of medical seeking is for the most part only available to patients who already enjoy the privileges associated with wealth and the social position that it confers.

23. Much has been written about the gray market in drugs and how many institutions do avail themselves of this source of supply (Liang and Mackey 2012; Donaldson 2010; Mitka 2012; Rosenthal 2012; Duffy 2012). However, given the ongoing problems with counterfeit medications, even in the absence of shortages, it seemed a safer course to avoid accessing this potential stock. While it could potentially partly relieve the scarcity, permitting us to treat patients we might otherwise not be able to treat, the possible risk of exposure to adulterated, out-of-date, or otherwise less-than-effective or even dangerous concoctions was one we did not wish to pursue. Moreover, the 2012 exposé of the real hazards of using commercial, poorly regulated compounding pharmacies to obtain drugs demonstrated the conservative wisdom of our decision. For example, see http://www.cdc.gov/HAI/outbreaks/currentsituation/index.html.

24. While perhaps a too overt political document, some of the points made in a report from the U.S. House of Representatives Committee on Oversight and Government Reform bear closer analysis. This is especially true of the suggestion that a section of the Medicare Modernization Act (2003) that limited price markups for all drugs administered in doctors' office (thus severely curtailing the ability of generic manufacturers to make more than a marginal profit) may have inadvertently contributed to making a festering problem much worse. (The report is available at http://oversight.house.gov/report/fdas-contribution-to-the-drug-shortage-crisis/. Also see Gupta and Huang 2013.) Another suggestion might be to take an approach analogous to that used to expand the number of vaccine manufacturers, which had become vanishingly small due in large part to the huge liability threat posed by people seeking compensation for alleged injury from immunization. In 1986 Congress enacted the National Childhood Vaccine Injury Act (NCVIA) of 1986 (42 U.S.C. §§300aa-1 to 300aa-34), which led the Department of Health and Human Services to create the National Vaccine Injury Compensation Program (NVICP), colloquially known as "Vaccine Court." This limited the liability of vaccine manufacturers, calming the market and enabling them to better predict their financial future. This created an incentive for more companies to get into the vaccine business and led to a surge of new vaccines

(for example, the multivalent anti–human papilloma virus vaccine, Gardasil®) (see Cook and Evans 2011). While the ability to predict the effects of such interference to the generic drug market on shortages is speculative at best, it may bear closer scrutiny and thought.

25. A very nice and concise history and analysis of the Oregon Health Plan is offered in a document published by the Oregon Department of Human Service (available at www.oregon.gov/oha/healthplan/data_pubs/ohpoverview0706.pdf; see also Hadorn 1991 and Oberlander 2007).

26. In truth, the actual way the negotiations worked was not nearly as "clean" as this description suggests. There was a brokered deal that was a compromise between being too generous and too miserly based on what could be on the list of covered treatment-condition pairs.

27. See also Cookson, McCabe, and Tsuchiya 2008, as well as Jenni and Loewenstein 1997.

28. See Daniels 1991, Hadorn 1991, and Oberlander, Marmor, and Jacobs 2001. This is not to say that TMJ pain does not produce suffering, sometimes significantly so. It's just that very few people die from these conditions, while they can and do perish from inattention to a burst appendix. That being said, there are many life-threatening conditions for which the treatment is straightforward and relatively cheap for the outcome frequently achieved. For instance, many kinds of very expensive chemotherapy regimens for advanced cancer can prolong life but at enormous cost. (See Pirker et al. 2009; De Bono et al. 2011; O'Shaughnessy et al. 2011.)

29. http://www.reuters.com/article/2010/10/13/us-chile-miners -idUSN0925972620101013. At the same time, the distribution of benefits to those we believe do not deserve them—especially if they prevent more "deserving" people from gaining access or receiving them, as with organ transplants for convicted and incarcerated felons—seems to offend our sensibilities and evoke an emotional response the opposite of that suggested by the rule of rescue. I discuss this at length, together with the implications it has for the limits of tolerability of any rationing scheme, in chapter 6.

30. I mentioned this story briefly in chapter 1.

31. I realize that this account differs from that given in chapter 1 where I introduced this story. The "fact" about the money shortfall in the first description was obtained from medical literature reports whereas this current version appeared in a local newspaper around the time of the events. The two can perhaps be reconciled by noting that while the full amount of funding was apparently raised eventually, the amount available at the time that Coby would have been able to benefit from the transplant was insufficient to cover the cost (presumably by $30,000).

32. This can also play out on a grand scale, as shown by the rather sad tale of the therapy of bone marrow ablation by megadose chemotherapy followed by autologous stem cell rescue for advanced breast cancer. Because of the paucity of evidence supporting the efficacy of this treatment, insurers initially refused to pay for it. But a major public relations campaign was initiated by patient advocacy groups, crushing all opposition in their wake by accusing the monolithic

and heartless insurance companies of killing ill women. The ultimate irony was that once sufficient scientific will was generated to actually perform double-blind clinical trials comparing this therapy with standard treatment, the results not only showed there was no advantage to the experimental treatment, but it was more toxic with greater side effects. (See Rosoff 2004; Antman 2002; Kolata and Eichenwald 2000; Mackenzie, Chapman, Salkeld, and Holding 2008; Mello and Brennan 2001; Angell and Kassirer 1994; Rettig, Jacobson, Farquhar, and Aubry 2007.)

33. Although not completely, as the story of Sarah Murnaghan, a child with cystic fibrosis whose lungs were failing. Her only chance at life was a lung transplant. However, the then existing rules for organ allocation precluded her from having access to the much larger donor pool of adult organs and relegated her to the smaller pool of pediatric organs, thus lowering her chances of receiving a transplant. Her parents took to the internet to publicize her case, the story went viral and she not only received a set of lungs, but when those failed, she got another set. See   http://www.reuters.com/article/2013/08/27/us-usa-transplant-pennsylvania -idUSBRE97Q14A20130827 and Halpern 2013.

34. Of course, if the benefit—small as it may be—was also very cheap, then it may not matter all that much if it were offered. However, the overwhelming majority of interventions that provide marginal benefits are also quite expensive, both individually and for what they usually entail as accessory treatments. For example, mechanical ventilation in a patient with advanced-stage lung cancer who is also in heart failure is itself reasonably costly. But this is magnified by the fact that it must be administered in an intensive-care unit along with many expensive medications.

35. See Fleck's discussion and in-depth analysis of democratic deliberation and decision making for what is reasonable in a rationing plan (Fleck 2009).

36. A seemingly insurmountable problem (although we will have to try to solve it) is that the plethora of disease-specific interest groups means that there are legions of committed, desperate patients and their families whose focused, determined, and blinkered devotion to their singular aim makes them unable or unwilling to abandon or even moderate their cause, especially if it means that they might not receive the attention they think they deserve. As an example, if we are trying to be generous in what we will reasonably pay for as well as holding total healthcare costs down, we will have to make difficult decisions about whether to fund hugely expensive treatments for metastatic, end-stage, incurable cancer to extend life for four to six months versus other priorities. The patients with end-stage, incurable cancer will undoubtedly protest, as will the few hundred families whose children have Fabry's disease, treated with the orphan drug Fabrazyme® at about $200,000 per year (http://www.ranker.com/list/world_s-most-expensive -drugs/doctor-baker), if a final rationing plan doesn't pay for their treatment. I realize this may sound harsh, but maybe that is okay, because with the savings we could afford to pay for primary care for everyone or prenatal care for all women. However, this could be a moot point even if we have the resolve to actually get this done. For the moment patients or their families feel that they should get something they have been denied (even if it was the result of a publicly debated

and accepted decision) and they go public, as Coby Howard's mother and friends did, the rule of rescue will become activated and the whole rationing plan could be threatened.

37. For example, unlike in 1989 when the initial law(s) were passed creating the OHP, the State House of Representatives was evenly divided between Republicans and Democrats. Indeed , there were even two Speakers (as of 2011).

38. David Corn, "SECRET VIDEO: Romney Tells Millionaire Donors What He REALLY Thinks of Obama Voters," *Mother Jones*, September 17, 2012, http:// www.motherjones.com/politics/2012/09/secret-video-romney-private-fundraiser.

39. That being said, at least one survey suggests that adults covered by the OHP are satisfied with it, or at least not dissatisfied (Mitchell, Haber, Khatutsky, and Donohughue 2002).

40. http://www.oregon.gov/oha/healthplan/pages/meetings/main.aspx. However, I should note that I could not find direct evidence either for or against this claim, because I could not discover attendance records for these meetings. I also could not find any data or surveys that attempt to assess the popularity (or lack thereof) of the program. It also bears mentioning that the initial effort to solicit and assess public input and opinion occurred prior to the first meetings of the Health Services Commission. However, as far as I could determine, there was no requirement that a specified number of potential recipients of the OHP would have to be present and have their views aired for the process to be considered legitimate and acceptable by this important group. (See Fox and Leichter 1991.) Of course, one could argue that since the original rules governing how the OHP would work were the product of deliberation and a majority vote of the state legislature, then the people (including those who would be affected by the plan as recipients) were represented by their elected officials. However, it would be specious to think that the views of potential beneficiaries were adequately and forcefully expressed on their behalf during the deliberations.

41. The OHP still exists but in a form considerably different from its original iteration. It has now folded in the expansion of Medicaid under the Affordable Care Act (see http://www.oregon.gov/oha/healthplan/Pages/index.aspx).

Chapter 3

1. For readers perhaps not familiar with the term *Hobson's choice* or its derivation, it refers to a situation in which there is the appearance of free choice but there is actually none at all. It is eponymously named after Thomas Hobson, a stable owner in late sixteenth-, early seventeenth-century London. He was known for offering prospective customers the ability to rent any horse in his livery so long as it was the one in the first stall (http://oxforddictionaries.com/us/definition/ american_english/Hobson%27s-choice?q=hobson%27s choice). A more recent example involves Henry Ford. In his autobiography, he first made the statement which is often taken as apocryphal but is true—about the color choices available in his Model T car: "Salesmen always want to cater to whims instead of acquiring sufficient knowledge of their product to be able to explain to the customer

with the whim that what they have will satisfy his every requirement—that is, of course, provided what they have will satisfy these requirements. Therefore in 1909 I announced one morning, without any previous warning, that in the future we were going to build only one model, that the model was going to be 'Model T,' and that the chassis would be exactly the same for all cars, and I remarked: 'any customer can have a car painted any colour that he wants so long as it is black'" (Ford 1922, 72).

2. Jonsen and colleagues (1993) have suggested that this committee and the ethical challenges it faced represented the "birth of bioethics." It is worth noting that the main dilemmas considered at this "birthing" were those of allocating critically scarce resources. Also see Darrah 1987 for an account by a member of the Seattle "God Committee."

3. The political story is beautifully summarized by Blagg (2007). The only caveat was that patients had to be U.S. citizens or permanent residents (holders of a green card) in the United States. As the program has grown almost exponentially (and has at the same time become a very big business for nephrologists and commercial providers of dialysis equipment, care, and associated supplies) the original budget estimates have exploded, so that recent data (from 2009) record ESRD expenditures at about $25 billion with about 10–11 percent growth per year (the latest data is for 2009). (See http://www.usrds.org/2011/view/v2_11.asp, figures 11.4 and 11.5. I discussed this briefly in the previous chapter.)

4. Blagg (2007, 492) paraphrases part of the behind-the-scenes discussion on the development of this program in this way: "Among Finance Committee staff, James Mongan, a physician, argued persuasively that an amendment to this effect should be included because chronic kidney failure was the only situation where money separated individuals from life or death."

5. Kidneys may be a different matter since almost everyone is born with two and can have a reasonably good life with just one. Some people have argued that the way to increase the supply of kidneys for transplant (and the treatment of renal failure with transplantation is considerably more cost-effective than dialysis) is to create a market for kidneys (Friedman and Friedman 2006; Erin and Harris 2003). However, there are powerful arguments against this idea, most notably those that hold that people who might be motivated to sell a kidney are the most exploitable and vulnerable populations in the world (see Satz 2010, chap. 9).

6. Acceptable to those both in and not in the line.

7. I discuss this point later in this chapter as well as in chapter 5, when I discuss a major flaw of the Oregon rationing plan for Medicaid recipients.

8. Both of these infections are common complications in the severely cognitively disabled and frail.

9. For example, see Humphrey 2006 and Henrich et al. 2010. Closely related (if not inextricably intertwined) with the concept of an innate sense of justice is the idea that humans also have inherent tendencies toward altruistic behavior; see Bowles and Gintis 2011. In addition, some have suggested that we also possess what might be labeled the other side of the fairness or altruism coin, a so-called cheater-detection module in our brains. This mechanism presumably prevents us

from all becoming chumps, although we can assume it may not be enormously effective, as demonstrated by some financial scandals in the United States (e.g., Bernard Madoff; for a review, see Machery 2008).

10. In this case Smith was using the term *justice* in a manner indistinguishable from what I am perhaps more coloquially referring to as *fairness*.

11. This assumption was the basis of Rawls's "original position," in which he postulated the state of affairs people would choose if they came together to discuss how to set up the general rules of society without knowledge of their own positions in society or any other facts about their capabilities. Thus, they would be unable to take advantage of the situation to privilege themselves or their location or standing in the eventual setup (Rawls 1999).

12. *Oxford English Dictionary*, http://www.oed.com/.

13. O'Reilly 2009.

14. UNOS still permits patients to be listed at multiple centers under some restrictions, but it does not appear that these restrictions would have prevented Steve Jobs from moving to Memphis and being listed both there (as his primary site) and in California. (See UNOS policy 4, §3.2.2 and §3.2.3, http://optn.transplant.hrsa.gov/policiesAndBylaws/policies.asp.)

15. "Yakuza: Japan's Not-So-Secret Mafia," http://www.cbsnews.com/2100-18560_162-5484118.html.

16. As I discuss in detail in chapter 6, UNOS policy clearly permits non–U.S. citizens or permanent residents to be listed for transplants, up to a maximum of 5 percent of the total, with the proviso that they are not coming to the United States for what they term "transplant tourism." It is arguable whether the Yakuza chieftains who came to California for their liver transplants met the criteria for being transplant tourists. UNOS also does not discriminate against incarcerated or convicted felons, following Supreme Court rulings (this subject is also discussed in chapter 6). (See UNOS policy 6, available at http://optn.transplant.hrsa.gov/policiesAndBylaws/policies.asp, and the UNOS Ethics Committee Position Statement, available at http://optn.transplant.hrsa.gov/resources/bioethics.asp?index=3.)

17. This does not even include the large number of patients who fail to meet the eligibility criteria for "psychosocial" reasons, frequently due to not having sufficient funds to cover both the cost of the transplant itself and the enormous postoperative medication costs.

18. Tavaglione and Hurst 2012; see also Morreim 1991 and Regis 2004. Interestingly, Oberlander and his colleagues have suggested one of the reasons why they and others have concluded that the Oregon Health Plan is not such a terrific model for a comprehensive healthcare rationing plan is that the system is "leaky." Physicians have figured out ways to game the system to avoid strict compliance with the list of covered condition-treatment pairs. In their words:

Establishing an explicit limit on service coverage is much more difficult in practice than in theory. Although the Oregon legislature has drawn a line across the list of prioritized services, that line has been rather fuzzy. Put simply, many Medicaid recipients continue to receive services that are supposedly excluded by the OHP. In large part, this can be attributed to the reticence of providers when it comes to abiding by the rules. The OHP pays for all diagnostic visits and procedures even if treatment is not covered, and physicians have taken advantage of this loop-hole to provide uncovered medical services. Patients presenting with comorbidities have also been diagnosed with conditions covered by the list in efforts by physicians to secure patients' access to services below the line. (Oberlander, Marmor, and Jacobs 2001, 1585)

19. Admittedly, over the past twenty years or so many private insurance companies, Medicare, and Medicaid have placed some restrictions on the ability of doctors to have free rein in prescribing, operating, implanting, and so on, but the truth of the matter is that physicians still retain significant leverage over what gets offered (sold) to patients. Not surprisingly, such influence, when combined with the traditional and still prevalent fee-for-service system of physician payment, can lead to a significant increase in costs due to perhaps inappropriate use. (See the references in the text as well as Cook et al. 2011; Gawande, Jha, Orav, and Joynt 2013; Lenzer 2012; and Rao and Levin 2012.) I discuss this topic further in chapter 7, when I consider a multifaceted approach to controlling healthcare costs within a generalized rationing scheme that calls for generous benefits.

20. The study by Werner and colleagues (2004) also suggested that more than 20 percent of patients thought that gaming the system was acceptable. An important caveat should be noted. No reasonable person could credibly claim that the U.S. healthcare system as it exists today is even remotely fair to any of its participants. These surveys were obviously performed with present-day patients and doctors who deal with the system as it stands. It would be only speculation to suggest that a fair system would inspire more confidence and be viewed as more legitimate, but it is certainly plausible to hold this belief. Certainly legitimacy is a prerequisite for acceptability. It can only be guessed whether doctors and their patients will agree to abide by decisions they wish were otherwise; if they do not, then gaming or other forms of deception and cheating will no doubt continue.

21. Of course, this is a very idealistic view, because it is well known that doctors often subordinate the interests of their patients to their own or at least find a way to serve both of their interests (i.e., everyone wins). One of the most publicized examples is in the area of recommending and prescribing drugs, when physicians will go out of their way to prescribe a treatment manufactured by a company in which they have a financial stake. Or a medical school faculty member may receive research funds from a drug company, or be a member of their paid speakers' bureau and not be completely honest in disclosing this information to patients or other stakeholders. (See Brennan et al. 2006; Campbell et al. 2007; Gray, Hlubocky, Ratain, and Daugherty 2007; Raad and Appelbaum 2012; Werner et al. 2004; Wynia et al. 2000.)

22. This does not mean that the application of fair rules always occurs fairly. That is why Daniels and Sabin included a provision for reasonable appeals of adverse decisions in their procedure; see below. However, Tavaglione and Hurst raise an interesting question: What is a conscientious doctor to do if she wishes to obey the "internal morality of medicine," as they put it, and attempt to ensure that

her patients get what she thinks they need. Should all doctors simply try to game the system when it doesn't given their patients what they want? Or are there more constructive ways of going about trying to *reform* the system? Consider what happens in the psychology of transplant doctors (not just in the story of Steve Jobs where, considering his personality, it seems likely that he may have been the driving force behind manipulating the system). For a report on National Public Radio (NPR) in early 2012, transplant surgeons were interviewed about how they were tempted to misrepresent the severity of their patients' disease in attempts to move them higher on the list to improve their chances of receiving a lung, liver, or other organ. This was not a case of lying to an evil insurance company. It was purposely misrepresenting how sick one's patient was in order to get an organ for her rather than have it go to someone else. Two quotes are instructive: "'I care more about my patients than I care about patients in another city,' says Dr. William Carey, a liver specialist at the Cleveland Clinic. 'And it clearly is in the interest of my patient to get transplanted however I can make that happen.'"; "'That patient is everything,' Budev says. 'And that's why I think we can't be trusted'" (http://www.nepr.net/news/who-decides-whether-26-year-old-woman-gets-lung -transplant).

Now, Tavaglione and Hurst dispute this, and refer to concerns about the overall functioning of a healthcare *system* as a consequentialist criticism of gaming (my emphasis). Furthermore, they stipulate that the healthcare system in their essay is sui generis unjust (but they don't tell us what they mean by this). But by focusing on the individual physician-patient interaction and giving it primacy, they fail to give due deference to other responsibilities physicians have outside of their offices. For example, it may be very respectful of the patient's privacy to not reveal that he has tuberculosis, but it is bad public health policy. Like the allocation decisions transplant doctors make every day, attempting to balance the competing requirements of utility for society (making sure the organ has the best chance of extending life for as long as possible) and the individual (any chance at life), doctors must always keep in mind that they do not practice in a moral or social vacuum. If that practice takes place in a coherent, comprehensive healthcare system in which rationing decisions have been made reasonably and vetted appropriately with suitable avenues for contesting unjust application of the rules, then there are no grounds for lying or gaming the system. The only justification for doing so must be holding the view that one patient (mine) is more important than another (yours), which is untenable both morally and practically. To take another example of a profession with its own "internal morality," the law, how would the admittedly far-from-perfect procedural justice of our court system continue to function if lawyers felt perfectly free to bribe the jury on the grounds that this best served their clients' interests? Interestingly, these authors finally argue that the best way for gaming the system to work on behalf of deprived patients is for doctors to openly coordinate their actions, presumably in some sort of organized protest against the limitations of the system. This removes the taint of subterfuge and deception when it is done "in the closet" as it were, and indeed seems to resemble an appeals process for the injustice of benefit denials. If the system were set up (even nonideally) so that principled objections to benefit denials could be made, then the need for gaming might be greatly diminished, if not eliminated altogether.

The position I am championing takes a larger view of the professional responsibilities of the practicing physician. In a sense, it is a version of a communitarian ethic, mixing the individualistic and personal duties of the doctor to her patient with those to the society in which medical practice exists. It recognizes that the societal rules under which doctors practice coexist with those that govern the private therapeutic encounter. Which has precedence (if one must be so designated) in any given situation is determined by the circumstances and the flexibility of the rules. As in my prior example of the patient with a reportable communicable disease, most physicians would agree that the needs of society outweigh those of patient confidentiality or privacy. Other situations may not be so clearcut or may not have achieved consensus among medical professionals.

Many, if not most, practicing physicians in the United States (myself included) have experienced what we readily diagnose as the obstinate and irrational stupidity of health insurance companies when they deny a patient something we think is essential. When tempers cool, however, several points could be made about this situation. First, the insurance company may actually be right. For instance, in the 1980s and 1990s when they initially denied coverage for high-dose myeloablative chemotherapy with autologous stem cell rescue for advanced breast cancer on the grounds that there was no good evidence for efficacy, there was an enormous hue and cry and public backlash until they were forced to back down. Unfortunately, when the clinical trials were finally done they showed no advantage (and increased toxicity) of the treatment over conventional therapy, so they were proved correct (Rosoff 2004). Second, they could be wrong. In this case, a reasonable system would allow timely appeals that were not simply public relations window dressing so that a good argument could prevail and the rejection could be overturned. Third, the treatment that is desired but rejected could be of such marginal benefit that it is debatable that it should be supported. In this case, with societal rationing in place, it would be a matter of public discussion and discourse about where to draw the line of how little a chance is too little, and doctors will have to accept this for their patients. I discuss line drawing or cutoffs in detail in chapter 4.

23. Cheaters and those who game the system are essentially free riders, people (and their enablers, such as doctors) who reap the benefits the system has to offer but suffer none of the responsibilities required by the system. A good example of this is those parents who refuse to vaccinate their children against infectious disease for whatever (in my view, indefensible) reasons they offer. So long as sufficient numbers of other parents agree to vaccination of their children, the unvaccinated kids are protected by the phenomenon of herd immunity (Luyten, Vandevelde, Van Damme, and Beutels 2011; Bauch, Bhattacharyya, and Ball 2010).

24. For example, see this story in the *New York Times* about how health insurance companies may be trying to buff up their poor public image (http://www.nytimes.com/2012/06/22/us/politics/insurance-companies-are-trying-to-soften-their-image.html?pagewanted=all).

25. Furthermore, if the system had a reliable and accessible mechanism for submitting and expeditiously adjudicating appeals that all (or at least most) of us bought into from the beginning, and not just because we had to, then gaming would be considerably less attractive or "necessary." On the other hand, in the

quasi-free-market system we currently have, doctors and hospitals also manipulate the system for personal gain, such as with the phenomenon of "upcoding" (Silverman and Skinner 2004). Morreim (1991, 445) makes a similar point about stealing from the common-resource pool.

26. *Sacramento Bee*, June 9, 2012, http://www.sacbee.com/2012/06/09/4549499/uc-davis-student-wins-coverage.html.

27. *Boise Weekly*, July 18, 2012, http://www.boiseweekly.com/boise/cancer-patient-fights-insurance-company-for-care-coverage/Content?oid=2687113. Avastin® is the trade name for bevacizumab, a biologic drug that interferes with new blood vessel formation, an antiangiogenic agent. Both of these cases take advantage of what Jonsen called the "rule of rescue," in which we have great sympathy for identifiable lives at risk as opposed to anonymous statistical lives (Jonsen 1986; Largent and Pearson 2012). Hence, we will spare no expense and rush enormous resources to save the five-year-old who has fallen into the well, but will not spend a comparative pittance to save all the nameless five-year-olds from hunger or infectious disease preventable by vaccination.

28. For examples, see Bryant, Worjoloh, Caughey, and Washington 2010; Trivedi, Grebla, Wright, and Washington 2011; and Robbins, Siegel, and Jemal 2012. Of course, it does not necessarily follow that those who receive more interventions or treatments or laboratory tests do better than those who do not. There are downsides to getting extra lab tests (like unnecessary surgery for false-positive results), invasive interventions and drugs that have unintended negative side effects, and the like. However, if the intervention is known to be effective for a specific indication and it is not offered for nonmedical reasons (such as race, poverty, immigration status, and the like), then it is not unreasonable to expect that patients will not do as well (as a group) as those who receive the intervention.

29. For example, Mechanic (1995, 1658) relates the following personal anecdote, which is telling:

In 1961, while teaching at the University of Washington Medical School, I was lunching with the chief nephrologist, a pioneer in establishing the first chronic dialysis unit for patients with end stage renal disease. The unit had developed an evaluation process in which community representatives participated to allocate the scarce places available on the artificial kidney. There was much criticism of the procedures used, but it was the process then in place. During lunch the chief was informed that the state's senior senator, a powerful figure in Washington and a strong friend and promoter of the medical school, was insistent that a friend with kidney failure should have dialysis, though it was unclear that he could receive this service through the usual process. While we sat there a plan was made to bypass the allocation committee by giving this patient dialysis as a research subject. I suspect that the rich and powerful if sufficiently motivated will always find ways to circumvent explicit criteria.

This is an extremely important observation. Some people will always be better situated to obtain things they want because of who or what they are: white, rich, the winning football coach, the cousin of the hospital's CEO, a powerful politician, and so forth. The point is whether that should matter. If an allocation system is to have legitimacy for all, it must be inclusive and not embrace "special" people.

30. Caplan 1995.

31. While it would appear to be unquestionable that an essential component of the human condition is that we are all susceptible to disease, old age, and death, it is also true that this susceptibility is not equally distributed (at least for the first of the three). It is clear that some people, whether by virtue of a genetic predisposition and/or their living conditions such as poverty, environmental exposures, and the like, are more at risk than others for suffering the burdens of illness. While there may be the rare individual who appears to live a charmed life seemingly free of all ailments and complaints, the more common—if not ubiquitous—state of affairs is the opposite. Until relatively recently our ability to predict who would stand a greater chance of contracting illnesses compared to others was based on epidemiology. For example, it has been well known that extreme poverty places persons at jeopardy to a number of diseases that are almost unheard of (unless by accident) in people with more privileged living circumstances. However, the advent of the fine-grained dissecting of the human genome has made it increasingly likely that there will be an enhanced ability to predict risk factors for numerous illnesses for individuals. This places even greater stress on the notion that we have a shared susceptibility to disease, as noted in the Swedish report and in most conceptions of justice in healthcare. Indeed, it was in recognition of the potential for injustice and bias that the U.S. Congress passed the Genetic Information Nondiscrimination Act of 2008 (GINA), which specifically prohibits employment and health insurance discrimination based on one's genetic information (see http://www.eeoc.gov/laws/statutes/gina.cfm). And a popular component of the Affordable Care Act has been the elimination of the ability of health insurance companies to deny coverage to patients with preexisting conditions, an obvious hallmark of further risk for disease. The point is that we can no longer take for granted this somewhat naive approach to de novo equality that is often viewed as the basis for discussions of fairness. Rather, it should be taken as a given that one's genetic endowment, while most often not a guarantee of one's future, can be seen as a Sword of Damocles hanging over one's potential well-being and should therefore inspire measures to counteract its corrosive effects on justice.

32. This is an extremely important point because it means that using strict cost-effectiveness analysis (CEA)—as the Oregon Health Commission started out doing and discovered (to their dismay) that it had some unpredicted consequences that were unacceptable (see chapter 2)—may be untenable by itself. Thus any approach in which this kind of thinking is incorporated must be tempered by other considerations, as embodied in the other two principles. (See Brock 2006; Cookson, McCabe, and Tsuchiya 2008; Walker and Siegel 2002; Eddy 1992a, 1992c, 1992b.)

33. The phrase "physiologically futile" refers to treatments or interventions that couldn't possibly work, given our knowledge of human biology, pathophysiology, and other specialties. For example, if someone has a cold caused by an adenovirus and demands treatment with an antibacterial antibiotic like amoxicillin, this could reasonably be refused on the grounds that it was physiologically useless (futile) (Schneiderman, Jecker, and Jonsen 1990; Bernat 2005). On the other hand, there could be a legitimate debate on anything else, so long as there was some reason to believe that there was even a theoretical chance of success. The argument will be over how little a chance is too little, and this will be a substantive compo-

nent of any discussion about limitations in available healthcare interventions in rationing. I discuss this in greater detail in chapters 4 and 6.

34. Leonard Fleck (2009) calls this imperfect form of justice achieved by democratic consensus "just enough."

35. If nothing is done to slow down the current annual rise in total U.S. healthcare costs, it is projected to reach 20 percent of GDP by the year 2020. In 2011 it was about 18 percent. (See Berwick and Hackbarth 2012; Keehan et al. 2011.)

36. A study by the Institute of Medicine estimates that up to a third of U.S. healthcare dollars may be attributable to waste, overhead, fraud, and so on and could be cut without appreciably affecting the quality of care. The report is available at http://iom.edu/Reports/2012/Best-Care-at-Lower-Cost-The-Path-to-Continuously-Learning-Health-Care-in-America.aspx.

37. It is interesting to observe that if we were ever able to achieve a universal system that was generous and fair and that restricted some forms of healthcare interventions, many people would have access to types of care that were never available to them before. Others, of course, might find themselves denied interventions that they had previously enjoyed or to which they felt entitled. However, I would hope and perhaps expect that they would still be able to purchase these services privately and I would imagine that a robust and flourishing market would emerge to satisfy these desires. The point is that most people would be either extremely pleased with what was newly obtainable or not notice much difference between what was on the "menu" then and now.

38. In some ways this echoes the approach taken by Scanlon when he speaks of options that people have "no reason to reject," a somewhat softer view than the stronger, affirmative one used by Daniels and Sabin (Scanlon 1998).

39. This may be thought to be a potentially controversial principle since it implies that people believe they have been mistreated as a result of a misapplication of the rules. (Or, presumably, they believe that the rules themselves may be unfair or inappropriate, although it may be assumed that this kind of argument would be hashed out before the final rules were adopted by some form of consensus agreement.) Under our current adversarial civil legal system in the United States, this translates into the ability of patients to sue healthcare providers (mostly doctors, as well as the institutions for which they work) for malpractice claims. Careful thought must be given to how this might work under a comprehensive rationing system. I discuss this in greater detail in chapter 6.

40. Quoted from Rosoff 2012b, 2, which was adapted from Daniels and Sabin 2008, 45. These are similar to the six criteria essential to procedural justice listed by Tsuchiya et al. 2005.

41. See the first scenario I described above, as well as my discussion of wealthy people gaming the transplant system for their own benefit. Of course prominent people not infrequently have prominent doctors who are better situated to game the system on their behalf, so it may not take something as blatantly obvious as a bribe to get things moving.

42. As Paul Starr (1982, chap. 4) pointed out in his monumental history of the development of modern American medicine (and physicians), after the emergence of scientific medicine, the hospital evolved from a place where the poor went to be

sick and die to one where increasingly more prominent and influential members of society sought care and cures. In the early part of this evolution most wards were teaching departments where patients received free care (often their only opportunity to receive medical care at all) in return for which they were cases that medical students and house staff could study. Obviously, what was learned could then be put to good use by treating paying patients elsewhere. As late as the 1970s and early 1980s when I began my career, university teaching hospitals still could be segregated into "private" patients and "ward" patients, the latter often being poor and ethnic minorities.

43. There is evidence that suggests that VIPs who are receiving "special" treatment may not do as well as regular garden-variety, everyday folks. For example, a relatively naive VIP patient might think that he wants the chair of the department to insert his intravenous line or perform his ECG, not realizing that it may have been years since that physician actually performed those procedures, compared with the highly skilled staff who do them hundreds of times a week. (See Diekema 1996; Guzman, Sasidhar, and Stoller 2011; Smally et al. 2011.)

44. As it does for organ transplants: but there are other issues that complicate the execution of this principle that I discuss in chapter 6.

45. Fleck 2009, chap. 1.

46. In the debate about healthcare insurance and reform it is common to hear the accusation that members of Congress should be at least as generous to the public in bestowing coverage benefits as they are to themselves, with their "gold-plated" and "Cadillac" insurance package. See http://www.washingtonpost.com/blogs/federal-eye/post/health-care-for-congress-examined/2012/05/07/gIQAFZZi8T_blog.html.

47. Indeed, it was in part the apparent secrecy and lack of transparency, as well as a failure to engage the public, that contributed to the failure of the Clinton health plan process (Yankelovich 1995; Thomas 1995–1996; Disch 1996).

48. The purposeful adjustment of the truth, imparting a sheen or veneer of sincerity and veracity to what is, at bottom, a mendacious effort to coldly manipulate how the uninformed view a specific process, is an artful example of Frankfurt's explication of bullshit (Frankfurt 2005). Of course, one could argue that a successful transmission of "spin" (or bullshit) could effectively fool people into thinking that a rationing scheme was good for them, but it is likely that sooner or later the truth would be discovered, producing both a sense of betrayal and even more distrust of decision making than previously existed. (See also Lenzer 2003.)

49. I discuss this last point in much greater detail in chapter 6.

50. Bratton, Chavin, and Baliga 2011; Creecy and Wright 1990; Davidson and Devney 1991.

51. U.S. Renal Data System (USRDS), *2012 Annual Data Report: Atlas of Chronic Kidney Disease and End-Stage Renal Disease in the United States*, National Institutes of Health, National Institute of Diabetes and Digestive and Kidney Diseases, Bethesda, MD, 2012, http://www.usrds.org/adr.aspx.

52. In chapter 7 I discuss (in general terms) how this approach, combined with other cost-saving measures, could help stem the escalation in healthcare expen-

ditures and perhaps actually reduce the amount of GDP devoted to healthcare, at the same time producing better health outcomes similar to those obtained in Western Europe and Japan.

53. As I discuss in greater detail elsewhere, mistrust in the decisions by members of the healthcare system, be they individual doctors or institutions, can have a significant distorting and corrosive effect on present-day decisions by patients. For example, ample data demonstrate that African Americans choose significantly more aggressive care at the end of life than other ethnic groups. This is seen from a variety of data, including Medicare costs in the last six months of life and responses to surveys. A significant contributor to this state of affairs is the sordid history of rampant discrimination against African Americans in access to many forms of medical care. A suspicion that doctors who wish to remove life support from patients, even if a dispassionate view would agree with such a decision (for instance, being blinded to the ethnicity of the patient), may be partially grounded in the belief that this action is being recommended *because of* the patient's race. In this view, the role of the family is to guard against discriminatory actions. While most ICU doctors (and others often involved in the care of dying patients) would no doubt argue that their decisions are made solely on the medical evidence, irrespective of other features of the patient, there is a large amount of data that disputes this. For instance, African Americans are much less likely to receive certain high-tech treatments than non–African Americans. Resolving these prejudices (in both directions) will be a major challenge for any future rationing scheme. That said, as I discuss in the next chapter, that resolution may have been at least partially accomplished with organ transplantation. (See Blackhall et al. 1999; Brandon, Isaac, and LaVeist 2005; Fairrow, McCallum, and Messinger-Rapport 2004; Harris, Gorelick, Samuels, and Bempong 1996; Jacobs et al. 2006; McKinley, Garrett, Evans, and Danis 1996; Shavers, Lynch, and Burmeister 2000, 2001; Bickell et al. 2006; Farmer et al. 2009; Gregory, LaVeist, and Simpson 2006; Barnato et al. 2009; Farjah et al. 2009; Hanchate et al. 2009.)

Chapter 4

1. As I have discussed in earlier chapters, I suspect that the only plausible way in which Americans would accept a comprehensive rationing plan would be if it were quite generous, perhaps to a fault. Thus, the savings to be realized would most likely be derived from eliminating "waste" in the system (administration, unnecessary tests, etc.), no longer covering marginally beneficial or non-evidence-based care, offering coverage to the vast numbers of people who currently have no insurance (especially primary care), and changing physician reimbursement models, to mention a few. Nevertheless, to "sell" such as approach, Americans would have to believe that they were receiving a good deal, equal to or better than that they have at present. This would include all of the above considerations as well as those ensuring that the deficiencies of less well-funded comprehensive healthcare systems—such as long waiting times for some kinds of elective surgery (such as joint replacements or nonemergency coronary artery surgery) and minimizing choice in doctors and hospitals be reduced to a tolerable level.

2. I do not mean to deny that there would be a formidable array of interest groups—both industrial and patient/disease-based—aligned against any kind of plan that would or could be interpreted as causing them to lose something to which they believed themselves entitled. No doubt these forces would represent the most significant practical obstacles to approval and implementation of this kind of healthcare reform. I discuss these challenges in more detail in chapter 7.

3. I consider what might be called the downside of this approach in chapter 6, where the opinions of the public could engender less-than-noble impulses involving gross prejudice. Indeed, one form of cutoff that I do not consider in this chapter concerns the limit of permissibility of morally unjustifiable restrictions in any publically funded and endorsed scheme of benefits (such as healthcare).

4. In the original and subsequent formulations of this idea in the 1980s and later, it was suggested that a full lifespan would be about seventy years. With the expansion of life expectancy in the developed, industrialized world to eighty years and beyond, one wonders if this should be revised. If so, it has practical implications for the age range in which we would consider someone to be eligible for some types of healthcare resources. Callahan (1987, 1990, 2009) also speaks to this when he writes about older adults who have already lived a long life not needing expensive new medical technologies or treatments at the expense of the young or society in general.

5. I also suspect that these cases will be those that will commonly be publicized and evoke the "rule of rescue," as discussed in chapter 3.

6. The problem of lingering uncertainty in prognostication for many and perhaps most conditions is usually due to the difficulty of assigning definitive predictions to an individual patient that are abstracted from population data. This can often be distilled into the vignette of the doctor stating to the patient that she has a 50 percent chance of recovery or cure, but the patient wanting to know "but what does that mean for *me*; what are *my* chances?" Of course the answer is unknown because the initial probability estimate came from comparing the patient with a similar group—similar, but not identical. Moreover, for rare disorders, population data may be lacking and it is the physician's best estimate (guess) that may be the arbiter. Finally, there are always outliers, such as the proverbial patient who has a fatal disease and then lives. This kind of uncertainty raises the question of whether we should continue to commit untold amounts of money to try to save everyone with a "fatal" condition, when in fact we may only be able to cure extraordinarily few individuals (and, unfortunately, we do not know which of the many who are treated fall into this category). Most people reasonably say no until it is a loved one who is very sick.

7. Of course, it also depended on what made it onto the list and where it was located. This in turn was based on the methods employed to analyze medical situations and their efficacy and cost.

8. As I have suggested, my bet is that because the decisions were being created by the payers for those who were the payees (so to speak), and the former were not affected directly by the outcome of the choices made, the representatives really didn't have any "skin in the game" and their self-interest was not at stake. How-

ever, if all were affected—meaning everyone was covered by a universal health plan—my suspicion is that it would be considerably more generous (as, for example, Medicare is) than the OHP. That does not mean that cutoffs would not need to be constructed, and how that might be done is the main subject of this chapter, but both the budget period–to–budget period variability and the pain felt by those who might think their condition-treatment pair was not being covered, would be minimized.

9. A current example of a program that does it differently is the End-Stage Renal Disease program, a component of Medicare. Here the number of patients being prescribed dialysis (and kidney transplantation) dictates the annual budget. This is not to say that a generous funding of this program with a preset budget determining how many patients could then receive dialysis would not be either preferable or ethical, but the existing approach avoids hard decisions and rationing.

10. It is this attribute of much population data, including IQ, that inspired Hernstein and Murray to entitle their book *The Bell Curve* (1994). Aside from the many methodological problems with their analysis (ably summarized by Stephen J. Gould in *The Mismeasure of Man* [1981] and more modestly by me [Rosoff 2010]), they have failed to acknowledge one of the most important and inherent characteristics of measurements such as IQ (i.e., such measurements are determined by the way the tests were/are created and scored). Importantly, IQ also varies continuously, meaning that it is somewhat arbitrary to draw discrete borders and make cutoffs between, say, cognitively disabled people and those just above them on the distribution curve. To be more specific, the Gaussian curve is more formally known as a "continuous probability distribution." As Rosner (2000, 117) puts it, "Many random variables, such as the distribution of birth weights or blood pressures in the general population, tended to approximately follow a normal distribution. In addition, many random variables that are not themselves normal are closely approximated by a normal distribution when summed many times."

11. Medicine does this routinely with laboratory values or constellations of symptoms and physical signs that help in distinguishing between the sick and the not-sick or diseased and well, or someone with liver disease and someone with a normal liver. With lab test values, abnormal results are frequently defined as +/- 2 standard deviations from the mean, with the mean being established in the population of interest. This latter point is important because in heterogeneous populations, the mean can vary. For example, a significant percentage of African Americans have a lower mean white blood cell count than European Americans. This is without clinical importance. But if one used the same standard-value blood counts for everyone in the United States, one might conclude that large numbers of African Americans had a blood disorder when they in fact do not (Hsieh et al. 2007; Reed and Diehl 1991; Reich et al. 2009).

12. Though perhaps not. Virtually all of the published surveys of public opinions about age preference in distributing important goods (such as solid organs for transplant, pandemic flu vaccines, etc.) have approached the problem by using scenarios with large dichotomous differences between the two age examples, thus avoiding the cutoff issue.

13. For example, see Chen, Cohen, and Chen 2007; Dawson and Weiss 2012; and Streiner 2002. And for a practical example of the inherent problems and dramatic effects this issue can have on clinical care, see Courdi et al. 1988.

14. One would think so, but it is indeed ironic and perhaps indicative of the dysfunction of our confused and heterogeneous healthcare system that the budgets for Medicare and Medicaid are not truly fixed and are dependent upon how much medical care is dispensed.

15. Richard S. Foster (Chief Actuary, Centers for Medicare and Medicaid Services), testimony to the House (U.S.) Committee on the Budget, February 28, 2012, p. 3 (http://budget.house.gov/uploadedfiles/fostertestimony_2-28-22012.pdf).

16. Some would also argue that we should limit access to massive amounts of healthcare resources to the very young as well, especially extremely premature infants and babies under one year of age who have severe and/or multiple congenital defects. The rationale for the former is that many of these infants have significant complications, often requiring lifelong care for serious disabilities, while the latter is additionally grounded on the belief that such young people have not yet had the opportunity to establish consequential connections or a foothold in life (to the extent that older children have) and hence their loss is less of a tragedy (and thus not worth the cost compared with other claims on the money) than that of an older child. Not surprisingly, many people regard such views with skepticism, if not downright horror and hostility. (See Dworkin 1993.)

17. For example, Rawls (1999) might suggest that it is just these people, the less fortunate, who should deserve more attention than their similarly aged peers who have been more advantaged or have been able to accomplish more both by their own efforts and because their station in life might have predisposed them to success. Of course, one could observe that the time to make amends is not near the end of people's lives when their ability to accomplish goals is minimized by the toll of years; rather, interventions should be designed to even the playing field in their youth.

18. "Given the importance that Eskimos attached to the aged, it is surprising that so many Westerners believe that they systematically eliminated elderly people as soon as they became incapable of performing the duties related to hunting or sewing. It is true that, in some regions, when a famine was in progress, an aged person might voluntarily venture out into a storm or into bitter cold weather to starve or freeze to death in order to leave what food there was for younger family members. Or sometimes, when people were moving to new hunting grounds, a heavy load, poor traveling conditions or infirmity might contribute to an elderly person's decision to be left behind without food or shelter. But Eskimos believed that death was just a temporary phase of life, a recycling of the soul from one body to another that would appear in due course. When, during a period of great hunger, an old woman quietly went out to meet certain death in the midst of a raging storm, everyone understood that her soul would return soon in the form of a baby. When a child was born, her name would be bestowed upon it, and within weeks people would notice how this and that trait of the old woman was beginning to emerge in its form and movements. Infanticide, or the systematic execution of babies, is similarly misunderstood. It was indeed practiced in a few

Eskimo groups from time to time. It was most common in regions where life was particularly harsh, but even there it normally occurred only during an extreme shortage of food" (Burch 1988, 21).

19. For example, see Chasteen and Madey 2003.

20. Perhaps ironically and certainly counter to this widely held view, the United States continues to spend an overwhelming amount of its healthcare dollars on care for older adults, a trend that is only expected to increase as the baby-boom generation becomes eligible for Medicare (Keehan et al. 2008; Agency for Healthcare Research and Quality 2006, http://www.ahrq.gov/research/ria19/expendria.htm).

21. The length of this normal life is often expressed by the authors, perhaps more for stylistic purposes, as "three score and ten" (Daniels 1983, 1988; Callahan 1987, 1990, 2009). But the truth of the matter is that life expectancy has continued to increase, and even if we examine the amount of time people can live independently, this too, has lengthened. Admittedly, the rate of increase has slowed, but a person born today in the United States can expect to live quite a bit longer, all things being equal, than his and especially her grandparents. Of course there are many confounding variables, the most important of which may be the social and economic circumstances into which one has been born. For example, the differential life expectancy between Caucasian and African-American men continues to be significant and can only be partially explained by reference to socioeconomic status (Arias, Rostron, and Tejada-Vera 2010; Geruso 2012).

22. Many people, certainly cardiologists and cardiothoracic surgeons, would also argue that for those patients who may not be heart transplant candidates for one reason or another or who are waiting for a transplant, an alternative therapy now exists that may be palatable, namely, left ventricular assist devices or LVADs. Now that they are quite small with portable battery packs, they can permit many patients to lead somewhat normal (albeit restricted) lives while they are either waiting for a heart or not. The main drawback, aside from the usual clinical toxicities associated with implantable cardiac devices, is their extremely high cost. However, because Medicare has approved these machines, almost all the cost is borne by the government; in 2009 the annual cost for an LVAD was more than $200,000 per patient (Mulloy et al. 2012; also see Lund, Matthews, and Aaronson 2010; Slaughter, Meyer, and Birks 2011; Johri, Damschroder, Zikmund-Fisher, and Ubel 2005; Parr et al. 2010).

23. The prototype for the latter class of interventions might be continued intensive-care life support for someone who meets the criteria for whole-brain death and is thus legally dead. These cases are far less common that those with some minimal ongoing, expected, or hoped for benefit.

24. It is interesting to note that the somewhat insidious ways often-expensive new medical technologies increase market share in the United States also tend to feed the desires of people to obtain them. For example, it is quite common for novel devices that have been FDA approved for a fairly narrow use (analogous to FDA approval for drugs and their indications) to gradually expand their market share to include types of patients and conditions beyond what the original data would support. Not surprisingly, device companies and the doctors that use the devices (and are often employed by the companies as "consultants") find this

practice conducive to their mutual financial benefit, especially in a fee-for-service environment. The final linchpin in this cabalistic alliance is the generation of demand from patients or disease-representative groups, often without reference to any substantial body of data supporting the efficacy of the intervention.

25. Peppercorn et al. 2011; Jox, Schaider, Merckmann, and Borasio 2012; Coller 2011; Schneiderman 2011b; Meadow et al. 2012.

26. Berwick and Hackbarth 2012.

27. See McGlynn et al. 2003; for an interesting discussion from a business-efficiency point of view, see http://blogs.hbr.org/2009/08/how-effective-is-american-heal.

28. See www.pcori.org.

29. Perhaps most significant (if not sadly), PCORI was prevented from factoring costs into the data or the results they generated and hence into their recommendations. Thus, an intervention could pass muster from the standpoint of efficacy if it were demonstrated to be as effective as some other treatment, even if it were vastly more expensive: PCORI is prevented from recommending a (relatively) cheap therapy over a much more expensive one (Mortimer and Peacock 2012). A related agency is the U.S. Preventive Services Task Force, which issues periodic reports on the utility of various medical interventions. On the surface, it seems somewhat bland, but recent experience has demonstrated that it has the ability to provoke enormous controversy. For example, its recommendation to limit the use of routine screening mammography to women deemed high risk was met with a perfect storm of protest by women's groups, breast cancer advocacy groups, surgeons, radiologists, and others. Even though the report justified its suggestions with substantial data showing the risks of mammography (radiation exposure, false positives leading to excess unneeded surgeries, false negatives in younger women, enormous expense, etc.) as well as the minimal benefit of expansive screening, it didn't seem to matter. As I will discuss shortly, this episode (and others) should reveal the hazards ahead of using marginal benefit as a yardstick for reining in healthcare costs and as a rationing target. (See U.S. Preventive Services Task Force 2009; Hendrick and Helvie 2011; Squiers et al. 2011; Volk and Wolf 2011; and a *USA Today* story on the hullabaloo: http://usatoday30.usatoday.com/news/health/story/2012-07-14/health-task-force-mammograms-psa/56205978/1.)

30. Indeed, if one undertakes a quick review of the groups that opposed the mammography recommendations, chief among them were radiologists and surgeons whose practice income would be directly affected (lowered) if the guidelines were followed. The problem of physician conflicts of interest pervades the creation of clinical guidelines, and indeed FDA expert committees as well, with many members being recognized for their expertise by drug and device companies that employ them as outside consultants. Hence, it is often difficult to find enough specialists who are authorities in their field and who can serve as unbiased members of committees charged with setting standards or providing advice for clinical practice on the use of various therapies and diagnostics. (See Guyatt et al. 2010; Neuman 2011; Norris, Homer, Ogden, and Burda 2011.)

31. An objection may be made to my assertion about drugs. After all, aren't all prescription medications in the United States approved by the FDA as both "safe and effective"? That is undoubtedly true. However, the bar for efficacy can sometimes be surprisingly low. For example, Brentuximab vedotin (Adcetris®) is approved for use in relapsed Hodgkin's disease and another rare form of lymphoma (anaplastic large-cell lymphoma), which have the protein "CD30" on the surface of their malignant cells. It was approved after testing (no randomized controlled clinical trials) in fewer than 200 patients. It can cost up to $100,000 for one course of treatment (http://www.medicalnewstoday.com/articles/233141.php).

32. Buyx, Friedrich, and Schöne-Seifert 2011. For another way of looking at this issue, see Hoffman and Pearson 2009.

33. An example of the first case might be the use of the drug erlotinib in combination with another, older chemotherapy agent for treatment of advanced pancreatic cancer, an almost uniformly fatal disease. This combination increases *average* survival by 0.4 months (less than 2 weeks) compared to the standard drug alone (http://www.cancer.gov/cancertopics/druginfo/fda-erlotinib-hydrochloride#Anchor-Pancreati-44285), and costs almost $17,000 (in 2006; Grubbs, Grusenmyer, Petrelli, and Gralla 2006). An example of the second case might be the treatment of Pompe disease (acid alpha-glucosidase deficiency) with glucosidase (Myozyme®). This is a very rare genetic disorder that is often fatal if untreated. This drug costs between $100,000 and $300,000 per patient per year, depending on the size of the person (http://www.forbes.com/2010/02/19/expensive-drugs-cost-business-healthcare-rare-diseases_2.html).

34. On the other hand, if the 1 percent chance of cure in the six-year-old actually works, then that lucky child goes on to live a full lifespan (presumably), but if the same cure occurred in the eighty-year-old, the number of years gained by that success would be constrained by the actuarial life expectancy of someone at that age (presumably less that the now-cured six-year-old). Not factored into this analysis is what the other 99 percent of patients who are treated (unsuccessfully) must go through in order to have the chance of a cure; it is not at all uncommon for there to be significant suffering from side effects and other unwanted events in the search for the restoration of health, and it is not at all clear that it such experiences are worthwhile either for society or for the individual. In an often-cited article, Schneiderman and his colleagues attempted to define what is meant by futile care, technically indicating that some form of desired or existing intervention can't work. While they distinguish true physiological futility (absolutely no chance of working as defined by biology such as cardiopulmonary resuscitation in someone who is actually dead) as unique, something different is most often encountered in the hospital and clinic. They proposed using an arbitrary cutoff on less than a 1 percent chance of achieving the stated goals (whatever they might be) as a practical, workable definition. They qualified their proposal by suggesting that the "data" or information used to create this performance assessment could come from the literature or personal clinical experience, thus leaving it wide open to potential bias. (See Schneiderman, Jecker, and Jonsen 1990, 1996, as well as Rosoff 2012b for my critique Schneiderman and policies derived from his proposal.)

35. Not surprisingly (at least to me, but I have been associated with academic medical centers and intensive-care units for many years), many ICU directors make these kinds of allocation decisions all the time. (See Courtwright 2012.)

36. It is difficult to imagine that cynical players of all stripes would not resort to "rule-of-rescue" publicity to obtain funding for their particular disease or condition and thus place it above the cutoff line. If this were the case, then we might find ourselves in a bind: we think marginally beneficial treatments should be covered, because we are struck by the pathos of Coby Howard stories, but then we realize that we actually don't want to pay for these treatments. I would not venture a guess as to which side in this emotional and economic tug of war would win out.

37. Indeed, the most recent updated data suggests that this trend is not decreasing. As Teno and her coauthors note, "Although the CDC reports that decedents aged 65 years and older are more likely to die at home, our results are not consistent with the notion that there is a trend toward less aggressive care. Between 2000 and 2009, the ICU utilization rate, overall transition rate, and number of late transitions in the last 3 days of life increased" (Teno et al. 2013, 476; for another perspective, see Lenzer 2012).

38. As a good explanation of this problem in the terminal cancer situation, see Smith and Hillner 2010. Unfortunately, these authors do not address the question of whether interventions that offer only incremental or marginal benefit should be available at all. They prefer to lay out the information to patients and let them make the decision. In other words, everything is on the menu, and the role of the oncologist is to guide the decision. However, while by no means impugning the motivation of these authors (or anyone else involved in the care of cancer patients), it should be pointed out that the current reimbursement structure for chemotherapy is such that much of an oncologist's income is derived from prescribing and administering chemotherapy. Thus there might be an inherent conflict of interest: doctors who dispense less chemotherapy get paid less.

39. This proposal turns out to be more challenging that one might think on initial reflection, because many "experts" turn out to also be considered as such by the pharmaceutical and medical device industries, which pay them hefty fees for consulting and other services. Thus avoiding these inherent conflicts of interest is quite difficult in practice, other than by avoiding the use of experts at all, which seems self-defeating. This situation has led some commentators to question how untainted or unbiased many clinical guidelines may actually be. (See Steinbrook 2009; Guyatt et al. 2010; Mendelson et al. 2011; Jones et al. 2012.)

40. http://www.nice.org.uk/; http://www.ahrq.gov/clinic/uspstfix.htm.

41. Countering this pessimism is our experience with drug shortages in which we have found surprisingly little resistance—if not outright acceptance—of the rationing plan. Perhaps the fact that it is a medical staff policy endorsed by physicians has contributed to its (so far) benign integration into practice (Rosoff et al. 2012). Furthermore, the decreasing accounts of transplant doctors manipulating the priority lists to favor their own patients also attest to some optimism that this sort of behavior might minimized under a favorable rationing plan with generous benefits. Admittedly, the situation may have improved with transplants in large

part due to a greater reliance on laboratory data and auditing of individual institutions, but this should not diminish the hope that similar perspicacity could limit the well-intentioned mendacity of some overly enthusiastic doctors.

42. Doctors also remain fond of anecdotal reports from either their own practice experience or that of others (Aronson 2003; Butterworth 2009; Cochrane et al. 2007; Baiardini et al. 2009).

43. Aronson 2003; Butterworth 2009; Cochrane et al. 2007; Hamann et al. 2005; McKinstry et al. 2006; Melis et al. 2010; Qaseem et al. 2010; Lugtenberg, Zegers–Van Schaick, Westert, and Burgers 2009. While guidelines can be very effective in informing doctors of the state of the art, they are far from perfect, dependent as they are on "experts" who themselves may have significant challenges (see Shaneyfelt and Centor 2009 as well as Guyatt et al. 2010).

44. Gerber, Patashnik, Doherty, and Dowling 2010. This was a very interesting study since it could break respondents down into subgroups depending on their professed political party allegiance, whether they voted in the 2008 election, and various demographic features (age, ethnicity, etc.). It showed that there were significant differences in attitudes between these various groups, which could have a major effect on how any national rationing plan were "sold" to a heterogeneous populace. For example, as discussed in chapters 1 and 2, trust that the system is fair and equitable, and that it is not necessarily taking something important away from individuals that they already possess (or think they do) or want, may be largely dependent on preformed and deeply held beliefs about the role and trustworthiness of the government in peoples' lives. This study demonstrates that there are clear divisions along political lines, with people who profess to be Republicans having much less confidence in the reliability of the government (and its representatives) than those who claim to be Democrats. Of interest was the observation that a statement that doctors endorse comparative-effectiveness research persuaded a large majority of respondents to support it, validating the weight patients often give to the opinions of physicians. However, what people say and then do may be discordant, because individuals who professed to be violently opposed to programs run by the federal government (especially healthcare programs) also did not want anyone messing with their Medicare or Social Security benefits: "At a recent town-hall meeting in suburban Simpsonville [South Carolina], a man stood up and told Rep. Robert Inglis (R-SC) to 'keep your government hands off my Medicare.' I had to politely explain that, 'Actually, sir, your health care is being provided by the government,' Inglis recalled. 'But he wasn't having any of it'" (Rucker 2009, available at http://www.washingtonpost.com/wp-dyn/content/article/2009/07/27/AR2009072703066.html?hpid=topnews&sid =ST2009072703107).

45. One of the most notorious of these was the long-held belief that bone marrow replacement after megadose chemotherapy (so-called autologous bone marrow transplant or ABMT, an obvious oxymoron, but in widespread use) would be effective treatment for advanced breast cancer. This idea took root and blossomed based on some small, Phase 2 (nonrandomized controlled) clinical trials that showed some promising results. A combination of desperate patients, few

effective alternatives, and hopeful (and biased) physicians led to a groundswell of approval and support for this approach, overwhelming the few voices who objected to the flimsiness of the evidence. Insurance companies were initially reluctant to pay for this expensive and unproven therapy, but due to a public relations blitz and accompanying political support, they were forced to comply. Eventually, sufficient concern was raised that several clinical trials were started to actually address the question of whether this therapy offered any advantage over the standard approach. Unfortunately, due to the common "understanding" that there was no question that ABMT of course had to be superior, enrollment of subjects on these trials was very slow, because both patients and their doctors were reluctant to undergo randomization and the 50 percent chance they would be assigned to the control arm of the study. Eventually the trials were completed and showed that there was no survival advantage for the more expensive and toxic ABMT. But between its introduction and almost wholesale acceptance by breast cancer patients and the medical community, thousands of women had been subjected to an unproven treatment. (See Rosoff 2004 as well as Rosoff and Coleman 2011, 668n71, for a more complete explanation and primary references.)

46. There is little dispute that these are the "gold standard," but it is important to note that they may not be possible to perform in some situations for very practical reasons. For example, some diseases or conditions are so uncommon that it wouldn't be feasible to attempt to perform a statistically powered trial to provide an answer to a reasonable therapeutic question. In other cases, prior trials have produced such successful treatments that it would take inordinate numbers of patients to enroll in the trial to be able to answer the question. For instance, in childhood "low-risk" acute lymphoblastic leukemia, the cure rate is greater than 90 percent, so to demonstrate an improvement to 95 percent would take many hundreds of patients to enroll in each arm of the study. This could take years due to the relative rarity of the disease. In these cases, there may be acceptable alternatives, albeit less satisfactory than the RCT.

47. See the discussion above concerning how statistical knowledge may be related to individual instantiations of disease. The entire premise of the doctor's consideration for a single patient's well-being is that she has the skill and the art to be able to distinguish the particular from the general. While it may be quite reasonable to question the validity of this view, it seems to be considered unimpeachable by patients and doctors. The former wishes to feel special and unique (and of course, he is) and not part of the faceless crowd, and there may be no better way to evoke this sensation than to be the recipient of a customized treatment plan that only applies to *me*. We should not underestimate the power this holds.

48. I will have more to say about marginally beneficial interventions in the next chapter when I discuss people who consider themselves losers under rationing.

49. Of course, this is a bias in favor of not providing marginally beneficial interventions, but if that were not palatable, one could also use age or some other metric as a cutoff. My guess is that the former would prove to be the most acceptable, or more realistically, the least objectionable to the most people.

Chapter 5

1. I discussed this challenge in the previous chapter.

2. Recall from my discussion in chapter 3 that one of the hallmarks of a procedurally fair system of rationing would be the enshrining of a formal ability to appeal a decision that one believed to be unfair. However, I purposely did not address there—and will only briefly touch on it here in this chapter—how this could feasibly be accomplished. (Also see Daniels 1993, 2000, 2008; Daniels and Sabin 2008.)

3. I would like to thank Dr. Thomas Gehrig (Duke University Medical Center Department of Medicine, Division of Cardiology) for his advice and assistance in constructing this clinical vignette and ensuring its clinical accuracy.

4. A poignant and relevant example of this is the case of Sunny von Bülow, a wealthy New York woman who lived at Columbia Presbyterian Hospital for almost thirty years in a permanent vegetative state, possibly induced after injections of insulin. Her husband—Claus von Bülow—was tried several times for trying to kill her, eventually being acquitted after sensational trials (sensational enough to inspire a dramatic film based on the story) (http://www.nytimes.com/2008/12/07/ nyregion/07vonbulow.html?pagewanted=all&_r=0). Nevertheless, the point is that her fortune enabled her—or what remained of her—to live in this condition for an extraordinarily long time. It is unlikely that those of us with more modest means would remain biologically alive for so long, irrespective if we wanted to or not. However, as I discuss in more detail in chapter 7, it is likely that any plausible rationing plan that could be acceptable in this country would continue to permit these kinds of choices for those who could afford to make them and so long as there were those willing to offer them.

5. Alpers and Lo 1999; Baily 2011; Davis 2008; Luce 2010.

6. While it is certainly true that some patients receive more and others receive less, even from the same physician and often for the same conditions (as I discussed in chapter 2), these disparities are not similar to a contest where it is "winner take all" or there is something of less or dubious value bestowed as a second or third prize. As I will discuss a bit later in this chapter, the classic healthcare contest in the United States (and other wealthy, developed nations)—in the truest sense of the word—is the competition for solid organs for transplantation. Since there is an absolute limit to the quantity available at any given time, and the number of patients vying for an organ that could truly be to their benefit vastly exceeds that amount, the recipients win and the rest unavoidably lose. The point is that in this kind of a contest, there can only be a binary outcome, and whatever consolation we might offer the "loser" (such as palliative, end-of-life care) pales in comparison to what has been "won" by someone else.

7. The caveat here is that this describes actual situations in which all have access to needed healthcare and it is only the alterations in these baseline conditions that set up the possibility for there to be winners and losers. Of course, in real life, there are massive structural and social barriers that prevent many people from

gaining effective entry into the healthcare system or receiving what they need even if they get their feet in the door, all of which result in enormous disparities in common medical outcomes.

8. One other point about pennies and healthcare deserves to be mentioned. Pennies, like money in general, are summative in the sense that their existence is not time dependent (although their relative value may be due to inflation) and that once I collect sufficient numbers of them I possess something of real value. But healthcare interventions are substantively different because they can rarely—if ever—be added together to get something that is the sum of their parts. They are also not static and very often are both time and context dependent. Notwithstanding these significant distinctions, the analogy is still reasonable to explain my point about relative value.

9. To recall my analogy to the penny or the quarter or the $10 bill on the floor, the futile—or worthless—intervention would equate with either something that looked like a penny, but wasn't, or a single penny on the floor when the least expensive thing that could be bought costs much more (and will not be available in time for someone to save up by picking up lots of pennies). The truly beneficial intervention (as judged by most people) would clearly be similar to the $10 bill, because most people would think it valuable and want to pick it up. The problem is the remainder, ranging from more than a penny up to the $10. This, of course, is a classic example of a cutoff problem, as I discussed in chapter 4.

10. It is not for nothing that in the preantibiotic era pneumonia—specifically that caused by this organism—was referred to as the "old man's friend" due to its predilection for afflicting older people. As Osler (with the later assistance of Mc-Crae) put it: "'Pneumonia may well be called the friend of the aged. Taken off by it in an acute, short, not often painful illness, the old escape those 'cold gradations of decay' that make the last stage of all so distressing" (Osler and McCrae 1912, 75; also see Kaplan et al. 2003).

11. Many people would argue that such care should not be available even if money is not an object, because these interventions don't really help people in a substantive way. (Also see Fleck 2009, 256–259.) The significance of public agreement in this context is worth stressing. As I discussed in chapter 2, the legitimacy of any acceptable and tolerable plan that restricts or limits access to some interventions is based—at least in part—on the fact that the people who it affects (presumably, everyone) would have been persuaded that it is both fair and reasonable, and hence acceptable on those grounds. It is likely that pre-approval discussion about what benefits should and should not be included (and therefore not paid for) would also include a debate on the issue of what is of value to most people if they were in the situation of needing (wanting) a particular intervention. As an example, I suspect that most people would not wish to be kept (biologically) alive if they were in a permanent vegetative state with no expectation of recovering conscious brain function, even though there are a small minority who would. Thus, a "vote" on whether to cover life support for these kinds of patients would presumably be negative. Lest one think that people who are presumed to have closed minds are immune to changing their views about these types of things, it would be worthwhile to review the history of the adoption of the Texas

Advance Directives Act in 1999 by Robert Fine. Fine (2001) recounts how the commission that was empowered to create a draft legislative proposal was at loggerheads until one side was able to be enlightened to the reality of the medical situations of the kinds of patients they were considering. Of note, I and others have recorded our objections to this law (but not for this reason) (Rosoff 2012a; Truog 2007, 2009a).

12. Of course, there is a potential trap even in this fairly simple statement, since it is all relative. If we have unlimited amounts of money to buy unlimited (medical) resources that we can give to anyone who wants them, then the only restriction might be a moral one, whereby we would hesitate to provide the antibiotic for the viral illness because it can't work and there is no reason to satisfy peoples' whims for irrational treatments. On the other hand, where we draw the bottom line for treatments that have the potential for some benefit, even if it's not very much, would depend on how much of the resource we have available. Whether it's dollars or livers, the calculation is the same.

13. It is important to note that a cardinal tenet of a just and ethical allocation system is that similar cases should be treated similarly. If there are two clinically indistinguishable patients and there is only enough medicine (for example) for one, then a method must be used in which there is an equivalent chance of each obtaining the vital resource (see Rosoff 2012b). A critical component of this view is how to judge that cases are similar enough to be considered identical (the operative term in real-life circumstances is "close enough"). Most people are likely to view their own situation as unique and special, hence deserving of greater concern than someone else who an impartial observer would evaluate as "close enough." They would thus deny identity of the relevant clinical conditions. This would only serve to enhance or exacerbate any feelings of loss at not receiving some benefit to which they felt entitled because they deserved it more than the other person with whom they competed for it. The result is a disavowal of the essential fairness of the rationing plan itself. In many ways this is the essential challenge for the development and implementation of just healthcare rationing.

14. The voluntariness of participants in this kind of competition may be debatable. Certainly there are patients who have failing hearts or livers who, while eligible for an organ transplant, choose not to have themselves listed for some reason. Perhaps they do not wish to live with the possibility of another chronic illness (i.e., chronic immunosuppression), or they are relatively young and understand that transplanted organs often have a finite lifespan and they may not wish to need to go through the entire process again in some unknown number of years, or they do not want to jeopardize their family's financial security due to the huge ancillary costs. But if one wants a liver in order to live, one has little choice but to submit to the process and all that it entails. The other point that should be made here is one that I have alluded to previously, and will discuss in some detail shortly: the validity of appeals for redress of perceived wrongful treatment (this should be distinguished from malpractice or negligence, which is an entirely different form of patient mistreatment). Presumably, one would be able to take advantage of an appeals process to plead one's case. It is easy to imagine that this system could be overwhelmed in short order with angry and disgruntled patients,

most of whom do not have legitimate disputes. Having a method to adjudicate warranted grievances and differentiating them from frivolous complaints would be of primary importance. Only the former would be worthy of further consideration for assessment of whether a true loss had occurred.

15. Or someone made a big donation to the transplant program in an attempt to influence their chances of getting an organ: see "Yakuza: Japan's Not-So-Secret Mafia," http://www.cbsnews.com/2100-18560_162-5484118.html. I also described this problem in chapter 3 when discussing fairness.

16. While I have argued that any conceivable and plausible comprehensive healthcare rationing plan in the United States would need to be both just *and* generous to stand a chance of being accepted by the public, this may be variable depending on the population covered by the plan. In Oregon there was initially no attempt to limit the funding of the OHP such that the recipients could be severely affected by the sparse number of healthcare interventions available to them. But it would be relatively simple to imagine scenarios in which a national legislature in thrall to wealthy and well-endowed interest groups representing say, rich people and large corporations wishing to maintain low tax rates, might well limit the funding—therefore increasing the severity of rationing—for a national insurance plan that they could easily supplement with added, purchased policies to make up any difference.

17. The recent revelation that a former dean of the Emory University School of Dentistry permitted Jewish students to enter and matriculate but then expelled them for made-up "academic reasons" solely on the basis of their religion or ethnicity, is an example of this (http://www.nytimes.com/2012/10/07/education/emory-confronts-legacy-of-bias-against-jews-in-dental-school.html?_r=0).

18. For example, in Atlanta, Georgia, Grady Memorial Hospital (the public, municipal institution) was providing chronic dialysis for a large number of illegal (undocumented) immigrants, paying for it out of their own funds. The financial burden threatened to become overwhelming, thus endangering other important clinical programs (including dialysis for the large indigent, native population that Grady has traditionally served). Ironically, end-stage renal disease care is one of the few types of medical intervention almost completely unrationed in the United States by either design or financial happenstance, due to its complete coverage under Medicare (but it only covers American citizens or permanent residents). The attempted resolution to this problem was to give these patients a choice: a time limit at the end of which they would be cut loose from the program or an open offer to repatriate them back to their home countries. Of course, in many cases the latter course of action would have led to the patients' death due to the general lack of availability of this therapy in their countries of origin. Perhaps surprisingly, given the negative public discourse about the treatment of undocumented immigrants, the plan generated a great deal of controversy, eventually leading to a modified approach by the hospital. However, in the interim several patients went back to their homes to an unknown fate. While this situation did not meet the classic definition of rationing, it was certainly the product of a tragic choice that had to be made due to scarce resources. The patients who were to have had their dialysis stopped would definitely be losers. And the fact that care had to be

terminated for these people solely due to their immigration status was relevant to denoting them as such.

19. What qualifies as "fault" may need to be described in greater detail. There are many diseases that are commonly viewed as "failures of personal will," such as alcoholism, nicotine addiction via smoking, obesity, and so on. While ample research has shown that the causes and maintenance of these conditions are considerably more complex, the popular conception is that people bring these disorders on themselves and have only themselves to blame for their predicaments. Therefore, it may be very difficult to achieve a social consensus that these patients are owed anything extra as "losers" in a healthcare rationing scheme for specific therapies (such as organs or other resources that could be needed because of their prior condition).

20. Although there have been several examples of retrospective compensation for past injuries due to bias or discriminatory acts committed by society. For example, the Civil Liberties Act of 1988 (Pub. L. 100–383) stated that surviving American citizens of Japanese ancestry interned during World War II were entitled to compensation as reparations for past injustices. More recently, North Carolina's Eugenics Compensation Task Force voted to provide compensation for surviving victims of that state's eugenics sterilization law and policies dating from the 1920s through 1974 (see http://www.newsobserver.com/2012/01/11/1768861/panel-pay-eugenics-victims-50000.html).

21. Of course, the practical challenge to immediately adjudicating and rectifying many cases of mistreatment due to poor or even malicious misinterpretation or application of otherwise fair rules, may bedevil any form of reasonable and workable appeals process. It is worthwhile mentioning that there is a substantial psychological difference between patients (or their families) who judge themselves to be losers of one type or another, and those judged by an independent or neutral board to be such. For this component of the rationing program to be impartially assessed as unbiased, it will have to scrutinize these types of complaints very seriously. But doing so and giving them their due may very well bog down the process to the point where it grinds to a halt, overcome by both the sheer number of allegations and grievances and the cumbersomeness of the process required to resolve them in a satisfactory manner. It may well be that some form of prescreening procedure—perhaps binding arbitration—would be necessary to streamline the system such that only the most egregious appeals would reach the final "supreme court."

22. A relevant and poignant example comes from the organ transplant field. It is common practice to include an evaluation of the socioeconomic wherewithal and features of the potential transplant candidate and her support systems before deeming her eligible for listing (Dew et al. 2007; Dobbels et al. 2009; Flamme, Terry, and Helft 2008; Kemmer, Alsina, and Neff 2011). This is due to the tremendous cost of the procedure and its aftermath (even when things go well), the intense surgical and medical follow-up required to ensure an optimum outcome (a functioning organ in a functional patient), and the influence of a stable and supportive home environment on transplant success. Not surprisingly, the presence of these positive factors—while certainly justifiable from the point of view of maximizing

the efficiency and efficacy of the transplant process—will disproportionately favor those patients who already possess more than their "fair" share of the material and social advantages in life. Poor and disadvantaged patients in organ failure often fail to meet eligibility criteria, not from a medical point of view, but because of the facts about their impoverished lives. Thus, the system exacerbates already existing inequities. But doing otherwise—for example, by giving an organ to someone whose social situation is such that he cannot "take care of it"—would not only not serve him well but would tend to "waste" an organ that could potentially save someone else's life.

23. Of course, when money is not the primary scarce resource—such as with organ transplantation—a similar situation exists. Some patients still win and others lose, just for different reasons.

24. The MELD score has made the system significantly fairer after a patient is *accepted* as a suitable transplant candidate, but has done nothing to ease the societal problems of major disparities in income and social resources that diminish or eliminate patients' ability to be considered for eligibility for transplant. This is compounded by the fact that the diseases that destroy livers, kidneys, and hearts are also not evenly distributed throughout the population. For example, see U.S. Renal Data System (USRDS) 2011, vol. 2, chap. 1, figure 1a. This figure shows the overrepresentation of African Americans in the population with end-stage kidney disease and who are thus at least nominally eligible for transplantation (available at http://www.usrds.org/2011/view/v2_01.asp).

Chapter 6

1. A remark made by Otto von Bismarck, August 11, 1867; available at http://www.quotationspage.com/search.php3?homesearch=politics+is+the+art+of+the+possible&startsearch=Search.

2. This epigraph is conventionally interpreted as saying that duties or obligations have force on an individual or agent only if they can actually be accomplished. The dictum is attributed to Kant in his *Critique of Pure Reason*. While there are many interpretations of what he meant (or should have meant), for my purposes I want to quote it more colloquially simply to indicate that under everyday conditions, especially in the public policy sphere, it more closely reflects Bismarck's view than anything else more philosophically complex. (See also Brown 1977; Sinnott-Armstrong 1984.)

3. I have relied for most of this information on the critically important book edited by Keith Wailoo and colleagues and the various chapters therein, especially chapter 1 by Susan E. Morgan, Tyler R. Harrison, Lisa Volk Chewning, and Jacklyn C. Habib (pp. 19–45) (see Wailoo, Livingston, and Guarnaccia 2006; also see Resnick 2003 for more historical detail).

4. http://optn.transplant.hrsa.gov/policiesAndBylaws/policies.asp, policy 6.

5. http://abcnews.go.com/Health/HeartHealth/convicted-rapist-kenneth-pike-line-organ-transplant/story?id=13454565#.UJkmDYU1aBo (April 26, 2011).

6. Steve Wiegand, "State Inmate Gets a New Heart," *Sacramento Bee*, January 25, 2002.

7. Indeed, some evidence suggests that these individuals donate more organs than they receive: presumably the excess goes to U.S. citizens or permanent residents. (See Goldberg, Simmerling, and Frader 2007, as well as Shankar Vedantam "US Citizens Get More Organs Than They Give; Donations from Foreign Residents on the Rise," *Washington Post*, March 3, 2003, section A, p. A03.)

8. The U.S. Supreme Court ruled in 1976 that it was unconstitutional to bar people in prison from receiving healthcare that they would have been free to obtain for themselves had they not been incarcerated; doing so would be a form of double punishment, because the principal penalty for their conviction was loss of liberty. (See *Estelle et al. v. Gamble* 1976.) It is interesting to note, however, that UNOS does not advertise their egalitarian approach to this topic (in the same way they do for transplant to non–U.S. nationals, which is an actual formal policy). It is a "white paper" that is not easy to find on the UNOS/OPTN website (http://optn.transplant.hrsa.gov/resources/bioethics.asp?index=3).

9. http://abcnews.go.com/US/story?id=90611&page=1#.UKOpMoU1aBo.

10. The Court's reasoning was based on the idea that incarceration or the deprivation of personal liberty is the primary punishment for a crime. In that state, prisoners are incapable of freely attending to their own healthcare needs, as in seeing a doctor or a nurse (it was considered irrelevant whether they actually would do so, or whether they would have the financial or others means to do so). Hence, depriving them of this necessity due to their incarcerated status would amount to a form of secondary, extrajudicial punishment not meted out by a judge or jury, and hence a violation of the Eighth Amendment's prohibition on inflicting cruel and unusual punishment.

11. Of course for abortion, the mistake about this approach is that the polls have consistently shown that the majority of people in the United States favor elective pregnancy termination with some restrictions.

12. And with the highest incarceration rate in the world in the United States, it is not surprising to find people who fall into this category.

13. One of the more distasteful accusations made against undocumented immigrants is that women come to the United States while pregnant so that they can give birth on American soil, thus instantly creating an American citizen; these children have been given the offensive label "anchor babies." While it is no doubt true that some women emigrate to the United States solely for this purpose, it is difficult to believe that it is a widespread practice. Nonetheless, these stories have entered common parlance and are often repeated as if it were gospel. (See Huang 2008; Castro 2009–2010.)

14. See http://www.politicalchips.org/profiles/blogs/hb-2192-repealing-instate-tuition-for-illegal-immigrants, http://www.nilc.org/basic-facts-instate.html, and http://blog.heritage.org/2011/12/06/morning-bell-illegal-aliens-in-state-tuition-and-the-law.

15. Baker and Strosberg 1992 and World Medical Association, "Regulations in Time of World Conflict," §11: "In emergencies, physicians are required to render immediate attention to the best of their ability. Whether civilian or combatant, the sick and wounded must receive promptly the care they need. No distinction shall be made between patients except those based upon clinical need" (adopted

1956 and updated numerous times, the most recent being 2012: http://www.wma
.net/en/30publications/10policies/a20/; see also Swan and Swan 1996, 451; for a
completely contrary view, see Adams 2008). However, the point should be made
that there may be a sharp distinction between what is written down as the "rules"
and what actually happens on a battlefield under extremely stressful conditions. It
would not be surprising (and indeed, perhaps understandable) that under real-life
circumstances a military surgeon would show a preference for treating his or her
own soldiers over injured prisoners from the other side, if a choice must be made.
It would be less justifiable if there were no competitive choices to be made and a
military doctor simply refused to treat a prisoner because he was an "enemy" (or
more correctly, *had been* an enemy).

16. In a number of the stories I have related in this chapter, I have either alluded
to the role of the media or quoted directly from news sources that are generally
considered to be either respected (or respectable) or "mainstream." By this I mean
that I have avoided using sources usually thought of as sensationalistic, such as
the *National Enquirer*. But it would be both naive and wrong to dismiss the central function of the news media in publicizing stories and then inflaming public
responses to them. This is not only relevant to the "murderer gets a heart transplant while pregnant mom dies waiting" type of stories, but to the integral role
they have played and continue to play in how the narrative of government policy
is portrayed. This was as true in the Santillan case as it was in the "Harry and
Louise" commercials that significantly swayed public opinion against the Clinton
healthcare plan in the early 1990s (Goldsteen, Goldsteen, Swan, and Clemeña
2001). This is certainly the case with the vast array of organizations who have
rolled out a public relations juggernaut both against and (less so) supporting the
Affordable Care Act. And, as I discuss in the final chapter, the practical challenges
to getting any centralized, national rationing plan enacted and implemented
would include, perhaps first and foremost, the formidable forces of "selling" the
plan (or its defeat) to the public (Gross et al. 2012; Frakes 2012).

17. However, the U.S. Supreme Court, in ruling the law constitutional but striking down the Medicaid "stick" by which the federal government could withhold
a state's federal Medicaid funds if the state did not expand its Medicaid rolls as
called for in the law, could threaten the ability to expand reasonable coverage
to as many people as it otherwise would have done (see *National Federation of
Independent Business v. Sebelius* 2012).

18. For example, see the enormous problems and less-than-laudatory partial resolution to this problem at Grady Memorial Hospital in Atlanta, a publicly funded
institution (Campbell, Sanoff, and Rosner 2010; Rodriguez 2010).

19. By way of an example, it is worth examining the recent laws enacted by the
legislature in North Carolina (where I live) to severely restrict the availability, the
amount, and the length of time one can receive unemployment benefits. Much of
the rhetoric of the Republican Representatives and Senators responsible for passing this legislation centered on the prior supposed generosity of these benefits,
which was reported to provide an incentive to not work. Hence, it was reasoned, a
more draconian approach would stimulate both the recently and long-term unemployed to get work. It can be inferred, then, that North Carolina's almost-highest-

in-the-country unemployment rate was almost entirely due to the shiftlessness of the unemployed (http://www.newsobscrver.com/2013/06/08/2948000/70000 -long-term-unemployed-in.html).

20. It is certainly conceivable that in the minds of many, Mitt Romney's infamous "47%" could qualify for less than an equal share of the healthcare pie. (See http:// www.motherjones.com/politics/2012/09/secret-video-romney-private-fundraiser.)

21. I wish to distinguish these kinds of complaints or grievances that are objections to either the applications of the procedure or possibly to the unfairness of the rules themselves from those that arise from the practice of bad medicine— that is, classic negligence or malpractice. Other than parallel attempts at tort or malpractice reform, those would remain separate from what I have in mind here.

22. If we assume that there are about 12 million undocumented immigrants in the United States at the time of this writing, with a total population estimated at almost 315 million, their proportion comes to about 3.8 percent (the total includes the undocumented). (See http://www.census.gov/population/www/ popclockus.html for up-to-date numbers and projections.)

23. While the Patient Protection and Affordable Care Act of 2010 (also known colloquially as "Obamacare" or simply as the "ACA") was presumably designed to offer affordable health insurance to the majority of those Americans who lacked it (by expanding Medicaid and offering subsidies to others), it was never expected—even under optimal conditions—to cover everyone. Unfortunately, the execution has been anything but optimal, starting with the Supreme Court ruling in *National Federation of Independent Business v. Sebelius* (2012), which voided the requirement that states expand Medicaid. Moreover, the ACA only covers American citizens or permanent residents and not undocumented immigrants, a majority of whom lack health insurance (see Wallace et al. 2013). Therefore, we are far from achieving even near-universal health insurance.

24. Schneiderman and Jecker 1996, 39. A lot would depend on who "counted" as having a say for purposes of appointing representatives to devise the plan. I have difficulty imagining that it would include people who do not have the legal right to vote, which would exclude minors, the undocumented, permanent residents, and incarcerated, convicted felons (and, in many jurisdictions, many out on parole and beyond).

25. Herd immunity is the epidemiological concept that once the percentage of immune individuals in a communicative population reaches a certain level, even the nonimmune are covered by the "herd." Of course, this includes both people who cannot be immunized for good medical reasons such as an underlying disease process (like cancer undergoing active treatment with chemotherapy), and those who chose—for whatever reason—to not be immunized; the latter can also be thought of as "free riders." (See Fine, Eames, and Heymann 2011; Quadri-Sheriff et al. 2012; and Bauch, Bhattacharyya, and Ball 2010.)

26. See Rosoff and Decamp 2011 for a discussion of this issue and historical references.

27. This is true for organ transplantation as well, although most of the arguments center on urging living-donor transplants of kidneys, thus not removing an organ from the communal donor pool (see Linden, Cano, and Coritsidis 2012).

28. Although it should be mentioned that a challenge to one of the basic components of the law, section 5, was recently decided (*Shelby County, Alabama v. Holder* 2013) and, for all intents and purposes, eliminated this section. There are some who believe that this was one of the most effective mechanisms for upholding the voting rights of members of minority groups that have historically (and, some would say, currently) been the victims of discrimination and voter suppression (See also http://www.naacpldf.org/case-issue/voting-rights-act-reauthorization-2006.)

Chapter 7

1. Woolf and Laudan (2013) available at http://books.nap.edu/openbook.php?record_id=13497. It is interesting that it is quite common to refer to technologically sophisticated and wealthy countries (for the most part in North America and Western Europe, with some exceptions such as Japan, Singapore, and Australia) as "advanced." Undoubtedly this refers to their financial and industrial capacities and complex economic systems. With respect to what might be called the moral development of a society/country, there seems to be an implicit understanding that technological and manufacturing advances and morality are somehow intertwined. This report, as many others prior to it have also demonstrated, provides ample evidence that in measures of good health the United States lags far behind what are thought to be its peers. Thus, to paraphrase the IOM report, wealth does not necessarily equate with health, when there is little attention paid to spending that money either equitably or wisely in a manner that could improve health outcomes for all residents of the country. In short, "advanced" clearly does not refer to the level of moral development, as we commonly understand it. Otherwise, we could not explain the indefensible disparities in healthcare access and delivery (which equate with outcomes) between the various populations in the country, particularly those with reasonable jobs and incomes and those without. Even the very poor, who are often touted as having cradle-to-grave coverage provided by state and federal government insurance programs, suffer from these inequities.

2. Currie 2012; Medicaid figures for 2010 are available from the U.S. Census Bureau at http://www.census.gov/compendia/statab/2012/tables/12s0146.pdf; Medicare data have been obtained from http://kff.org/medicare/state-indicator/total-medicare-beneficiaries.

3. It is certainly plausible that policymakers could decide to partially reform and remake the healthcare system, with rationing affecting only those who already receive some sort of comprehensive, government-supplied health insurance such as Medicaid or Medicare. This approach has already been used "successfully" (see my discussion of DRGs in chapter 1). But doing so would entail the same ethical problems I examined in chapter 2 with the Oregon Health Plan. While a noble experiment, the OHP was impaired by the fact that most of the decisions were reasonably opaque and made by those who were not subject to their effects. The same kind of strategy would undoubtedly be attempted if something similar were attempted with Medicaid and Medicare at the national level, but with the

cautionary proviso that older adults vote, which could put a halt to any major overhaul. If rationing affected everyone, this might blunt the individual, particularistic, and parochial objections of smaller subgroups of the entire population. But that conclusion must remain speculative at this time.

4. I realize that this is a normative claim and a debatable one at that. But it seems reasonable from both a philosophical and practical point of view to make the effort to more closely align needs and desires.

5. Available at www.huffingtonpost.com/2009/08/07/palin-obamas-death-panel _n_254399.html.

6. Palin might be comforted to know that in the considerably more resource-poor organ transplant system, children with Down syndrome (or others with cognitive disabilities) are not a priori or arbitrarily excluded from access to organs and hence condemned to death.

7. The population in the 1940 census was 131,669,275; table 1, p. 6, United States Summary, http://www2.census.gov/prod2/decennial/documents/33973538v1ch02 .pdf.

8. It is also worth noting that for many Americans the allotments under wartime rationing were not all that different from what they had become accustomed to during the Depression. This is relevant to my argument throughout this book that any conceivable centralized healthcare rationing in the United States would necessarily be quite generous. Thus, for many people who have no insurance or are underinsured—which may be a significant portion of the entire population, if not the majority if we include those whose sole insurance is Medicare—benefits under rationing may actually be an improvement compared to what they have now. If we can get past the dual psychological barriers posed by "socialized medicine" and "rationing," we could expect an avid embracing of the program. Indeed, one might also see a parallel with the overwhelming acceptance of Medicare by American doctors (including the American Medical Association) after their initial opposition, when it became apparent what a boon to their practices (and income) the program would be (Blumenthal 1995; Marmor 2000a, chaps. 2 and 3).

9. However, it bears mentioning that not all was harmonious and rosy patriotism. There were periodic strikes and walkouts protesting a variety of issues, including discrimination against African-American shipyard workers (Nelson 1993). Even though there was a "no-strike pledge" by the American Federation of Labor, there were numerous walkouts and slowdowns due to a variety of grievances (Atleson 1998).

10. See National Hospice and Palliative Care Organization, *NHPCO Facts and Figures: Hospice Care in America* (2012 ed.), http://www.nhpco.org/sites/default/ files/public/Statistics_Research/2012_Facts_Figures.pdf.

11. This could perhaps be accomplished via a program similar to the federal capitation grants made to medical schools in the 1970s as authorized via the Comprehensive Health Manpower Training Act of 1971 (Matlack 1972).

12. Indeed, promoting the use of honest and forthright discussions of end-of-life care planning by physicians with their patients (and their families), with the increased utilization of advance directive documents, can only decrease the reliance

on intensive care and other marginally beneficial interventions for dying patients or those with fatal diseases (Bullock 2006; Song et al. 2009; Sudore and Fried 2010; Tulsky, Fischer, Rose, and Arnold 1998). Of course, this is not as simple to accomplish as both common sense and the data would dictate, as the experience with the Affordable Care Act and the attempt to provide Medicare reimbursement for doctors having these conversations would indicate: there was a huge fight over the prospect of doctors telling their patients that they would have to forgo certain types of care because they were too old or had cancer, and so on. Needless to say, this rather straightforward and sensible approach was axed from the final bill (though it was restored by Executive Order a bit later) (Tinetti 2012).

13. Of course, some would argue that Jobs's life was worth more than many others in much the same way as many argue that law-abiding people should not have to share their access to transplant organs with convicted felons who are "worth less." Carving up society into tiers of worthiness could be the death knell of any rationing scheme that wishes to claim fairness as a central tenet. By the same token, I have also argued in chapter 6 that there may be limits to the kind of fairness that is tolerable in a pluralistic, democratic society.

14. An enormous amount has been written about what might constitute a "basic minimum" of healthcare, ranging from specific interventions such as comprehensive childhood (and now adult) vaccinations, preventive healthcare services, prophylactic dental care, and so forth. Some writers have also endorsed the concept that good health can only be achieved when the social determinants of health are addressed as well. This would include the standard components of public health such as clean water and sanitation, but also such things as good housing, safe neighborhoods, and a clean environment. I do not wish to engage in a discussion of what a wealthy nation like the United States could conceivably offer its residents in this way, but I suspect that if one totaled up the overall amount of money spent in all these areas and distributed it more equitably, the range of benefits offered as a baseline would be generous indeed.

15. At the end of 2011, almost 2.5 million people were in detention in the United States, and "about 2.9% of adults in the U.S. (or 1 in every 34 adults) were under some form of correctional supervision" (this includes probation). While this sounds like a huge number, amazingly "The correctional supervision rate observed in 2011 marked the lowest rate of adults in the U.S. under correctional supervision since 2000. The 2011 rate was comparable to the correctional supervision rate observed in 1998 (1 in every 34 adults) when about one million fewer offenders were under correctional supervision (5.9 million in 1998)" (see *Correctional Populations in the United States, 2011*, available at http://bjs.ojp.usdoj.gov/index.cfm?ty=pbdetail&iid=4537).

16. Unfortunately, there is no similar Supreme Court ruling stating that people who are not in prison and who are undocumented have a "right" to healthcare stemming from their status as fellow human beings (of course, there is no such right for citizens, either). The mandate that requires prisoners to receive standard-of-care medical treatments does not exist for the undocumented. While I can imagine a reluctant acceptance of comprehensive healthcare reform (encompassing rationing) that includes prisoners—as long as law-abiding citizens are not de-

prived of something, such as an organ, because it has been given to a prisoner—it remains highly unlikely that such generosity, even if we can afford it, would be extended to immigrants so long as they remain "illegal aliens" for many people.

17. Or, to use Callahan's words, the "beloved beast" (Callahan 2009).

18. The text of Truman's speech can be found at http://www.presidency.ucsb.edu/ws/?pid=13293.

References

Aaron, Henry J., William B. Schwartz, and Melissa Cox. 2005. *Can We Say No? The Challenge of Rationing Health Care*. Washington, DC: Brookings Institution Press.

Acharya, A., T. Adam, R. Baltussen, D. Evans, R. Hutubessy, C. J. L. Murray, and T. Tan Torres. 2003. *Making Choices in Health: WHO Guide to Cost-Effectiveness Analysis*. Geneva: World Health Organization.

Adams, Marcus P. 2008. Triage priorities and military physicians. In Fritz Allhoff, ed., *Physicians at War*, 215–236. Heidelberg: Springer Netherlands.

Agency for Healthcare Research and Quality (AHRQ). 2006. *The high concentration of U.S. health care expenditures*. Washington, DC: Agency for Healthcare Research and Quality.

Aggarwal, Praveen, Sung Youl Jun, and Jong Ho Huh. 2011. SCARCITY MESSAGES: A consumer competition perspective. *Journal of Advertising* 40 (3): 19–30.

Akinniyi, D. C., and P. W. Payne. 2011. Bidil lessons: Cardiologists' views of a race-based personalized medicine. *Journal of the American College of Cardiology* 57 (14): E1926.

Alden, D. L., and A. H. Cheung. 2000. Organ donation and culture: A comparison of Asian American and European American beliefs, attitudes, and behaviors. *Journal of Applied Social Psychology* 30 (2): 293–314.

Alexander, S. 1962. They decide who lives, who dies. *Life (Chicago)* 53 (November): 102–125.

Allen, Steve, Daniel Holena, Maureen McCunn, Benjamin Kohl, and Babak Sarani. 2011. A review of the fundamental principles and evidence base in the use of extracorporeal membrane oxygenation (ECMO) in critically ill adult patients. *Journal of Intensive Care Medicine* 26 (1): 13–26. doi:10.1177/0885066610384061.

Almond, Christopher S., Tajinder P. Singh, Kimberlee Gauvreau, Gary E. Piercey, Francis Fynn-Thompson, Peter T. Rycus, Robert H. Bartlett, and Ravi R. Thiagarajan. 2011. Extracorporeal membrane oxygenation for bridge to heart transplantation among children in the United States / clinical perspective. *Circulation* 123 (25): 2975–2984. doi:10.1161/circulationaha.110.991505.

Alpers, A., and B. Lo. 1999. Avoiding family feuds: Responding to surrogate demands for life-sustaining interventions. *Journal of Law, Medicine & Ethics* 27 (1): 74–80.

Amaral, Sandra, Rachel E. Patzer, Nancy Kutner, and William McClellan. 2012. Racial disparities in access to pediatric kidney transplantation since Share 35. *Journal of the American Society of Nephrology* 23 (6): 1069–1077. doi:10.1681/asn.2011121145.

Anderson, Christopher J., and Yuliya V. Tverdova. 2001. Winners, losers, and attitudes about government in contemporary democracies. *International Political Science Review* 22 (4): 321–338. doi:10.1177/0192512101022004003.

Angell, M., and J. P. Kassirer. 1994. Setting the record straight in the breast-cancer trials. *New England Journal of Medicine* 330 (20): 1448–1450. doi:10.1056/NEJM199405193302010.

Angus, D. C., A. E. Barnato, W. T. Linde-Zwirble, L. A. Weissfeld, R. S. Watson, T. Rickert, and G. D. Rubenfeld. 2004. Use of intensive care at the end of life in the United States: An epidemiologic study. *Critical Care Medicine* 32 (3): 638–643.

Antman, K. 2002. Randomized trials of high-dose chemotherapy in breast cancer: Fraud, the press and the data (or lessons learned in medical policy governing clinical research). *Transactions of the American Clinical and Climatological Association* 113:56–66, discussion 66–67.

Arias, E., B. L. Rostron, and B. Tejada-Vera. 2010. United States life tables, 2005. *National Vital Statistics Reports: From the Centers for Disease Control and Prevention, National Center for Health Statistics. National Vital Statistics System* 58 (10): 1–132.

Aronson, J. K. 2003. Anecdotes as evidence. *BMJ (Clinical Research Ed.)* 326 (7403): 1346.

Atleson, James B. 1998. *Labor and the Wartime State: Labor Relations and Law during World War II.* Urbana: University of Illinois Press.

Auwaerter, Paul G., Johan S. Bakken, Raymond J. Dattwyler, J. Stephen Dumler, John J. Halperin, Edward McSweegan, Robert B. Nadelman, et al. 2011. Antiscience and ethical concerns associated with advocacy of Lyme disease. *Lancet Infectious Diseases* 11 (9): 713–719. doi:10.1016/s1473-3099(11)70034-2.

Avolio, A. W., U. Cillo, M. Salizzoni, L. De Carlis, M. Colledan, G. E. Gerunda, V. Mazzaferro, et al. 2011. Balancing donor and recipient risk factors in liver transplantation: The value of D-MELD with particular reference to HCV recipients. *American Journal of Transplantation: Official Journal of the American Society of Transplantation and the American Society of Transplant Surgeons* 11 (12): 2724–2736. doi:10.1111/j.1600-6143.2011.03732.x.

Axelrod, D. A., M. K. Guidinger, S. Finlayson, D. E. Schaubel, D. C. Goodman, M. Chobanian, and R. M. Merion. 2008. Rates of solid-organ wait-listing, transplantation, and survival among residents of rural and urban areas. *Journal of the American Medical Association* 299 (2): 202–207. doi:10.1001/jama.2007.50.

Ayanian, J. Z., P. D. Cleary, J. H. Keogh, S. J. Noonan, J. A. David-Kasdan, and A. M. Epstein. 2004. Physicians' beliefs about racial differences in referral for renal transplantation. *American Journal of Kidney Diseases: The Official Journal of the National Kidney Foundation* 43 (2): 350–357.

Baiardini, Ilaria, Fulvio Braido, Matteo Bonini, Enrico Compalati, and Giorgio Walter Canonica. 2009. Why do doctors and patients not follow guidelines? *Current Opinion in Allergy and Clinical Immunology* 9 (3): 228–233. doi:10.1097/ACI.0b013e32832b4651.

Baicker, K., A. Chandra, and J. S. Skinner. 2012. Saving money or just saving lives? Improving the productivity of US health care spending. *Annual Review of Economics* 4 (4): 3–66. doi:10.1146/Annurev-Economics-080511-110942.

Baicker, Katherine, and Amy Finkelstein. 2011. The effects of Medicaid coverage—learning from the Oregon experiment. *New England Journal of Medicine* 365 (8): 683–685. doi:10.1056/NEJMp1108222.

Baily, Mary Ann. 1984. "Rationing" and American health policy. *Journal of Health Politics, Policy and Law* 9 (3): 489–501. doi:10.1215/03616878-9-3-489.

Baily, Mary Ann. 2011. Futility, autonomy, and cost in end-of-life care. *Journal of Law, Medicine & Ethics* 39 (2): 172–182. doi:10.1111/j.1748-720X.2011.00586.x.

Baker, R., and M. Strosberg. 1992. Triage and equality: An historical reassessment of utilitarian analyses of triage. *Kennedy Institute of Ethics Journal* 2 (2): 103–123.

Barnato, Amber, Denise Anthony, Jonathan Skinner, Patricia Gallagher, and Elliott Fisher. 2009. Racial and ethnic differences in preferences for end-of-life treatment. *Journal of General Internal Medicine* 24 (6): 695–701. doi:10.1007/s11606-009-0952-6.

Barnato, Amber E., Chung-Chou H. Chang, Max H. Farrell, Judith R. Lave, Mark S. Roberts, and Derek C. Angus. 2010. Is survival better at hospitals with higher "end-of-life" treatment intensity? *Medical Care* 48 (2): 125–132. doi:10.1097/MLR.0b013e3181c161e4.

Barry, J. M. 2004. *The Great Influenza: The Epic Story of the Deadliest Plague in History*. New York: Viking Press.

Bartels, Andrew H. 1983. The Office of Price Administration and the legacy of the New Deal, 1939–1946. *Public Historian* 5 (3): 5–29. doi:10.2307/3377026.

Basu, Anirban, Anupam B. Jena, and Tomas J. Philipson. 2011. The impact of comparative effectiveness research on health and health care spending. *Journal of Health Economics* 30 (4): 695–706. doi:http://dx.doi.org/10.1016/j.jhealeco.2011.05.012.

Basu, Rituparna, Luisa Franzini, Patrick M. Krueger, and David R. Lairson. 2010. Gender disparities in medical expenditures attributable to hypertension in the United States. *Women's Health Issues* 20 (2): 114–125. doi:http://dx.doi.org/10.1016/j.whi.2009.12.001.

Bauch, Chris T., Samit Bhattacharyya, and Robert F. Ball. 2010. Rapid emergence of free-riding behavior in new pediatric immunization programs. *PLOS ONE* 5 (9): e12594. doi:10.1371/journal.pone.0012594.

Baughn, D., S. M. Auerbach, and L. A. Siminoff. 2010. Roles of sex and ethnicity in procurement coordinator–family communication during the organ donation discussion. *Progress in Transplantation (Aliso Viejo, CA)* 20 (3): 247–255.

Baumer, Amanda M., Angela M. Clark, David R. Witmer, Shirley B. Geize, Lee C. Vermeulen, and Joseph H. Deffenbaugh. 2004. National survey of the impact of drug shortages in acute care hospitals. *American Journal of Health-System Pharmacy* 61 (19): 2015–2022.

Bearman, P. 2009. Just-so stories: Vaccines, autism, and the single-bullet disorder. *Social Psychology Quarterly* 73:112–115. doi:10.1177/0190272510371672.

Bentley, Amy. 1998. *Eating for Victory: Food Rationing and the Politics of Domesticity*. Urbana: University of Illinois Press.

Bergan, Daniel, and Genevieve Risner. 2012. Issue ads and the health reform debate. *Journal of Health Politics, Policy and Law* 37 (3): 513–549. doi:10.1215/03616878-1573103.

Berkman, Lisa F. 2009. Social epidemiology: Social determinants of health in the United States: Are we losing ground? *Annual Review of Public Health* 30 (1): 27–41. doi:10.1146/annurev.publhealth.031308.100310.

Bernat, J. L. 2005. Medical futility: Definition, determination, and disputes in critical care. *Neurocritical Care* 2 (2): 198–205.

Bernier, R. H., and E. K. Marcuse. 2005. *Citizen Voices on Pandemic Flu Choices: A Report of the Public Engagement Project on Pandemic Influenza*. Keystone, CO: Keystone Center.

Berwick, D. M., and A. D. Hackbarth. 2012. Eliminating waste in US health care. *Journal of the American Medical Association* 307 (14): 1513–1516. doi:10.1001/jama.2012.362.

Bickell, N. A., J. J. Wang, S. Oluwole, D. Schrag, H. Godfrey, K. Hiotis, J. Mendez, and A. A. Guth. 2006. Missed opportunities: Racial disparities in adjuvant breast cancer treatment. *Journal of Clinical Oncology* 24 (9): 1357–1362.

Birks, E. J. 2010. Left ventricular assist devices. *Heart (British Cardiac Society)* 96 (1): 63–71. doi:10.1136/hrt.2007.130740.

Bishop, T. F., A. D. Federman, and S. Keyhani. 2010. Physicians' views on defensive medicine: A national survey. *Archives of Internal Medicine* 170 (12): 1081–1083. doi:10.1001/archinternmed.2010.155.

Blackhall, L. J., G. Frank, S. T. Murphy, V. Michel, J. M. Palmer, and S. P. Azen. 1999. Ethnicity and attitudes towards life sustaining technology. *Social Science & Medicine* 48 (12): 1779–1789.

Blagg, Christopher R. 2007. The early history of dialysis for chronic renal failure in the United States: A view from Seattle. *American Journal of Kidney Diseases* 49 (3): 482–496. doi:10.1053/j.ajkd.2007.01.017.

Blais, André, and François Gélineau. 2007. Winning, losing and satisfaction with democracy. *Political Studies* 55 (2): 425–441. doi:10.1111/j.1467-9248.2007.00659.x.

Bloche, M. Gregg. 2012. Beyond the "R word"? Medicine's new frugality. *New England Journal of Medicine* 366 (21): 1951–1953. doi:10.1056/NEJMp1203521.

Block, Lauren D., Marian P. Jarlenski, Albert W. Wu, and Wendy L. Bennett. 2013. Mammography use among women ages 40–49 after the 2009 U.S. Preventive Services Task Force Recommendation. *Journal of General Internal Medicine* 28 (11):1447–1453. doi:10.1007/s11606-013-2482-5.

Blumenthal, David. 1995. Health care reform—past and future. *New England Journal of Medicine* 332 (7): 465–468. doi:10.1056/NEJM199502163320711.

Bonney, Glenn K., Mark A. Aldersley, Sonal Asthana, Giles J. Toogood, Stephen G. Pollard, J. Peter Lodge, and K. Rajendra Prasad. 2009. Donor Risk Index and MELD interactions in predicting long-term graft survival: A single-centre experience. *Transplantation* 87 (12): 1858–1863. doi:10.1097/TP.0b013e3181a75b37.

Boulis, Ann, Susan Goold, and Peter A. Ubel. 2002. Responding to the immunoglobulin shortage: A case study. *Journal of Health Politics, Policy and Law* 27 (6): 977–1000. doi:10.1215/03616878-27-6-977.

Boulware, L. E., L. E. Ratner, J. A. Sosa, L. A. Cooper, T. A. LaVeist, and N. R. Powe. 2002. Determinants of willingness to donate living related and cadaveric organs: Identifying opportunities for intervention. *Transplantation* 73 (10): 1683–1691.

Bowles, Samuel, and Herbert Gintis. 2011. *A Cooperative Species: Human Reciprocity and Its Evolution.* Princeton, NJ: Princeton University Press.

Bradley, Cathy J., Sabina Ohri Gandhi, David Neumark, Sheryl Garland, and Sheldon M. Retchin. 2012. Lessons for coverage expansion: A Virginia primary care program for the uninsured reduced utilization and cut costs. *Health Affairs* 31 (2): 350–359. doi:10.1377/hlthaff.2011.0857.

Brandon, D. T., L. A. Isaac, and T. A. LaVeist. 2005. The legacy of Tuskegee and trust in medical care: Is Tuskegee responsible for race differences in mistrust of medical care? *Journal of the National Medical Association* 97 (7): 951–956.

Brannstrom, Jon, Yngve Gustafson, Katarina Hamberg, Hugo Lovheim, and Lena Molander. 2011. Gender disparities in the pharmacological treatment of cardiovascular disease and diabetes mellitus in the very old: An epidemiological, cross-sectional survey. *Drugs & Aging* 28:993.

Bratton, C., K. Chavin, and P. Baliga. 2011. Racial disparities in organ donation and why. *Current Opinion in Organ Transplantation* 16 (2): 243–249. doi:10.1097/MOT.0b013e3283447b1c.

Braun, M. Miles, Sheiren Farag-El-Massah, Kui Xu, and Timothy R. Coté. 2010. Emergence of orphan drugs in the United States: A quantitative assessment of the first 25 years. *Nature Reviews Drug Discovery* 9 (7): 519–522. doi:http://www.nature.com/nrd/journal/v9/n7/suppinfo/nrd3160_S1.html.

Braun, Ursula, Rebecca Beyth, Marvella Ford, and Laurence McCullough. 2008. Voices of African American, Caucasian, and Hispanic surrogates on the burdens of end-of-life decision making. *Journal of General Internal Medicine* 23 (3): 267–274. doi:10.1007/s11606-007-0487-7.

Brennan, T. A., D. J. Rothman, L. Blank, D. Blumenthal, S. C. Chimonas, J. J. Cohen, J. Goldman, et al. 2006. Health industry practices that create conflicts of interest: A policy proposal for academic medical centers. *Journal of the American Medical Association* 295 (4): 429–433.

Brock, Dan W. 2006. Ethical issues in the use of cost effectiveness analysis for the prioritization of health care resources. In Sudhir Anand, Fabienne Peter, and Amartya Sen, eds., *Public Health, Ethics, and Equity*, 201–223. Oxford: Oxford University Press.

Brody, H., and L. D. Hermer. 2011. Professionally responsible malpractice reform. *Journal of General Internal Medicine* 26 (7): 806–809. doi:10.1007/s11606-011 -1635-7.

Brown, James. 1977. Moral theory and the ought-can principle. *Mind* 86 (342): 206–223. doi:10.2307/2253713.

Bryant, Allison S., Ayaba Worjoloh, Aaron B. Caughey, and A. Eugene Washington. 2010. Racial/ethnic disparities in obstetric outcomes and care: Prevalence and determinants. *American Journal of Obstetrics and Gynecology* 202 (4): 335–343. doi: 10.1016/j.ajog.2009.10.864.

Bullock, K. 2006. Promoting advance directives among African Americans: A faith-based model. *Journal of Palliative Medicine* 9 (1): 183–195. doi:10.1089/ jpm.2006.9.183.

Burch, Ernest S. 1988. *The Eskimos*. Ed. Werner Forman. Norman: University of Oklahoma Press.

Burgess, J. A. 1993. The great slippery-slope argument. *Journal of Medical Ethics* 19 (3): 169–174. doi:10.1136/jme.19.3.169.

Bustamante, A. V., H. Fang, J. Garza, O. Carter-Pokras, S. P. Wallace, J. A. Rizzo, and A. N. Ortega. 2012. Variations in healthcare access and utilization among Mexican immigrants: The role of documentation status. *Journal of Immigrant and Minority Health* 14 (1): 146–155. doi:10.1007/s10903-010-9406-9.

Butterworth, J. F. 2009. Case reports: Unstylish but still useful sources of clinical information. *Regional Anesthesia and Pain Medicine* 34 (3): 187–188. doi:10.1097/AAP.0b013e31819a2775.

Buyx, Alena M., Daniel R. Friedrich, and Bettina Schöne-Seifert. 2011. Ethics and effectiveness: Rationing healthcare by thresholds of minimum effectiveness. *BMJ (Clinical Research Ed.)* 342. doi:10.1136/bmj.d54.

Calabresi, Guido, and Philip Bobbitt. 1978. *Tragic Choices*. New York: Norton.

Callahan, Daniel. 1987. *Setting Limits: Medical Goals in an Aging Society*. New York: Simon and Schuster.

Callahan, Daniel. 1990. *What Kind of Life: The Limits of Medical Progress*. New York: Simon and Schuster.

Callahan, Daniel. 1998. *False Hopes: Why America's Quest for Perfect Health Is a Recipe for Failure*. New York: Simon and Schuster.

Callahan, Daniel. 2009. *Taming the Beloved Beast*. Princeton, NJ: Princeton University Press.

Campbell, E. G., J. S. Weissman, S. Ehringhaus, S. R. Rao, B. Moy, S. Feibelmann, and S. D. Goold. 2007. Institutional academic industry relationships. *Journal of the American Medical Association* 298 (15): 1779–1786.

Campbell, G. A., S. Sanoff, and M. H. Rosner. 2010. Care of the undocumented immigrant in the United States with ESRD. *American Journal of Kidney Diseases: The Official Journal of the National Kidney Foundation* 55 (1): 181–191. doi:10.1053/j.ajkd.2009.06.039.

Caplan, Arthur L. 1995. Straight talk about rationing. *Annals of Internal Medicine* 122 (10): 795–796. doi:10.7326/0003-4819-122-10-199505150-00011.

Carman, Kristin L., Maureen Maurer, Jill Mathews Yegian, Pamela Dardess, Jeanne McGee, Mark Evers, and Karen O. Marlo. 2010. Evidence that consumers are skeptical about evidence-based health care. *Health Affairs* 29 (7): 1400–1406. doi:10.1377/hlthaff.2009.0296.

Casalino, Lawrence P., Sean Nicholson, David N. Gans, Terry Hammons, Dante Morra, Theodore Karrison, and Wendy Levinson. 2009. What does it cost physician practices to interact with health insurance plans? *Health Affairs* 28 (4): w533–w543. doi:10.1377/hlthaff.28.4.w533.

Castro, John A. 2009–2010. Second-class citizens: The schism between immigration policy and children's health care. *Hastings Constitutional Law Quarterly* 37:199–224.

Chandra, Amitabh, David Cutler, and Zirui Song. 2011. Chapter Six—who ordered that? The economics of treatment choices in medical care. In Thomas G. McGuire, Mark V. Pauly, Pedro Barros, eds., *Handbook of Health Economics*, 397–432. Oxford: Elsevier.

Chasteen, Alison L., and Scott F. Madey. 2003. Belief in a just world and the perceived injustice of dying young or old. *Omega* 47 (4): 313–326.

Chen, Elsa Y. 2008. Impacts of "Three Strikes and You're Out" on crime trends in California and throughout the United States. *Journal of Contemporary Criminal Justice* 24 (4): 345–370. doi:10.1177/1043986208319456.

Chen, Henian, Patricia Cohen, and Sophie Chen. 2007. Biased odds ratios from dichotomization of age. *Statistics in Medicine* 26 (18): 3487–3497. doi:10.1002/sim.2737.

Childress, J. F. 1970. Who shall live when not all can live? *Soundings* 53:339–355.

Childress, J. F. 1989. Ethical criteria for procuring and distributing organs for transplantation. *Journal of Health Politics, Policy and Law* 14 (1): 87–113.

Chin, Lynda, Jannik N. Andersen, and P. Andrew Futreal. 2011. Cancer genomics: From discovery science to personalized medicine. *Nature Medicine* 17 (3): 297–303.

Cialdini, Robert B. 2009. *Influence: Science and Practice*. 5th ed. Boston: Pearson Education.

Clark, P. B., and F. M. Parsons. 1966. Routine use of the Scribner Shunt for haemodialysis. *British Medical Journal* 1 (5497): 1200–1202.

Clinard, Marshall B. 1946. Criminological theories of violations of wartime regulations. *American Sociological Review* 11 (3): 258–270. doi:10.2307/2087110.

Clinard, Marshall B. 1952. *The Black Market: A Study of White Collar Crime*. New York: Rinehart.

Cochrane, Lorna J., Curtis A. Olson, Suzanne Murray, Martin Dupuis, Tricia Tooman, and Sean Hayes. 2007. Gaps between knowing and doing: Understanding and assessing the barriers to optimal health care. *Journal of Continuing Education in the Health Professions* 27 (2): 94–102. doi:10.1002/chp.106.

Cohen, Alan B. 2012. The debate over health care rationing: Deja vu all over again? *Inquiry* 2012 (Summer): 90.

Colan, Steven B. 2006. Cardiomyopathies. In John F. Keane, Donald C. Fyler, and James E. Lock, eds., *Nadas' Pediatric Cardiology*, 415–458. Philadelphia: Saunders.

Coller, B. S. 2011. Realigning incentives to achieve health care reform. *Journal of the American Medical Association* 306 (2): 204–205. doi:10.1001/jama.2011.978.

Collins, Mike. 2010. Reevaluating the Dead Donor Rule. *Journal of Medicine and Philosophy* 35 (2): 154–179. doi:10.1093/jmp/jhq009.

Committee on Understanding and Eliminating Racial and Ethnic Disparities in Health Care. 2003. *Unequal Treatment: Confronting Racial and Ethnic Disparities in Health Care* [with CD], Brian D. Smedley, Adrienne Y. Stith, and Alan R. Nelson, eds. Washington, DC: National Academies Press.

Cook, Katherine M., and Geoffrey Evans. 2011. The National Vaccine Injury Compensation Program. *Pediatrics* 127 (Suppl. 1): S74–S77. doi:10.1542/peds.2010-1722K.

Cook, Nakela L., E. John Orav, Catherine L. Liang, Edward Guadagnoli, and S. Hicks LeRoi. 2011. Racial and gender disparities in implantable cardioverter-defibrillator placement: Are they due to overuse or underuse? *Medical Care Research and Review* 68 (2): 226–246. doi:10.1177/1077558710379421.

Cookson, Richard, and Paul Dolan. 1999. Public views on health care rationing: A group discussion study. *Health Policy (Amsterdam)* 49 (1–2): 63–74. doi:10.1016/s0168-8510(99)00043-3.

Cookson, R., C. McCabe, and A. Tsuchiya. 2008. Public healthcare resource allocation and the Rule of Rescue. *Journal of Medical Ethics* 34 (7): 540–544. doi:10.1136/jme.2007.021790.

Courdi, A., M. Hery, P. Chauvel, J. Gioanni, M. Namer, and F. Demard. 1988. Prognostic value of continuous variables in breast cancer and head and neck cancer: Dependence on the cut-off level. *British Journal of Cancer* 58 (1): 88–90.

Courtwright, Andrew. 2012. Who is "too sick to benefit"? *Hastings Center Report* 42 (4): 41–47. doi:10.1002/hast.51.

Crawshaw, R., M. Garland, and B. Hines. 1989. Organ transplants: A search for health policy at the state level. *Western Journal of Medicine* 150 (3): 361–363.

Creecy, R. F., and R. Wright. 1990. Correlates of willingness to consider organ donation among blacks. *Social Science & Medicine* 31 (11): 1229–1232.

Cropper, M. L., S. K. Aydede, and P. R. Portney. 1992. Rates of time preference for saving lives. *American Economic Review* 82 (2): 469–472.

Cropper, M. L., S. K. Aydede, and P. R. Portney. 1994. Preferences for life saving programs—how the public discounts time and age. *Journal of Risk and Uncertainty* 8 (3): 243–265. doi:10.1007/Bf01064044.

Cruz-Flores, S., A. Rabinstein, J. Biller, M. S. Elkind, P. Griffith, P. B. Gorelick, G. Howard, et al. 2011. Racial-ethnic disparities in stroke care: The American experience: A statement for healthcare professionals from the American Heart Association/American Stroke Association. *Stroke* 42 (7): 2091–2116. doi:10.1161/STR.0b013e3182213e24.

Cunningham, Peter J. 2010. The growing financial burden of health care: National and state trends, 2001–2006. *Health Affairs* 29 (5): 1037–1044. doi:10.1377/hlthaff.2009.0493.

Currie, Donya. 2012. US uninsurance rate falls, but 48.6 million still lack coverage: Affordable Care Act contributes to gains. *Nation's Health* 42 (9): 1, 14.

Daniels, Norman. 1983. Justice between age groups: Am I my parents' keeper? *Milbank Memorial Fund Quarterly: Health and Society* 61 (3): 489–522. doi:10.2307/3349870.

Daniels, Norman. 1988. *Am I My Parents' Keeper?* New York: Oxford University Press.

Daniels, Norman. 1991. Is the Oregon rationing plan fair? *Journal of the American Medical Association* 265 (17): 2232–2235. doi:10.1001/jama.1991.03460170086039.

Daniels, Norman. 1993. Rationing fairly—programmatic considerations. *Bioethics* 7 (2–3): 224–233. doi:10.1111/j.1467-8519.1993.tb00288.x.

Daniels, Norman. 2000. Accountability for reasonableness. *BMJ (Clinical Research Ed.)* 321 (7272): 1300–1301.

Daniels, Norman. 2008. *Just Health: Meeting Health Needs Fairly*. New York: Cambridge University Press.

Daniels, Norman, and James Sabin. 1997. Limits to health care: Fair procedures, democratic deliberation, and the legitimacy problem for insurers. *Philosophy & Public Affairs* 26 (4): 303–350.

Daniels, Norman, and James Sabin. 2008. *Setting Limits Fairly: Learning to Share Resources for Health*. 2nd ed. Oxford: Oxford University Press.

Darrah, John B. 1987. The Committee. *ASAIO Journal (American Society for Artificial Internal Organs)* 33 (4): 791–793.

Davidson, M. N., and P. Devney. 1991. Attitudinal barriers to organ donation among black Americans. *Transplantation Proceedings* 23 (5): 2531–2532.

Davies, A., D. Jones, M. Bailey, J. Beca, R. Bellomo, N. Blackwell, P. Forrest, et al. 2009. Extracorporeal membrane oxygenation for 2009 Influenza A(H1N1) Acute Respiratory Distress Syndrome. *Journal of the American Medical Association* 302 (17): 1888–1895. doi:10.1001/jama.2009.1535.

Davis, J. K. 2008. Futility, conscientious refusal, and who gets to decide. *Journal of Medicine and Philosophy* 33 (4): 356–373. doi:10.1093/jmp/jhn019.

Davis, K., S. Holtzman, R. Durand, P. J. Decker, B. Zucha, and L. Atkins. 2005. Leading the flock: Organ donation feelings, beliefs, and intentions among African American clergy and community residents. *Progress in Transplantation* 15 (3): 211–216.

Davis, Tonya N., Mark O'Reilly, Soyeon Kang, Russell Lang, Mandy Rispoli, Jeff Sigafoos, Giulio Lancioni, Daelynn Copeland, Shanna Attai, and Austin Mulloy. 2013. Chelation treatment for autism spectrum disorders: A systematic review. *Research in Autism Spectrum Disorders* 7 (1): 49–55. doi:10.1016/j.rasd.2012.06.005.

Dawson, Neal V., and Robert Weiss. 2012. Dichotomizing continuous variables in statistical analysis: A practice to avoid. *Medical Decision Making* 32 (2): 225–226. doi:10.1177/0272989x12437605.

De Bono, Johann S., Christopher J. Logothetis, Arturo Molina, Karim Fizazi, Scott North, Luis Chu, Kim N. Chi, Robert J. Jones, Oscar B. Goodman, Fred Saad, John N. Staffurth, Paul Mainwaring, Stephen Harland, Thomas W. Flaig, Thomas E. Hutson, Tina Cheng, Helen Patterson, John D. Hainsworth, Charles J. Ryan, Cora N. Sternberg, Susan L. Ellard, Aude Fléchon, Mansoor Saleh, Mark Scholz, Eleni Efstathiou, Andrea Zivi, Diletta Bianchini, Yohann Loriot, Nicole Chieffo, Thian Kheoh, Christopher M. Haqq, and Howard I. Scher. 2011. Abiraterone and increased survival in metastatic prostate cancer. *New England Journal of Medicine* 364 (21): 1995–2005. doi:10.1056/NEJMoa1014618.

De Jonge, Suzan, Robert J. de Vos, Adam Weir, Hans T. M. van Schie, Sita M. A. Bierma-Zeinstra, Jan A. N. Verhaar, Harrie Weinans, and Johannes L. Tol. 2011. One-year follow-up of platelet-rich plasma treatment in chronic Achilles tendonopathy. *American Journal of Sports Medicine* 39 (8): 1623–1629. doi:10.1177/0363546511404877.

Derose, Kathryn Pitkin,, Benjamin W. Bahney, Nicole Lurie, and José J. Escarce. 2009. Review: Immigrants and health care access, quality, and cost. *Medical Care Research and Review* 66 (4): 355–408. doi:10.1177/1077558708330425.

De Vos, R. J., A. Weir, H. M. van Schie, et al. 2010. Platelet-rich plasma injection for chronic Achilles tendonopathy: A randomized controlled trial. *Journal of the American Medical Association* 303 (2): 144–149. doi:10.1001/jama.2009.1986.

Dew, Mary Amanda, Andrea F. DiMartini, Annette De Vito Dabbs, Larissa Myaskovsky, Jennifer Steel, Mark Unruh, Galen E. Switzer, Rachelle Zomak, Robert L. Kormos, and Joel B. Greenhouse. 2007. Rates and risk factors for nonadherence to the medical regimen after adult solid organ transplantation. *Transplantation* 83 (7): 858–873. doi:10.1097/01.tp.0000258599.65257.a6.

De Wispelaere, Jurgen. 2012. Tacitly opting out of organ donation: Too presumptuous after all? *Journal of Medical Ethics* 38 (2): 73–74. doi:10.1136/medethics-2011-100252.

Diederich, Adele, Jeannette Winkelhage, and Norman Wirsik. 2011. Age as a criterion for setting priorities in health care? A survey of the German public view. *PLOS ONE* 6 (8): e23930. doi:10.1371/journal.pone.0023930.

Diekema, D. S. 1996. The preferential treatment of VIPs in the emergency department. *American Journal of Emergency Medicine* 14 (2): 226–229. doi:10.1016/S0735-6757(96)90137-0.

Disch, Lisa. 1996. Publicity-stunt participation and sound bite polemics: The health care debate 1993–94. *Journal of Health Politics, Policy and Law* 21 (1): 3–33. doi:10.1215/03616878-21-1-3.

Dobbels, Fabienne, Johan Vanhaecke, Lieven Dupont, Frederik Nevens, Geert Verleden, Jacques Pirenne, and Sabina de Geest. 2009. Pretransplant predictors of posttransplant adherence and clinical outcome: An evidence base for pretransplant psychosocial screening. *Transplantation* 87 (10): 1497–1504. doi:10.1097/TP.0b013e3181a440ae.

Donaldson, Andrew. 2010. "And the ones that mother gives you don't do anything at all": Combating counterfeit pharmaceuticals: The American and British perspectives. *New England Journal of International and Comparative Law* 16:145–168.

Dower, John W. 1986. *War without Mercy: Race and Power in the Pacific War.* New York: Pantheon Books.

Dranove, David. 2003. *What's Your Life Worth: Health Care Rationing … Who Lives? Who Dies? And Who Decides?* Upper Saddle River, NJ: Pearson Education.

Drug Gray Market. 2012. *Journal of the American Medical Association* 308 (10): 964.

Duffy, Erin. 2012. Drug shortage crisis resolution. *Journal of Pharmacy Practice* 25 (6): 619–620. doi:10.1177/0897190012460987

Dutkowski, Philipp, Christian E. Oberkofler, Ksenija Slankamenac, Milo A. Puhan, Erik Schadde, Beat Müllhaupt, Andreas Geier, and Pierre A. Clavien. 2011. Are there better guidelines for allocation in liver transplantation?: A novel score targeting justice and utility in the model for end-stage liver disease era. *Annals of Surgery* 254 (5): 745–754. doi:10.1097/SLA.0b013e3182365081.

Dworkin, Ronald. 1993. *Life's Dominion: An Argument about Abortion and Euthanasia.* New York: Knopf.

Eddy, D. M. 1983. Finding cancer in asymptomatic people: Estimating the benefits, costs and risks. *Cancer* 51 (12 Suppl.): 2440–2445.

Eddy, D. M. 1986. Setting priorities for cancer control programs. *Journal of the National Cancer Institute* 76 (2): 187–199.

Eddy, D. M. 1991. Oregon's methods: Did cost-effectiveness analysis fail? *Journal of the American Medical Association* 266 (15): 2135–2141.

Eddy, D. M. 1992a. Clinical decision making: From theory to practice—Applying cost-effectiveness analysis: The inside story. *Journal of the American Medical Association* 268 (18): 2575–2582.

Eddy, D. M. 1992b. Clinical decision making: From theory to practice—Cost-effectiveness analysis: Is it up to the task? *Journal of the American Medical Association* 267 (24): 3342–3348.

Eddy, D. M. 1992c. Clinical decision making: From theory to practice—Cost-effectiveness analysis: Will it be accepted? *Journal of the American Medical Association* 268 (1): 132–136.

Egan, T. M., S. Murray, R. T. Bustami, T. H. Shearon, K. P. McCullough, L. B. Edwards, M. A. Coke, et al. 2006. Development of the new lung allocation system in the United States. *American Journal of Transplantation* 6 (5 part 2): 1212–1227. doi:10.1111/j.1600-6143.2006.01276.x.

Ein-Dor, Tsachi, and Gilad Hirschberger. 2012. *Sore losers: On perceptions of defeat and displaced retaliation. Social Psychological and Personality Science.* doi: 10.1177/1948550612457957.

Eisenberg, Daniel, Gary L. Freed, Matthew M. Davis, Dianne Singer, and Lisa A. Prosser. 2011. Valuing health at different ages: Evidence from a nationally representative survey in the US. *Applied Health Economics and Health Policy* 9 (3): 149–156. doi:10.2165/11587340-000000000-00000.

Emanuel, E. J., and S. D. Pearson. 2012. Physician autonomy and health care reform. *Journal of the American Medical Association* 307 (4): 367–368. doi:10.1001/jama.2012.19.

Emanuel, E. J., and A. Wertheimer. 2006. Public health: Who should get influenza vaccine when not all can? *Science* 312 (5775): 854–855.

Erin, Charles A, and John Harris. 2003. An ethical market in human organs. *Journal of Medical Ethics* 29 (3): 137–138. doi:10.1136/jme.29.3.137.

Estelle et al. v. Gamble. 1976. Supreme Court of the United States.

Fairrow, A. M., T. J. McCallum, and B. J. Messinger-Rapport. 2004. Preferences of older African-Americans for long-term tube feeding at the end of life. *Aging & Mental Health* 8 (6): 530–534.

Farjah, F., D. E. Wood, N. D. Yanez III, T. L. Vaughan, R. G. Symons, B. Krishnadasan, and D. R. Flum. 2009. Racial disparities among patients with lung cancer who were recommended operative therapy. *Archives of Surgery* 144 (1): 14–18. doi:10.1001/archsurg.2008.519.

Farmer, Steven A., James N. Kirkpatrick, Paul A. Heidenreich, Jeptha P. Curtis, Yongfei Wang, and Peter W. Groeneveld. 2009. Ethnic and racial disparities in cardiac resynchronization therapy. *Heart Rhythm* 6 (3): 325–331. doi:10.1016/j.hrthm.2008.12.018.

Fedewa, S. A., S. B. Edge, A. K. Stewart, M. T. Halpern, N. M. Marlow, and E. M. Ward. 2011. Race and ethnicity are associated with delays in breast cancer treatment (2003–2006). *Journal of Health Care for the Poor and Underserved* 22 (1): 128–141. doi:10.1353/hpu.2011.0006.

Fine, Paul, Ken Eames, and David L. Heymann. 2011. "Herd immunity": A rough guide. *Clinical Infectious Diseases* 52 (7): 911–916. doi:10.1093/cid/cir007.

Fine, R. L. 2001. The Texas Advance Directives Act of 1999: Politics and reality. *HEC Forum* 13 (1): 59–81.

Fineberg, Harvey V. 2012. A successful and sustainable health system—how to get there from here. *New England Journal of Medicine* 366 (11): 1020–1027. doi:10.1056/NEJMsa1114777.

Flamme, N. E., C. L. Terry, and P. R. Helft. 2008. The influence of psychosocial evaluation on candidacy for liver transplantation. *Progress in Transplantation (Aliso Viejo, CA)* 18 (2): 89–96.

Fleck, Leonard M. 2009. *Just Caring: Health Care Rationing and Democratic Deliberation.* New York: Oxford University Press.

Flint, Kelsey M., Daniel D. Matlock, JoAnn Lindenfeld, and Larry A. Allen. 2012. Frailty and the selection of patients for destination therapy left ventricular assist device. *Circulation: Heart Failure* 5 (2): 286–293. doi:10.1161/circheartfailure.111.963215.

Flores, Glenn, and Sandra C. Tomany-Korman. 2008. Racial and ethnic disparities in medical and dental health, access to care, and use of services in US children. *Pediatrics* 121 (2): e286–e298. doi:10.1542/peds.2007-1243.

Ford, Henry, in collaboration with Samuel Crowther. 1922. *My Life and Work.* Garden City, NY: Garden City Publishing.

Forsythe, John. 2012. Debating the ethics of organ transplantation. *Lancet* 380 (9847): 1047. doi:10.1016/S0140-6736(12)61586-4.

Fox, D. M., and H. M. Leichter. 1991. Rationing care in Oregon: The new accountability. *Health Affairs* 10 (2): 7–27.

Fox, D. M., and H. Markel. 2010. Is history relevant to implementing health reform? *Journal of the American Medical Association* 303 (17): 1749–1750. doi:10.1001/jama.2010.556.

Fox, Erin R., and Linda S. Tyler. 2003. Managing drug shortages: Seven years' experience at one health system. *American Journal of Health-System Pharmacy* 60 (3): 245.

Fox, M. D. 2003. Stewards of public trust: Responsible transplantation. *American Journal of Bioethics (AJOB)* 3 (1): v–vii. doi:10.1162/152651603321611773.

Frader, Joel E. 2012. Re-evaluating the recipient criteria for organ transplants. *Pediatric Annals* 41 (4): 135–136. doi:10.3928/00904481-20120307-03.

Frakes, Vincent L. 2012. Partisanship and (un)compromise: A study of the Patient Protection and Affordable Care Act. *Harvard Journal on Legislation* 49:135–150.

Frankfurt, H. G. 2005. *On Bullshit.* Princeton: Princeton University Press.

Friedman, E. A., and A. L. Friedman. 2006. Payment for donor kidneys: Pros and cons. *Kidney International* 69 (6): 960–962.

Gabbay, Ezra, and Klemens B. Meyer. 2009. Identifying critically ill patients with acute kidney injury for whom renal replacement therapy is inappropriate: An exercise in futility? *NDT Plus* 2 (2): 97–103. doi:10.1093/ndtplus/sfn196.

Galarneau, C. 2011. Still missing: Undocumented immigrants in health care reform. *Journal of Health Care for the Poor and Underserved* 22 (2): 422–428. doi:10.1353/hpu.2011.0040.

Galbraith, John Kenneth. 1943. Price control: Some lessons from the first phase. *American Economic Review* 33 (1): 253–259. doi:10.2307/1819009.

Galbraith, John Kenneth. 1981. *A Life in Our Times: Memoirs.* Boston: Houghton Mifflin.

Gao, Hai-Nv, Hong-Zhou Lu, Bin Cao, Bin Du, Hong Shang, Jian-He Gan, Shui-Hua Lu, et al. 2013. Clinical findings in 111 cases of Influenza A (H7N9) virus infection. *New England Journal of Medicine* 368 (24): 2277–2285. doi:10.1056/NEJMoa1305584.

Garber, Alan M., and C. E. Phelps. 1997. Economic foundations of cost-effectiveness analysis. *Journal of Health Economics* 16 (1): 1–31.

Garber, Alan M., and Sean R. Tunis. 2009. Does comparative-effectiveness research threaten personalized medicine? *New England Journal of Medicine* 360 (19): 1925–1927. doi:10.1056/NEJMp0901355.

Gatesman, Mandy L., and Thomas J. Smith. 2011. The shortage of essential chemotherapy drugs in the United States. *New England Journal of Medicine* 365 (18): 1653–1655. doi:10.1056/NEJMp1109772.

Gawande, A. A., A. K. Jha, E. Orav, and K. E. Joynt. 2013. Contribution of preventable acute care spending to total spending for high-cost Medicare patients. *Journal of the American Medical Association* 309 (24): 2572–2578. doi:10.1001/jama.2013.7103.

Gehrett, B. K. 2012. A prescription for drug shortages. *Journal of the American Medical Association* 307 (2): 153–154. doi:10.1001/jama.2011.2000.

Gerber, Alan S., Eric M. Patashnik, David Doherty, and Conor Dowling. 2010. The public wants information, not board mandates, from comparative effectiveness research. *Health Affairs* 29 (10): 1872–1881. doi:10.1377/hlthaff.2010.0655.

Geruso, Michael. 2012. Black-white disparities in life expectancy: How much can the standard SES variables explain? *Demography* 49 (2): 553–574. doi:10.1007/s13524-011-0089-1.

Giacomini, Mita K., Deborah J. Cook, David L. Streiner, and Sonia S. Anand. 2001. Guidelines as rationing tools: A qualitative analysis of psychosocial patient selection criteria for cardiac procedures. *CMAJ: Canadian Medical Association Journal* 164 (5): 634.

Gill, P., and L. Lowes. 2008. Gift exchange and organ donation: Donor and recipient experiences of live related kidney transplantation. *International Journal of Nursing Studies* 45 (11): 1607–1617.

Golann, Dwight. 2011. Dropped medical malpractice claims: Their surprising frequency, apparent causes, and potential remedies. *Health Affairs* 30 (7): 1343–1350. doi:10.1377/hlthaff.2010.1132.

Goldberg, A. M., M. Simmerling, and J. E. Frader. 2007. Why nondocumented residents should have access to kidney transplantation: Arguments for lifting the federal ban on reimbursement. *Transplantation* 83 (1): 17–20. doi:10.1097/01.tp.0000247795.41898.55.

Goldfarb-Rumyantzev, Alexander S., James K. Koford, Bradley C. Baird, Madhukar Chelamcharla, Arsalan N. Habib, Ben-Jr Wang, Lin Shih-jui, Fuad Shihab, and Ross B. Isaacs. 2006. Role of socioeconomic status in kidney transplant outcome. *Clinical Journal of the American Society of Nephrology (CJASN)* 1 (2): 313–322. doi:10.2215/cjn.00630805.

Goldsteen, Raymond L., Karen Goldsteen, James H. Swan, and Wendy Clemeña. 2001. Harry and Louise and health care reform: Romancing public opinion. *Journal of Health Politics, Policy and Law* 26 (6): 1325–1352. doi:10.1215/03616878-26-6-1325.

Goldzwig, Steven R. 2003. LBJ, the rhetoric of transcendence, and the Civil Rights Act of 1968. *Rhetoric & Public Affairs* 6 (1): 25–53.

Gould, Stephen Jay. 1981. *The Mismeasure of Man.* 2nd ed. New York: Norton.

Govier, Trudy. 1982. What's wrong with slippery slope arguments? *Canadian Journal of Philosophy* 12 (2): 303–316. doi:10.2307/40231258.

Grande, David, Sarah E. Gollust, and David A. Asch. 2011. Polling analysis: Public support for health reform was broader than reported and depended on how proposals were framed. *Health Affairs* 30 (7): 1242–1249. doi:10.1377/hlthaff.2011.0180.

Gray, Alastair M., Philip M. Clarke, Jane L. Wolstenholme, and Sarah Wordsworth. 2011. *Applied Methods of Cost-Effectiveness Analysis in Healthcare.* Oxford: Oxford University Press.

Gray, S. W., F. J. Hlubocky, M. J. Ratain, and C. K. Daugherty. 2007. Attitudes toward research participation and investigator conflicts of interest among advanced cancer patients participating in early phase clinical trials. *Journal of Clinical Oncology* 25 (23): 3488–3494.

Grayson, Martha S., Dale A. Newton, and Lori F. Thompson. 2012. Payback time: The associations of debt and income with medical student career choice. *Medical Education* 46 (10): 983–991. doi:10.1111/j.1365-2923.2012.04340.x.

Gregory, P. C., T. A. LaVeist, and C. Simpson. 2006. Racial disparities in access to cardiac rehabilitation. *American Journal of Physical Medicine & Rehabilitation / Association of Academic Psychiatrists* 85 (9): 705–710. doi:10.1097/01.phm.0000233181.34999.3d.

Griffin, M. D., and M. Prieto. 2008. Case studies in transplant ethics. *Transplantation Reviews (Orlando, FL)* 22 (3): 178–183.

Griffin, Xavier L., David Wallace, Nick Parsons, and L. Costa Matthew. 2012. Platelet rich therapies for long bone healing in adults. *Cochrane Database of Systematic Reviews* (7). http://onlinelibrary.wiley.com/doi/10.1002/14651858.CD009496.pub2/abstract.

Gross, Liza. 2009. A broken trust: Lessons from the vaccine-autism wars. *PLOS Biology* 7 (5): e1000114.

Gross, Wendy, Tobias Stark, Jon Krosnick, Josh Pasek, Trevor Tompson, Jennifer Agiesta, and Dennis Junius. 2012. *Americans' Attitudes toward the Affordable Care Act: Would Better Public Understanding Increase or Decrease Favorability?* Stanford University. https://pprg.stanford.edu/wp-content/uploads/Health-Care-2012-Knowledge-and-Favorability.pdf.

Grubbs, S. S., P. A. Grusenmyer, N. J. Petrelli, and R. J. Gralla. 2006. Is it cost-effective to add erlotinib to gemcitabine in advanced pancreatic cancer? *Journal of Clinical Oncology* 24 (18S): 6048.

Grund, Christian, and Dirk Sliwka. 2005. Envy and compassion in tournaments. *Journal of Economics & Management Strategy* 14 (1): 187–207. doi:10.1111/j.1430-9134.2005.00039.x.

Gruttadauria, S., G. Grosso, A. Mistretta, D. Pagano, G. Scianna, G. B. Vizzini, D. Cintorino, M. Spada, F. Basile, and B. Gridelli. 2011. Impact of recipients' socio-economic status on patient and graft survival after liver transplantation:

The IsMeTT experience. *Digestive and Liver Disease: Official Journal of the Italian Society of Gastroenterology and the Italian Association for the Study of the Liver* 43 (11): 893–898. doi:10.1016/j.dld.2011.06.017.

Gupta, D. K., and S. M. Huang. 2013. Drug shortages in the United States: A critical evaluation of root causes and the need for action. *Clinical Pharmacology and Therapeutics* 93 (2): 133–135.

Guttmacher, Alan E., Amy L. McGuire, Bruce Ponder, and Kari Stefansson. 2010. Personalized genomic information: Preparing for the future of genetic medicine. *Nature Reviews: Genetics* 11 (2): 161–165.

Guttman, Nurit, Tamar Ashkenazi, Anat Gesser-Edelsburg, and Vered Seidmann. 2011. Laypeople's ethical concerns about a new Israeli organ transplantation prioritization policy aimed to encourage organ donor registration among the public. *Journal of Health Politics, Policy and Law* 36 (4): 691–716. doi:10.1215/03616878-1334686.

Guyatt, Gordon, Elie A. Akl, Jack Hirsh, Clive Kearon, Mark Crowther, David Gutterman, Sandra Zelman Lewis, Ian Nathanson, Roman Jaeschke, and Holger Schnemann. 2010. The vexing problem of guidelines and conflict of interest: A potential solution. *Annals of Internal Medicine* 152 (11): 738–741. doi:10.7326/0003-4819-152-11-201006010-00254.

Guzman, Jorge A., Madhu Sasidhar, and James K. Stoller. 2011. Caring for VIPs: Nine principles. *Cleveland Clinic Journal of Medicine* 78 (2): 90–94. doi:10.3949/ccjm.78a.10113.

Hadorn, D. C. 1991. Setting health care priorities in Oregon: Cost-effectiveness meets the rule of rescue. *Journal of the American Medical Association* 265 (17): 2218–2225.

Hall, Mark A., Wenke Hwang, and Alison Snow Jones. 2011. Model safety-net programs could care for the uninsured at one-half the cost of Medicaid or private insurance. *Health Affairs* 30 (9): 1698–1707. doi:10.1377/hlthaff.2010.0946.

Halpern, Neil A., and Stephen M. Pastores. 2010. Critical care medicine in the United States 2000–2005: An analysis of bed numbers, occupancy rates, payer mix, and costs. *Critical Care Medicine* 38 (1): 65–71. doi:10.1097/CCM.0b013e3181b090d0.

Halpern, Scott D. 2013. Turning wrong into right: The 2013 lung allocation controversy. *Annals of Internal Medicine* 159 (5): 358–359. doi:10.7326/0003-4819-159-5-201309030-00684.

Halpern, Scott D., and Robert D. Truog. 2010. Organ donors after circulatory determination of death: Not necessarily dead, and it does not necessarily matter. *Critical Care Medicine* 38 (3): 1011–1012. doi:10.1097/CCM.0b013e3181cc1228.

Hamann, J., G. Kolbe, R. Cohen, S. Leucht, and W. Kissling. 2005. How do psychiatrists choose among different antipsychotics? *European Journal of Clinical Pharmacology* 61 (11): 851–854.

Hamburg, Margaret A., and Francis S. Collins. 2010. The path to personalized medicine. *New England Journal of Medicine* 363 (4): 301–304. doi:10.1056/NEJMp1006304.

Hanchate, Amresh, Andrea C. Kronman, Yinong Young-Xu, Arlene S. Ash, and Ezekiel Emanuel. 2009. Racial and ethnic differences in end-of-life costs: Why do minorities cost more than whites? *Archives of Internal Medicine* 169 (5): 493–501. doi:10.1001/archinternmed.2008.616.

Harris, John. 1975. The survival lottery. *Philosophy (London)* 50 (191): 81–87.

Harris, John. 1980. *Violence and Responsibility*. London: Routledge & Kegan Paul.

Harris, John. 1985. *The Value of Life: An Introduction to Medical Ethics*. London: Routledge & Kegan Paul.

Harris, John. 1994. The survival lottery. In Bonnie Steinbock and Alastair Norcross, eds., *Killing and Letting Die*, 257–265. New York: Fordham University Press.

Harris, Y., P. B. Gorelick, P. Samuels, and I. Bempong. 1996. Why African Americans may not be participating in clinical trials. *Journal of the National Medical Association* 88 (10): 630–634.

Hartman, Micah, Anne B. Martin, Joseph Benson, Aaron Catlin, and the National Health Expenditure Accounts Team. 2013. National health spending in 2011: Overall growth remains low, but some payers and services show signs of acceleration. *Health Affairs* 32 (1): 87–99. doi:10.1377/hlthaff.2012.1206.

Haselton, Martie G., and Daniel Nettle. 2006. The paranoid optimist: An integrative evolutionary model of cognitive biases. *Personality and Social Psychology Review* 10 (1): 47–66. doi:10.1207/s15327957pspr1001_3.

Hendrick, R. Edward, and Mark A. Helvie. 2011. United States Preventive Services Task Force screening mammography recommendations: Science ignored. *American Journal of Roentgenology (AJR)* 196 (2): W112–W116. doi:10.2214/ajr.10.5609.

Henrich, Joseph, Jean Ensminger, Richard McElreath, Abigail Barr, Clark Barrett, Alexander Bolyanatz, Juan Camilo Cardenas, et al. 2010. Markets, religion, community size, and the evolution of fairness and punishment. *Science* 327 (5972): 1480–1484. doi:10.1126/science.1182238.

Herrnstein, R. J., and C. Murray. 1994. *The Bell Curve: Intelligence and Class Structure in American Life*. New York: Free Press.

Hippen, Benjamin E., J. Richard Thistlethwaite, and Lainie Friedman Ross. 2011. Risk, prognosis, and unintended consequences in kidney allocation. *New England Journal of Medicine* 364 (14): 1285–1287. doi:10.1056/NEJMp1102583.

Hochberg, Mark S., Carolyn D. Seib, Russell S. Berman, Adina L. Kalet, Sondra R. Zabar, and H. Leon Pachter. 2011. Perspective: Malpractice in an academic medical center: A frequently overlooked aspect of professionalism education. *Academic Medicine* 86 (3): 365–368. doi:10.1097/ACM.0b013e3182086d72.

Hoffman, Ari, and Steven D. Pearson. 2009. "Marginal medicine": Targeting comparative effectiveness research to reduce waste. *Health Affairs* 28 (4): w710–w718. doi:10.1377/hlthaff.28.4.w710.

Hoffman, S. 2012. The drugs stop here: A public health framework to address the drug shortage crisis. *Food and Drug Law Journal* 67 (1): 1–21.

Howard, Daniel L., April P. Carson, N. Holmes DaJuanicia, and Jay S. Kaufman. 2009. Consistency of care and blood pressure control among elderly African Americans and whites with hypertension. *Journal of the American Board of Family Medicine* 22 (3): 307–315. doi:10.3122/jabfm.2009.03.080145.

Hsieh, Matthew M., James E. Everhart, Danita D. Byrd-Holt, John F. Tisdale, and Griffin P. Rodgers. 2007. Prevalence of neutropenia in the U.S. population: Age, sex, smoking status, and ethnic differences. *Annals of Internal Medicine* 146 (7): 486–492. doi:10.7326/0003-4819-146-7-200704030-00004.

Hu, Yue-Yung, Alvin C. Kwok, Wei Jiang, Nathan Taback, Elizabeth T. Loggers, Gladys V. Ting, Stuart R. Lipsitz, Jane C. Weeks, and Caprice C. Greenberg. 2012. High-cost imaging in elderly patients with stage IV cancer. *Journal of the National Cancer Institute* 104 (15): 1165–1173. doi:10.1093/jnci/djs286.

Huang, Priscilla. 2008. Anchor babies, over-breeders, and the population bomb: The reemergence of nativism and population control in anti-immigration policies. *Harvard Law and Policy Review* 2:385–406.

Humphrey, Nicholas. 2006. Introduction: Science looks at fairness. *Social Research* 73 (2): 345–347.

Hurst, S. A., and M. Danis. 2007. A framework for rationing by clinical judgment. *Kennedy Institute of Ethics Journal* 17 (3): 247–266.

Hynes, Denise M., Kevin T. Stroupe, Michael J. Fischer, Domenic J. Reda, Willard Manning, Margaret M. Browning, Zhiping Huo, Karen Saban, James S. Kaufman, and the ESRD Cost Study Group. 2012. Comparing VA and private sector healthcare costs for end-stage renal disease. *Medical Care* 50 (2): 161–170. doi:10.1097/MLR.0b013e31822dcf15.

Iglehart, John K. 1982. New Jersey's experiment with DRG-based hospital reimbursement. *New England Journal of Medicine* 307 (26): 1655–1660. doi:10.1056/NEJM198212233072632.

Iltis, A. S., M. A. Rie, and A. Wall. 2009. Organ donation, patients' rights, and medical responsibilities at the end of life. *Critical Care Medicine* 37 (1): 310–315. doi:10.1097/CCM.0b013e3181928ff8.

Institute of Medicine, Committee on Increasing Rates of Organ Donation. 2006. *Organ Donation: Opportunities for Action*, Committee on Increasing Rates of Organ, Donation, James F. Childress, and Catharyn T. Liverman, eds. Washington, DC: National Academies Press, c.

Jacobs, E. A., I. Rolle, C. E. Ferrans, E. E. Whitaker, and R. B. Warnecke. 2006. Understanding African Americans' views of the trustworthiness of physicians. *Journal of General Internal Medicine* 21 (6): 642–647. doi:10.1111/j.1525-1497.2006.00485.x.

Jacobs, Meg. 1997. "How about some meat?": The Office of Price Administration, consumption politics, and state building from the bottom up, 1941–1946. *Journal of American History* 84 (3): 910–941. doi:10.2307/2953088.

Jenni, K. E., and G. Loewenstein. 1997. Explaining the "identifiable victim effect." *Journal of Risk and Uncertainty* 14 (3): 235–257.

Jensen, Valerie, and Bob A. Rappaport. 2010. The reality of drug shortages—the case of the injectable agent propofol. *New England Journal of Medicine* 363 (9): 806–807. doi:10.1056/NEJMp1005849.

Jha, A. K., D. O. Staiger, F. L. Lucas, and A. Chandra. 2007. Do race-specific models explain disparities in treatments after acute myocardial infarction? *American Heart Journal* 153 (5): 785–791.

Johannesson, Magnus, and Per-Olov Johansson. 1996. The economics of ageing: On the attitude of Swedish people to the distribution of health care resources between the young and the old. *Health Policy (Amsterdam)* 37 (3): 153–161. doi:10.1016/s0168-8510(96)90022-6.

Johnson, E. J., and D. G. Goldstein. 2004. Defaults and donation decisions. *Transplantation* 78 (12): 1713–1716.

Johri, Mira, Laura J. Damschroder, Brian J. Zikmund-Fisher, and Peter A. Ubel. 2005. The importance of age in allocating health care resources: Does intervention-type matter? *Health Economics* 14 (7): 669–678. doi:10.1002/hec.958.

Jones, D. J., A. N. Barkun, Y. Lu, R. Enns, P. Sinclair, M. Martel, I. Gralnek, M. Bardou, E. J. Kuipers, and J. Sung. 2012. Conflicts of interest ethics: Silencing expertise in the development of international clinical practice guidelines. *Annals of Internal Medicine* 156 (11): 809–816. doi:10.1059/0003-4819-156-11-201206050-00008.

Jonsen, Albert R. 1986. Bentham in a box: Technology assessment and health care allocation. *Law, Medicine & Health Care* 14 (3–4): 172–174.

Jonsen, Albert R., Shana Alexander, Judith P. Swazey, Warren T. Reich, Robert M. Veatch, Daniel Callahan, Tom L. Beauchamp, et al. 1993. Special supplement: The birth of bioethics. *Hastings Center Report* 23 (6): S1–S16.

Joshi, Shivam, Jeffrey J. Gaynor, Stephanie Bayers, Giselle Guerra, Ahmed Eldefrawy, Zoila Chediak, Lazara Companioni, Junichiro Sageshima, Linda Chen, Warren Kupin, David Roth, Adela Mattiazzi, George W. Burke III, and Gaetano Ciancio. 2013. Disparities among blacks, Hispanics, and whites in time from starting dialysis to kidney transplant waitlisting. *Transplantation* 95 (2): 309–318. doi:10.1097/TP.0b013e31827191d4.

Jox, Ralf J., Andreas Schaider, Georg Marckmann, and Gian Domenico Borasio. 2012. Medical futility at the end of life: The perspectives of intensive care and palliative care clinicians. *Journal of Medical Ethics* 38 (9): 540–545. doi:10.1136/medethics-2011-100479.

Kaakeh, Rola, Burgunda V. Sweet, Cynthia Reilly, Colleen Bush, Sherry DeLoach, Barb Higgins, Angela M. Clark, and James Stevenson. 2011. Impact of drug shortages on U.S. health systems. *American Journal of Health-System Pharmacy* 68 (19): 1811–1819. doi:10.2146/ajhp110210.

Kachalia, Allen, and Michelle M. Mello. 2011. New directions in medical liability reform. *New England Journal of Medicine* 364 (16): 1564–1572. doi:10.1056/NEJMhpr1012821.

Kahn, J. 2003. The ethics of organ transplantation for prisoners. *Seminars in Dialysis* 16 (5): 365–366.

Kahneman, Daniel. 2011. *Thinking, Fast and Slow*. New York: Farrar, Straus and Giroux.

Kamerow, Douglas. 2011. PCORI: Odd name, important job, potential trouble. *BMJ* 342. doi:10.1136/bmj.d2635.

Kamm, F. M. 1993. *Death, and Whom to Save from It*. Vol. 1: *Morality, Mortality*. New York: Oxford University Press.

Kaplan V, Clermont G. Griffin M. F., and et al. 2003. "Pneumonia: Still the old man's friend?" *Archives of Internal Medicine* 163 (3):317–323. doi: 10.1001/archinte.163.3.317.

Keating, Nancy L., Mary Beth Landrum, Selwyn O. Rogers, Susan K. Baum, Beth A. Virnig, Haiden A. Huskamp, Craig C. Earle, and Katherine L. Kahn. 2010. Physician factors associated with discussions about end-of-life care. *Cancer* 116 (4): 998–1006. doi:10.1002/cncr.24761.

Keehan, Sean, Andrea Sisko, Christopher Truffer, Sheila Smith, Cathy Cowan, John Poisal, M. Kent Clemens, the National Health Expenditure Accounts Projections Team, Centers for Medicare, and Baltimore Medicaid Services, Maryland. 2008. Health spending projections through 2017: The baby-boom generation is coming to Medicare. *Health Affairs* 27 (2): w145–w155. doi:10.1377/hlthaff.27.2.w145.

Keehan, Sean P., Andrea M. Sisko, Christopher J. Truffer, John A. Poisal, Gigi A. Cuckler, Andrew J. Madison, Joseph M. Lizonitz, and Sheila D. Smith. 2011. National health spending projections through 2020: Economic recovery and reform drive faster spending growth. *Health Affairs* 30 (8): 1594–1605. doi:10.1377/hlthaff.2011.0662.

Kemmer, N., A. Alsina, and G. W. Neff. 2011. Social determinants of orthotopic liver transplantation candidacy: Role of patient-related factors. *Transplantation Proceedings* 43 (10): 3769–3772. doi:10.1016/j.transproceed.2011.08.076.

Kershnar, Stephen. 1999. Are the descendants of slaves owed compensation for slavery? *Journal of Applied Philosophy* 16 (1): 95–101. doi:10.1111/1468-5930.00111.

Kesselheim, A. S., J. A. Myers, and J. Avorn. 2011. Characteristics of clinical trials to support approval of orphan vs nonorphan drugs for cancer. *Journal of the American Medical Association* 305 (22): 2320–2326. doi:10.1001/jama.2011.769.

Khushf, George. 2010. A matter of respect: A defense of the dead donor rule and of a "whole-brain" criterion for determination of death. *Journal of Medicine and Philosophy* 35 (3): 330–364. doi:10.1093/jmp/jhq023.

Kilner, John F. 1990. *Who Lives? Who Dies?* New Haven, CT: Yale University Press.

Kirklin, James K., David C. Naftel, Robert L. Kormos, Lynne W. Stevenson, Francis D. Pagani, Marissa A. Miller, Karen L. Ulisney, J. Timothy Baldwin, and James B. Young. 2011. Third INTERMACS Annual Report: The evolution of destination therapy in the United States. *Journal of Heart and Lung Transplantation* 30 (2): 115–123. doi:10.1016/j.healun.2010.12.001.

Kitzhaber, John A. 1993. Prioritising health services in an era of limits: The Oregon experience. *British Medical Journal* 307 (6900): 373–377.

Klevit, Harvey D., Alan C. Bates, Tina Castanares, E. Paul Kirk, Paige R. Sipes-Metzler, and Richard Wopat. 1991. Prioritization of Health Care Services: A Progress Report by the Oregon Health Services Commission. *Archives of Internal Medicine* 151 (5): 912–916. doi:10.1001/archinte.1991.00400050062012.

Kohn, L. T., J. M. Corrigan, and M. S. Donaldson. 2000. *To Err Is Human: Building a Safer Health System.* Washington, DC: National Academy Press.

Kohn, R., G. D. Rubenfeld, M. M. Levy, P. A. Ubel, and S. D. Halpern. 2011. Rule of rescue or the good of the many? An analysis of physicians' and nurses' preferences for allocating ICU beds. *Intensive Care Medicine* 37 (7): 1210–1217. doi:10.1007/s00134-011-2257-6.

Kolata, G., and K. Eichenwald. 2000. Insurer drops a therapy for breast cancer. *New York Times*, February 16, 2000, 24.

Koppes, Clayton R. 1987. *Hollywood Goes to War: How Politics, Profits, and Propaganda Shaped World War II Movies*, Gregory D. Black, ed. New York: Free Press.

Kotlyar, David S., Anne Burke, Mical S. Campbell, and Robert M. Weinrieb. 2008. A critical review of candidacy for orthotopic liver transplantation in alcoholic liver disease. *American Journal of Gastroenterology* 103 (3): 734–743.

Kovacs, Pamela J., Nathan Perkins, Elizabeth Nuschke, and Norman Carroll. 2012. How end-stage renal disease patients manage the Medicare Part D coverage gap. *Health & Social Work* 37 (4): 225–233. doi:10.1093/hsw/hls031.

Kravitz, Richard L., and Mitchell D. Feldman. 2010. From the Editors' Desk: Confronting costs of care at the end of life. *Journal of General Internal Medicine* 25 (10): 997. doi:10.1007/s11606-010-1474-y.

Krimsky, Sheldon. 2012. The short life of a race drug. *Lancet* 379 (9811): 114–115.

Kroeker, K. I., V. G. Bain, T. Shaw-Stiffel, T. L. Fong, and E. M. Yoshida. 2008. Adult liver transplant survey: Policies towards eligibility criteria in Canada and the United States 2007. *Liver International* 28 (9): 1250–1255.

Kucirka, L. M., M. E. Grams, K. S. Balhara, B. G. Jaar, and D. L. Segev. 2012. Disparities in provision of transplant information affect access to kidney transplantation. *American Journal of Transplantation* 12 (2): 351–357. doi:10.1111/j.1600-6143.2011.03865.x.

Kwak, Eunice L., Yung-Jue Bang, D. Ross Camidge, Alice T. Shaw, Benjamin Solomon, Robert G. Maki, Sai-Hong I. Ou, Bruce J. Dezube, Pasi A. Jänne, Daniel B. Costa, Marileila Varella-Garcia, Woo-Ho Kim, Thomas J. Lynch, Panos Fidias, Hannah Stubbs, Jeffrey A. Engelman, Lecia V. Sequist, WeiWei Tan, Leena Gandhi, Mari Mino-Kenudson, Greg C. Wei, S. Martin Shreeve, Mark J. Ratain, Jeffrey Settleman, James G. Christensen, Daniel A. Haber, Keith Wilner, Ravi Salgia, Geoffrey I. Shapiro, Jeffrey W. Clark, and A. John Iafrate. 2010. Anaplastic lymphoma kinase inhibition in non-small-cell lung cancer. *New England Journal of Medicine* 363 (18): 1693–1703. doi:10.1056/NEJMoa1006448.

Kwok, Alvin C., Marcus E. Semel, Stuart R. Lipsitz, Angela M. Bader, Amber E. Barnato, Atul A. Gawande, and Ashish K. Jha. 2011. The intensity and variation of surgical care at the end of life: A retrospective cohort study. *The Lancet* 378 (9800): 1408–1413. doi:10.1016/S0140-6736(11)61268-3.

Ladin, K., and D. W. Hanto. 2011. Rational rationing or discrimination: Balancing equity and efficiency considerations in kidney allocation. *American Journal of Transplantation* 11 (11): 2317–2321. doi:10.1111/j.1600-6143.2011.03726.x.

Lange, Beverly J., Franklin O. Smith, James Feusner, Dorothy R. Barnard, Patricia Dinndorf, Stephen Feig, Nyla A. Heerema, et al. 2008. Outcomes in CCG-2961, a Children's Oncology Group Phase 3 Trial for untreated pediatric acute myeloid leukemia: A report from the Children's Oncology Group. *Blood* 111 (3): 1044–1053. doi:10.1182/blood-2007-04-084293.

Lantos, J., and D. Matlock A. Wendler. 2011. Clinician integrity and limits to patient autonomy. *Journal of the American Medical Association* 305 (5): 495–499. doi:10.1001/jama.2011.32.

Largent, Emily A., and Steven D. Pearson. 2012. Which orphans will find a home? The rule of rescue in resource allocation for rare diseases. *Hastings Center Report* 42 (1): 27–34. doi:10.1002/hast.12.

Laugesen, Miriam J., and Sherry A. Glied. 2011. Higher fees paid to US physicians drive higher spending for physician services compared to other countries. *Health Affairs* 30 (9): 1647–1656. doi:10.1377/hlthaff.2010.0204.

Lavee, J., T. Ashkenazi, G. Gurman, and D. Steinberg. 2010. A new law for allocation of donor organs in Israel. *Lancet* 375 (9720): 1131–1133. doi:10.1016/S0140-6736(09)61795-5.

Lee, Seung Hyun, Cheol Hyun Chung, Jae Won Lee, Sung Ho Jung, and Suk Jung Choo. 2012. Factors predicting early- and long-term survival in patients undergoing extracorporeal membrane oxygenation (ECMO). *Journal of Cardiac Surgery* 27 (2): 255–263. doi:10.1111/j.1540-8191.2011.01400.x.

Leff, B., and T. E. Finucane. 2008. Gizmo idolatry. *Journal of the American Medical Association* 299 (15): 1830–1832. doi:10.1001/jama.299.15.1830.

Leff, Mark H. 1991. The politics of sacrifice on the American home front in World War II. *Journal of American History* 77 (4): 1296–1318. doi:10.2307/2078263.

Lenzer, Jeanne. 2003. Spin doctors soft pedal data on antihypertensives. *BMJ (Clinical Research Ed.)* 326 (7381): 170. doi:10.1136/bmj.326.7381.170.

Lenzer, Jeanne. 2012. Unnecessary care: Are doctors in denial and is profit driven healthcare to blame? *BMJ (Clinical Research Ed.)* 345. doi:10.1136/bmj.e6230.

Levenson, J. L., and M. E. Olbrisch. 1993. Psychosocial evaluation of organ transplant candidates: A comparative survey of process, criteria, and outcomes in heart, liver, and kidney transplantation. *Psychosomatics* 34 (4): 314–323.

Levin, Henry M., and Patrick J. McEwan. 2001. *Cost-Effectiveness Analysis: Methods and Applications*. 2nd ed. Thousand Oaks, CA: Sage.

Li, Meng, Jeffrey Vietri, Alison P. Galvani, and Gretchen B. Chapman. 2010. How do people value life? *Psychological Science* 21 (2): 163–167. doi:10.1177/0956797609357707.

Liang, Bryan A., and Tim K. Mackey. 2012. Online availability and safety of drugs in shortage: A descriptive study of Internet vendor characteristics. *Journal of Medical Internet Research* 14 (1): 27. doi:10.2196/jmir.1999.

Lichtman, Marshall A. 2001. Acute myelogenous leukaemia doi: 10.1002/9780470015902.a0002180.pub3.

Linden, Ellena A., Jeannette Cano, and George N. Coritsidis. 2012. Kidney transplantation in undocumented immigrants with ESRD: A policy whose time has come? *American Journal of Kidney Diseases* 60 (3): 354–359. doi:10.1053/j.ajkd.2012.05.016.

Lindsay, R. A. 2009. Oregon's experience: Evaluating the record. *American Journal of Bioethics* 9 (3): 19–27.

Link, Michael P., Karen Hagerty, and Hagop M. Kantarjian. 2012. Chemotherapy drug shortages in the United States: Genesis and potential solutions. *Journal of Clinical Oncology* 30 (7): 692–694. doi:10.1200/jco.2011.41.0936.

Liu, V., M. R. Zamora, G. S. Dhillon, and D. Weill. 2010. Increasing lung allocation scores predict worsened survival among lung transplant recipients. *American Journal of Transplantation* 10 (4): 915–920. doi:10.1111/j.1600-6143.2009.03003.x.

Luce, J. M. 2010. A history of resolving conflicts over end-of-life care in intensive care units in the United States. *Critical Care Medicine* 38 (8): 1623–1629. doi:10.1097/CCM.0b013e3181e71530.

Lugtenberg, M., J. M. Zegers–Van Schaick, G. P. Westert, and J. S. Burgers. 2009. Why don't physicians adhere to guideline recommendations in practice? An analysis of barriers among Dutch general practitioners. *Implementation Science (IS)* 4:54. doi:10.1186/1748-5908-4-54.

Lund, Lars H., Jennifer Matthews, and Keith Aaronson. 2010. Patient selection for left ventricular assist devices. *European Journal of Heart Failure* 12 (5): 434–443. doi:10.1093/eurjhf/hfq006.

Luyten, Jeroen, Antoon Vandevelde, Pierre Van Damme, and Philippe Beutels. 2011. Vaccination policy and ethical challenges posed by herd immunity, suboptimal uptake and subgroup targeting. *Public Health Ethics* 4 (3): 280–291. doi:10.1093/phe/phr032.

Ma, Junling, Jonathan Dushoff, and David J. D. Earn. 2011. Age-specific mortality risk from pandemic influenza. *Journal of Theoretical Biology* 288:29–34. doi:10.1016/j.jtbi.2011.08.003.

MacDorman, M. F., and T. J. Mathews. 2010. Behind international rankings of infant mortality: How the United States compares with Europe. *International Journal of Health Services* 40 (4): 577–588.

Machery, Edouard. 2008. Massive modularity and the flexibility of human cognition. *Mind & Language* 23 (3): 263–272. doi:10.1111/j.1468-0017.2008.00341.x.

Mackenzie, R., S. Chapman, G. Salkeld, and S. Holding. 2008. Media influence on Herceptin subsidization in Australia: Application of the rule of rescue? *Journal of the Royal Society of Medicine* 101 (6): 305–312. doi:10.1258/jrsm.2008.070289.

Marmor, Theodore R. 2000. *The Politics of Medicare: Social Institutions and Social Change*. 2nd ed. New York: Aldine de Gruyter.

Marshall, K. J., X. Urrutia-Rojas, F. S. Mas, and C. Coggin. 2005. Health status and access to health care of documented and undocumented immigrant Latino women. *Health Care for Women International* 26 (10): 916–936.

Masterton, G. 2000. Psychosocial factors in selection for liver transplantation: Need to be explicitly assessed and managed. *BMJ (Clinical Research Ed.)* 320 (7230): 263–264.

Matas, A. J. 2009. Allocation or rationing—word choice is crucial. *American Journal of Transplantation* 9 (1): 9–10. doi:10.1111/j.1600-6143.2008.02484.x.

Mathur, A. K., D. E. Schaubel, Q. Gong, M. K. Guidinger, and R. M. Merion. 2010. Racial and ethnic disparities in access to liver transplantation. *Liver Transplantation* 16 (9): 1033–1040. doi:10.1002/lt.22108.

Mathur, A. K., D. E. Schaubel, Q. Gong, M. K. Guidinger, and R. M. Merion. 2011. Sex-based disparities in liver transplant rates in the United States. *American Journal of Transplantation* 11 (7): 1435–1443. doi:10.1111/j.1600-6143.2011.03498.x.

Matlack, D. R. 1972. Changes and trends in medical education. *Academic Medicine* 47 (8): 612–619.

McCarthy, Ellen P., Michael J. Pencina, Margaret Kelly-Hayes, Jane C. Evans, Elizabeth J. Oberacker, Ralph B. D'Agostino, Risa B. Burns, and Joanne M. Murabito. 2008. Advance care planning and health care preferences of community-dwelling elders: The Framingham Heart Study. *Journals of Gerontology: Series A, Biological Sciences and Medical Sciences* 63 (9): 951–959.

McGlynn, Elizabeth A., Steven M. Asch, John Adams, Joan Keesey, Jennifer Hicks, Alison DeCristofaro, and Eve A. Kerr. 2003. The quality of health care delivered to adults in the United States. *New England Journal of Medicine* 348 (26): 2635–2645. doi:10.1056/NEJMsa022615.

McKinley, E. D., J. M. Garrett, A. T. Evans, and M. Danis. 1996. Differences in end-of-life decision making among black and white ambulatory cancer patients. *Journal of General Internal Medicine* 11 (11): 651–656.

McKinstry, B., R. E. Ashcroft, J. Car, G. K. Freeman, and A. Sheikh. 2006. Interventions for improving patients' trust in doctors and groups of doctors. *Cochrane Database of Systematic Reviews* 3:CD004134. doi:10.1002/14651858.CD004134.pub2.

McKneally, M. F., and R. M. Sade. 2003. The prisoner dilemma: Should convicted felons have the same access to heart transplantation as ordinary citizens? Opposing views. *Journal of Thoracic and Cardiovascular Surgery* 125 (3): 451–453.

Meadow, William, Sally Cohen-Cutler, Bridget Spelke, Anna Kim, Melissa Plesac, Kirsten Weis, and Joanne Lagatta. 2012. The prediction and cost of futility in the NICU. *Acta Paediatrica (Oslo, Norway)* 101 (4): 397–402. doi:10.1111/j.1651-2227.2011.02555.x.

Mechanic, David. 1995. Dilemmas in rationing health care services: The case for implicit rationing. *BMJ (Clinical Research Ed.)* 310 (6995): 1655–1659.

Meekings, Kiran N., Cory S. M. Williams, and John E. Arrowsmith. 2012. Orphan drug development: An economically viable strategy for biopharma R&D. *Drug Discovery Today* 17 (13–14): 660–664. doi:10.1016/j.drudis.2012.02.005.

Melis, Marcovalerio, Richard Karl, Sandra Wong, Murray Brennan, Jeffrey Matthews, and Kevin Roggin. 2010. Evidence-based surgical practice in academic medical centers: Consistently anecdotal? *Journal of Gastrointestinal Surgery* 14 (5): 904–909. doi:10.1007/s11605-010-1175-1.

Mello, M. M., and T. A. Brennan. 2001. The controversy over high-dose chemotherapy with autologous bone marrow transplant for breast cancer. *Health Affairs (Project Hope)* 20 (5): 101–117.

Mello, Michelle M., Amitabh Chandra, Atul A. Gawande, and David M. Studdert. 2010. National costs of the Medical Liability System. *Health Affairs* 29 (9): 1569–1577. doi:10.1377/hlthaff.2009.0807.

Melnitchouk, S., U. Jorde, H. Takayama, N. Uriel, P. Colombo, J. Yang, D. Mancini, and Y. Naka. 2011. 363 Continuous-Flow LVAD Destination Therapy versus orthotopic heart transplantation in patients above 65 years of age. *Journal of Heart and Lung Transplantation* 30 (4 Suppl.): S125–S126. doi:10.1016/j.healun.2011.01.371.

Meltzer, D. O., and A. S. Detsky. 2010. The real meaning of rationing. *Journal of the American Medical Association* 304 (20): 2292–2293. doi:10.1001/jama.2010.1671.

Mendelson, T. B., M. Meltzer, E. G. Campbell, A. L. Caplan, and J. N. Kirkpatrick 2011. Conflicts of interest in cardiovascular clinical practice guidelines. *Archives of Internal Medicine* 171 (6): 577–584. doi:10.1001/archinternmed.2011.96.

Merlo, Christian A., Eric S. Weiss, Jonathan B. Orens, Marvin C. Borja, Marie Diener West, John V. Conte, and Ashish S. Shah. 2009. Impact of U.S. Lung Allocation Score on survival after lung transplantation. *Journal of Heart and Lung Transplantation* 28 (8): 769–775. doi:10.1016/j.healun.2009.04.024.

Mills, Geofrey, and Hugh Rockoff. 1987. Compliance with price controls in the United States and the United Kingdom during World War II. *Journal of Economic History* 47 (1): 197–213. doi:10.2307/2121945.

Minniefield, W. J., and P. Muti. 2002. Organ donation survey results of a Buffalo, New York, African-American community. *Journal of the National Medical Association* 94 (11): 979–986.

Minniefield, W. J., J. Yang, and P. Muti. 2001. Differences in attitudes toward organ donation among African Americans and whites in the United States. *Journal of the National Medical Association* 93 (10): 372–379.

Mitchell, Janet B., Susan G. Haber, Galina Khatutsky, and Suzanne Donoghue. 2002. Impact of the Oregon Health Plan on access and satisfaction of adults with low-income. *Health Services Research* 37 (1): 19–39. doi:10.1111/1475-6773.00036.

Mitka, M. 2012. Drug Gray Market. *Journal of the American Medical Association* 308 (10): 964.

Mitton, C., and C. Donaldson. 2004. Health care priority setting: Principles, practice and challenge. *Cost Effectiveness and Resource Allocation* 2:3.

Morden, Nancy E., Chiang-Hua Chang, Joseph O. Jacobson, Ethan M. Berke, Julie P. W. Bynum, Kimberly M. Murray, and David C. Goodman. 2012. End-of-life care for Medicare beneficiaries with cancer is highly intensive overall and varies widely. *Health Affairs* 31 (4): 786–796. doi:10.1377/hlthaff.2011.0650.

Morgan, Susan E., Tyler R. Harrison, Lisa Volk Chewning, and Jacklyn G. Habib. 2006. America's angel or thieving immigrant? In Keith Wailoo, Julie Livingston, and Peter Guaraccia, eds., *A Death Retold: Jesica Santillan, the Bungled Transplant, and Paradoxes of Medical Citizenship*, 19–45. Chapel Hill: University of North Carolina Press.

Morgan, Susan E., Tyler R. Harrison, Walid A. Afifi, Shawn D. Long, and Michael T. Stephenson. 2008. In their own words: The reasons why people will (not) sign an organ donor card. *Health Communication* 23 (1): 23–33. doi:10.1080/10410230701805158.

Morreim, E. 1991. Gaming the system: Dodging the rules, ruling the dodgers. *Archives of Internal Medicine* 151 (3): 443–447. doi:10.1001/archinte.1991.00400030013003.

Morrison, R. S., and D. E. Meier. 2004. High rates of advance care planning in New York City's elderly population. *Archives of Internal Medicine* 164 (22): 2421–2426. doi:10.1001/archinte.164.22.2421.

Mortimer, Duncan, and Stuart Peacock. 2012. Social welfare and the Affordable Care Act: Is it ever optimal to set aside comparative cost? *Social Science & Medicine* 75 (7): 1156–1162. doi:10.1016/j.socscimed.2012.05.019.

Moseley, K. L., A. Church, B. Hempel, H. Yuan, S. D. Goold, and G. L. Freed. 2004. End-of-life choices for African-American and white infants in a neonatal intensive-care unit: A pilot study. *Journal of the National Medical Association* 96 (7): 933–937.

Moss, Alvin H. 2011. Ethical principles and processes guiding dialysis decision-making. *Clinical Journal of the American Society of Nephrology (CJASN)* 6 (9): 2313–2317. doi:10.2215/cjn.03960411.

Moylan, C. A., C. W. Brady, J. L. Johnson, A. D. Smith, J. E. Tuttle-Newhall, and A. J. Muir. 2008. Disparities in liver transplantation before and after introduction of the MELD score. *Journal of the American Medical Association* 300 (20): 2371–2378.

Moynihan, Ray. 2011. Surrogates under scrutiny: Fallible correlations, fatal consequences. *BMJ (Clinical Research Ed.)* 343. doi:10.1136/bmj.d5160.

Mulloy, Daniel P., Castigliano M. Bhamidipati, Matthew L. Stone, Gorav Ailawadi, Irving L. Kron, and John A. Kern. 2012. Orthotopic heart transplant versus left ventricular assist device: A national comparison of cost and survival. *Journal of Thoracic and Cardiovascular Surgery*. doi:10.1016/j.jtcvs.2012.10.034.

Murray, M. A., G. Brunier, J. O. Chung, L. A. Craig, C. Mills, A. Thomas, and D. Stacey. 2009. A systematic review of factors influencing decision-making in adults living with chronic kidney disease. *Patient Education and Counseling* 76 (2):149–158

National Federation of Independent Business v. Sebelius. 2012. In *United States Reports*: Supreme Court.

Nelson, Bruce. 1993. Organized labor and the struggle for black equality in Mobile during World War II. *Journal of American History* 80 (3): 952–988. doi:10.2307/2080410.

Neuberger, James. 2007. Public and professional attitudes to transplanting alcoholic patients. *Liver Transplantation* 13 (S2): S65–S68. doi:10.1002/lt.21337.

Neuberger, James. 2012. Rationing life-saving resources—how should allocation policies be assessed in solid organ transplantation? *Transplant International* 25 (1): 3–6. doi:10.1111/j.1432-2277.2011.01327.x.

Neuberger, James, David Adams, Paul MacMaster, Anita Maidment, and Mark Speed. 1998. Assessing priorities for allocation of donor liver grafts: Survey of public and clinicians. *BMJ (Clinical Research Ed.)* 317 (7152): 172–175. doi:10.1136/bmj.317.7152.172.

Neuberger, J., A. Gimson, M. Davies, M. Akyol, J. Grady, A. Burroughs, M. Hudson, for the Liver Advisory Group, UK Blood and Transplant. 2008. Selection of patients for liver transplantation and allocation of donated livers in the UK. *Gut* 57 (2): 252–257. doi:10.1136/gut.2007.131730.

Neuman, J. 2011. Prevalence of financial conflicts of interest among panel members producing clinical practice guidelines in Canada and United States: Cross sectional study. *British Medical Journal* 343. doi:10.1136/bmj.d7063.

Nord, Erik. 2005. Concerns for the worse off: Fair innings versus severity. *Social Science & Medicine* 60 (2): 257–263. doi:10.1016/j.socscimed.2004.05.003.

Norris, Keith C., and Lawrence Y. Agodoa. 2012. Reducing disparities in assessment for kidney transplantation. *Clinical Journal of the American Society of Nephrology (CJASN)* 7 (9): 1378–1381. doi:10.2215/cjn.07690712.

Norris, Susan L., Haley K. Holmer, Lauren A. Ogden, and Brittany U. Burda. 2011. Conflict of interest in clinical practice guideline development: A systematic review. *PLOS ONE* 6 (10): 1–6. doi:10.1371/journal.pone.0025153.

Novakovic, B. 1994. U.S. childhood cancer survival, 1973–1987. *Medical and Pediatric Oncology* 23 (6): 480–486.

Oberlander, J. 2007. Health reform interrupted: The unraveling of the Oregon Health Plan. *Health Affairs* 26 (1): w96–w105. doi:10.1377/hlthaff.26.1.w96.

Oberlander, J., T. Marmor, and L. Jacobs. 2001. Rationing medical care: Rhetoric and reality in the Oregon Health Plan. [CMAJ] *Canadian Medical Association Journal* 164 (11): 1583–1587.

Oberlander, J., and Joseph White. 2009. Public attitudes toward health care spending aren't the problem; prices are. *Health Affairs* 28 (5): 1285–1293. doi:10.1377/hlthaff.28.5.1285.

O'Leary, Paul M. 1945. Wartime rationing and governmental organization. *American Political Science Review* 39 (6): 1089–1106. doi:10.2307/1949657.

O'Reilly. Kevin B. 2012. Liver transplant for Apple CEO turns spotlight on organ transplant inequities. *American Medical News,* July 27, 2009. http://www .ama-assn.org/amednews/2009/07/27/prsa0727.htm.

Orens, Jonathan B., and Edward R. Garrity. 2009. General overview of lung transplantation and review of organ allocation. *Proceedings of the American Thoracic Society* 6 (1): 13–19. doi:10.1513/pats.200807-072GO.

Orszag, Peter R. 2011. How health care can save or sink America: The case for reform and fiscal sustainability. *Foreign Affairs* 90:42–56.

Orwell, G. 1996. *Animal Farm.* New York: Signet Classics.

O'Shaughnessy, Joyce, Cynthia Osborne, John E. Pippen, Mark Yoffe, Debra Patt, Christine Rocha, Ingrid Chou Koo, Barry M. Sherman, and Charles Bradley. 2011. Iniparib plus chemotherapy in metastatic triple-negative breast cancer. *New England Journal of Medicine* 364 (3): 205–214. doi:10.1056/NEJMoa1011418.

Osler, William, and Thomas McCrae. 1912. *The Principles and Practice of Medicine.* 8th ed. New York: D. Appleton & Company.

Osterholm, Michael T., Nicholas S. Kelley, Alfred Sommer, and Edward A. Belongia. 2012. Efficacy and effectiveness of influenza vaccines: A systematic review and meta-analysis. *The Lancet Infectious Diseases* 12 (1): 36–44. doi:10.1016/ S1473-3099(11)70295-X.

Øverland, Gerhard. 2007. Survival lotteries reconsidered. *Bioethics* 21 (7): 355–363. doi:10.1111/j.1467-8519.2007.00570.x.

Pace, Lydia E., Yulei He, and Nancy L. Keating. 2013. Trends in mammography screening rates after publication of the 2009 US Preventive Services Task Force recommendations. *Cancer.* doi:10.1002/cncr.28105.

Paoloni, Justin, Robert J. De Vos, Bruce Hamilton, George A. C. Murrell, and John Orchard. 2011. Platelet-rich plasma treatment for ligament and tendon injuries. *Clinical Journal of Sport Medicine* 21 (1): 37–45. doi:10.1097/ JSM.0b013e31820758c7.

Parr, J. D., B. H. Zhang, M. E. Nilsson, A. Wright, T. Balboni, E. Duthie, E. Paulk, and H. G. Prigerson. 2010. The influence of age on the likelihood of receiving end-of-life care consistent with patient treatment preferences. *Journal of Palliative Medicine* 13 (6): 719–726. doi:10.1089/jpm.2009.0337.

Patzer, R. E., S. Amaral, M. Klein, N. Kutner, J. P. Perryman, J. A. Gazmararian, and W. M. McClellan. 2012. Racial disparities in pediatric access to kidney transplantation: Does socioeconomic status play a role? *American Journal of Transplantation* 12 (2): 369–378. doi:10.1111/j.1600-6143.2011.03888.x.

Patzer, R. E., and S. O. Pastan. 2013. Measuring the disparity gap: Quality improvement to eliminate health disparities in kidney transplantation. *American Journal of Transplantation* 13 (2): 247–248. doi:10.1111/ajt.12060.

Pavia, Andrew T. 2013. Influenza A(H7N9): From anxiety to preparedness. *Annals of Internal Medicine.* doi:10.7326/0003-4819-159-3-201308060-00653.

Peppercorn, Jeffrey M., Thomas J. Smith, Paul R. Helft, David J. DeBono, Scott R. Berry, Dana S. Wollins, Daniel M. Hayes, Jamie H. Von Roenn, and Lowell E. Schnipper. 2011. American Society of Clinical Oncology Statement: Toward individualized care for patients with advanced cancer. *Journal of Clinical Oncology* 29 (6): 755–760. doi:10.1200/jco.2010.33.1744.

Persad, Govind, Alan Wertheimer, and Ezekiel J. Emanuel. 2009. Principles for allocation of scarce medical interventions. *Lancet* 373 (9661): 423–431. doi:10.1016/s0140-6736(09)60137-9.

Persad, Govind, Alan Wertheimer, and Ezekiel J. Emanuel. 2010. Standing by our principles: Meaningful guidance, moral foundations, and multi-principle methodology in medical scarcity. *American Journal of Bioethics* 10 (4): 46–48. doi:10.1080/15265161003650528.

Piemonte, Nicole M., and Laura Hermer. 2013. Avoiding a "death panel" redux. *Hastings Center Report* 43 (4): 20–28. doi:10.1002/hast.190.

Pirker, Robert, Jose R. Pereira, Aleksandra Szczesna, Joachim von Pawel, Maciej Krzakowski, Rodryg Ramlau, Ihor Vynnychenko, et al. 2009. Cetuximab plus chemotherapy in patients with advanced non-small-cell lung cancer (FLEX): An open-label randomised phase III trial. *Lancet* 373 (9674): 1525–1531.

Poli, Francesca, Mario Scalamogna, Massimo Cardillo, Eliana Porta, and Girolamo Sirchia. 2000. An algorithm for cadaver kidney allocation based on a multivariate analysis of factors impacting on cadaver kidney graft survival and function. *Transplant International* 13 (S1): S259–S262. doi:10.1111/j.1432-2277.2000.tb02032.x.

Pui, Ching-Hon, Charles G. Mullighan, William E. Evans, and Mary V. Relling. 2012. Pediatric acute lymphoblastic leukemia: Where are we going and how do we get there? *Blood* 120 (6): 1165–1174. doi:10.1182/blood-2012-05-378943.

Qaseem, Amir, Vincenza Snow, Douglas K. Owens, Paul Shekelle, and the Clinical Guidelines Committee of the American College of Physicians. 2010. The development of clinical practice guidelines and guidance statements of the American College of Physicians: Summary of methods. *Annals of Internal Medicine* 153 (3): 194–199. doi:10.1059/0003-4819-153-3-201008030-00010.

Quadri-Sheriff, Maheen, Kristin S. Hendrix, Stephen M. Downs, Lynne A. Sturm, Gregory D. Zimet, and S. Maria E. Finnell. 2012. The role of herd immunity in parents' decision to vaccinate children: A systematic review. *Pediatrics* 130 (3): 522–530. doi:10.1542/peds.2012-0140.

Quigley, Muireann, Linda Wright, and Vardit Ravitsky. 2012. Organ donation and priority points in Israel: An ethical analysis. *Transplantation* 93 (10): 970–973. doi:10.1097/TP.0b013e31824e3d95.

Quill, Timothy E., and Howard Brody. 1996. Physician recommendations and patient autonomy: Finding a balance between physician power and patient choice. *Annals of Internal Medicine* 125 (9): 763–769. doi:10.7326/0003-4819-125-9-199611010-00010.

Quinn, S. C., S. Kumar, V. S. Freimuth, K. Kidwell, and D. Musa. 2009. Public willingness to take a vaccine or drug under Emergency Use Authorization during the 2009 H1N1 pandemic. *Biosecurity and Bioterrorism: Biodefense Strategy, Practice, and Science* 7 (3): 275–290. doi:10.1089/bsp.2009.0041.

Quinton, W. E., D. H. Dillard, J. J. Cole, and B. H. Scribner. 1962. Eight months' experience with Silastic-Teflon bypass cannulas. *Transactions—American Society for Artificial Internal Organs* 8:236–245.

Raad, Raymond, and Paul S. Appelbaum. 2012. Relationships between medicine and industry: Approaches to the problem of conflicts of interest. *Annual Review of Medicine* 63 (1): 465–477. doi:10.1146/annurev-med-061410-121850.

Randall, V. R. 1996. Slavery, segregation and racism: Trusting the health care system ain't always easy! An African American perspective on bioethics. *Saint Louis University Public Law Review* 15 (2): 191–235.

Rao, Vijay M., and David C. Levin. 2012. The overuse of diagnostic imaging and the Choosing Wisely Initiative. *Annals of Internal Medicine* 157 (8): 574–576. doi:10.7326/0003-4819-157-8-201210160-00535.

Rawls, John. 1999. *A Theory of Justice*. Rev. ed. Cambridge, MA: Belknap Press of Harvard University Press.

Reed, W. W., and L. F. Diehl. 1991. Leukopenia, neutropenia, and reduced hemoglobin levels in healthy American blacks. *Archives of Internal Medicine* 151 (3): 501–505. doi:10.1001/archinte.1991.00400030063011.

Reese, Peter P., and Arthur L. Caplan. 2011. Better off living—the ethics of the new UNOS proposal for allocating kidneys for transplantation. *Clinical Journal of the American Society of Nephrology (CJASN)* 6 (9): 2310–2312. doi:10.2215/cjn.03310411.

Regis, Catherine. 2004. Physicians gaming the system: Modern-day Robin Hood? *Health Law Review* 2004 (Winter): 19.

Reich, D., M. A. Nalls, W. H. L. Kao, E. L. Akylbekova, A. Tandon, N. Patterson, J. Mullikin, et al. 2009. Reduced neutrophil count in people of African descent is due to a regulatory variant in the Duffy antigen receptor for chemokines gene. *PLOS Genetics* 5 (1). doi:10.1371/Journal.Pgen.1000360.

Reimers, David M. 1998. *Unwelcome Strangers: American Identity and the Turn against Immigration*. New York: Columbia University Press.

Rescher, Nicholas. 1969. The allocation of exotic medical lifesaving therapy. *Ethics* 79 (3): 173–186.

Resnick, David. 2003. The Jesica Santillan tragedy: Lessons learned. *Hastings Center Report* 33 (4): 15–20. doi:10.2307/3528375.

Rettig, Richard A., Peter D. Jacobson, Cynthia M. Farquhar, and Wade M. Aubry. 2007. *False Hope: Bone Marrow Transplantation for Breast Cancer*. New York: Oxford University Press.

Rhorer, Janelle, Christopher S. Ambrose, Stephanie Dickinson, Holli Hamilton, Napoleon A. Oleka, Frank J. Malinoski, and Janet Wittes. 2009. Efficacy of live attenuated influenza vaccine in children: A meta-analysis of nine randomized clinical trials. *Vaccine* 27 (7): 1101–1110. doi:10.1016/j.vaccine.2008.11.093.

Riggs, J. E., J. C. Hobbs, G. R. Hobbs, and T. H. Riggs. 2011. U.S. national health-care expenditures: Demonstration and explanation of cubic growth dynamics. *Theoretical Economics Letters* 1:105–110.

Riley, Gerald F., and James D. Lubitz. 2010. Long-term trends in Medicare payments in the last year of life. *Health Services Research* 45 (2): 565–576. doi:10.1111/j.1475-6773.2010.01082.x.

Robbins, Anthony S., Rebecca L. Siegel, and Ahmedin Jemal. 2012. Racial disparities in stage-specific colorectal cancer mortality rates from 1985 to 2008. *Journal of Clinical Oncology* 30 (4): 401–405. doi:10.1200/jco.2011.37.5527.

Robert, Nicholas J., Véronique Diéras, John Glaspy, Adam M. Brufsky, Igor Bondarenko, Oleg N. Lipatov, Edith A. Perez, Denise A. Yardley, Stephen Y. T. Chan, Xian Zhou, See-Chun Phan, and Joyce O'Shaughnessy. 2011. RIBBON-1: Randomized, double-blind, placebo-controlled, phase III trial of chemotherapy with or without bevacizumab for first-line treatment of human epidermal growth factor receptor 2-negative, locally recurrent or metastatic breast cancer. *Journal of Clinical Oncology* 29 (10): 1252–1260. doi:10.1200/jco.2010.28.0982.

Robinson, R. 1993. Cost-effectiveness analysis. *BMJ (Clinical Research Ed.)* 307 (6907): 793–795. doi:10.1136/bmj.307.6907.793.

Rockoff, Hugh. 1981. Price and wage controls in four wartime periods. *Journal of Economic History* 41 (2): 381–401. doi:10.2307/2120981.

Rodrigue, J. R., D. L. Cornell, and R. J. Howard. 2006a. Attitudes toward financial incentives, donor authorization, and presumed consent among next-of-kin who consented vs. refused organ. *Transplantation* 81:1249–1256.

Rodrigue, J. R., D. L. Cornell, and R. J. Howard. 2006b. Organ donation decision: Comparison of donor and nondonor families. *American Journal of Transplantation* 6 (1): 190–198.

Rodriguez, Daniel B., and Barry R. Weingast. 2002–2003. The positive political theory of legislative history: New perspectives on the 1964 Civil Rights Act and its interpretation. *University of Pennsylvania Law Review* 151:1417–1542.

Rodriguez, Rudolph A. 2010. The dilemma of undocumented immigrants with ESRD. *Dialysis & Transplantation* 39 (4): 141–143. doi:10.1002/dat.20437.

Roe v. Wade. 1973. In *United States Reports*: Supreme Court.

Rogers, Joseph G., Robin R. Bostic, Kuo B. Tong, Rob Adamson, Mark Russo, and Mark S. Slaughter. 2012. Cost-effectiveness analysis of continuous-flow left ventricular assist devices as destination therapy / clinical perspective. *Circulation: Heart Failure* 5 (1): 10–16. doi:10.1161/circheartfailure.111.962951.

Rosenblum, Amanda M., Lucy D. Horvat, Laura A. Siminoff, Versha Prakash, Janice Beitel, and Amit X. Garg. 2012. The authority of next-of-kin in explicit and presumed consent systems for deceased organ donation: An analysis of 54 nations. *Nephrology, Dialysis, Transplantation* 27 (6): 2533–2546. doi:10.1093/ndt/gfr619.

Rosenthal, Eric T. 2012. Frustration over gray-market drugs lingers throughout nation. *Journal of the National Cancer Institute* 104 (4): 264–267. doi:10.1093/jnci/djs129.

Rosner, Bernard. 2000. *Fundamentals of Biostatistics*. 5th ed. Pacific Grove, CA: Duxbury.

Rosoff, P. M. 2004. Can underpowered clinical trials be justified? *IRB* 26 (3): 16–19.

Rosoff, P. M. 2010. In search of the mommy gene: Truth and consequences in behavioral genetics. *Science, Technology & Human Values* 35 (2): 200–243.

Rosoff, P. M. 2012a. Institutional futility policies are inherently unfair. *HEC Forum* 25 (3): 1–19. doi:10.1007/s10730-012-9194-9.

Rosoff, P. M. 2012b. Unpredictable drug shortages: An ethical framework for short-term rationing in hospitals. *American Journal of Bioethics* 12 (1): 1–9.

Rosoff, P. M., and D. L. Coleman. 2011. The case for legal regulation of physicians' off-label prescribing. *Notre Dame Law Review* 86 (2): 649–691.

Rosoff, P. M., and M. Decamp. 2011. Preparing for an influenza pandemic: Are some people more equal than others? *Journal of Health Care for the Poor and Underserved* 22 (3 Suppl.): 19–35. doi:10.1353/hpu.2011.0098.

Rosoff, P. M., K. R. Patel, A. Scates, G. Rhea, P. W. Bush, and J. A. Govert. 2012. Coping with critical drug shortages: An ethical approach for allocating scarce resources in hospitals. *Archives of Internal Medicine* 172 (19): 1494–1499. doi:10.1001/archinternmed.2012.4367.

Rucker, Philip. 2009. Sen. DeMint of S.C. is voice of opposition to health-care reform. *Washington Post*, July 28.

Russell, E., D. H. Robinson, N. J. Thompson, J. P. Perryman, and K. R. Arriola. 2011. Distrust in the healthcare system and organ donation intentions among African Americans. *Journal of Community Health*. doi:10.1007/s10900-011-9413-3.

Russo, Mark J., Berhane Worku, Alexander Iribarne, Kimberly N. Hong, Jonathan A. Yang, Wickii Vigneswaran, and Joshua R. Sonett. 2011. Does lung allocation score maximize survival benefit from lung transplantation? *Journal of Thoracic and Cardiovascular Surgery* 141 (5): 1270–1277. doi:10.1016/j.jtcvs.2010.12.028.

Sandel, Michael J. 2012. *What Money Can't Buy: The Moral Limits of Markets*. New York: Farrar, Straus and Giroux.

Sanders, D., and J. Dukeminier Jr. 1968. Medical advance and legal lag: Hemodialysis and kidney transplantation. *UCLA Law Review* 15:357–413.

Sasaki, S., M. Sullivan, C. F. Narvaez, T. H. Holmes, D. Furman, N. Y. Zheng, M. Nishtala, et al. 2011. Limited efficacy of inactivated influenza vaccine in elderly individuals is associated with decreased production of vaccine-specific antibodies. *Journal of Clinical Investigation* 121 (8): 3109–3119. doi:10.1172/JCI57834.

Satz, Debra. 2010. *Why Some Things Should Not Be for Sale: The Moral Limits of Markets*. New York: Oxford University Press.

Scanlon, T. M. 1998. *What We Owe to Each Other*. Cambridge, MA: The Belknap Press of Harvard University Press.

Scheunemann, Leslie P., and Douglas B. White. 2011. The ethics and reality of rationing in medicine. *Chest* 140 (6): 1625–1632. doi:10.1378/chest.11-0622.

Schifrin, Barry S., and Wayne R. Cohen. 2012. The effect of malpractice claims on the use of caesarean section. *Best Practice & Research. Clinical Obstetrics & Gynaecology*. doi:10.1016/j.bpobgyn.2012.10.004.

Schilsky, Richard L. 2010. Personalized medicine in oncology: The future is now. *Nature Reviews: Drug Discovery* 9 (5): 363–366.

Schneiderman, L. J. 2011a. Defining medical futility and improving medical care. *Journal of Bioethical Inquiry* 8 (2): 123–131. doi:10.1007/s11673-011-9293-3.

Schneiderman, L. J. 2011b. Rationing just medical care. *American Journal of Bioethics* 11 (7): 7–14. doi:10.1080/15265161.2011.577511.

Schneiderman, L. J. 2011c. *Wrong Medicine: Doctors, Patients, and Futile Treatment*, Ann Silbergeld and Nancy Jecker, eds. 2nd ed. Baltimore: Johns Hopkins University Press.

Schneiderman, L. J., and N. S. Jecker. 1995. *Wrong Medicine: Doctors, Patients, and Futile Treatment*. Baltimore: Johns Hopkins University Press.

Schneiderman, L. J., and N. S. Jecker. 1996. Should a criminal receive a heart transplant? Medical justice vs. societal justice. *Theoretical Medicine* 17 (1): 33–44.

Schneiderman, L. J., N. S. Jecker, and Albert R. Jonsen. 1990. Medical futility: Its meaning and ethical implications. *Annals of Internal Medicine* 112 (12): 949–954. doi:10.1059/0003-4819-112-12-949.

Schneiderman, L. J., N. S. Jecker, and Albert R. Jonsen. 1996. Medical futility: Response to critiques. *Annals of Internal Medicine* 125 (8): 669–674. doi:10.1059/0003-4819-125-8-199610150-00007.

Schoen, Cathy, Robin Osborn, David Squires, Michelle M. Doty, Roz Pierson, and Sandra Applebaum. 2010. How health insurance design affects access to care and costs, by income, in eleven countries. *Health Affairs* 29 (12): 2323–2334. doi:10.1377/hlthaff.2010.0862.

Schroeder, Steven A., and William Frist. 2013. Phasing out fee-for-service payment. *New England Journal of Medicine* 368 (21): 2029–2032. doi:10.1056/NEJMsb1302322.

Schwartz, W. B., and D. N. Mendelson. 1992. Why managed care cannot contain hospital costs—without rationing. *Health Affairs* 11 (2): 100–107. doi:10.1377/hlthaff.11.2.100.

Secunda, Katharine, Elisa J. Gordon, Min W. Sohn, Laura A. Shinkunas, Lauris C. Kaldjian, Michael D. Voigt, and Josh Levitsky. 2012. A national survey of provider opinions on controversial characteristics of liver transplant candidates. *Liver Transplantation*. doi:10.1002/lt.23581.

Segev, D. L. 2009. Evaluating options for utility-based kidney allocation. *American Journal of Transplantation* 9 (7): 1513–1518. doi:10.1111/j.1600-6143.2009.02667.x.

Shaneyfelt, T. M., and R. M. Centor. 2009. Reassessment of clinical practice guidelines: Go gently into that good night. *Journal of the American Medical Association* 301 (8): 868–869. doi:10.1001/jama.2009.225.

Shavers, V. L., C. F. Lynch, and L. F. Burmeister. 2000. Knowledge of the Tuskegee study and its impact on the willingness to participate in medical research studies. *Journal of the National Medical Association* 92 (12): 563–572.

Shavers, V. L., C. F. Lynch, and L. F. Burmeister. 2001. Factors that influence African-Americans' willingness to participate in medical research studies. *Cancer* 91 (1 Suppl.): 233–236.

Sher, George. 2005. Transgenerational compensation. *Philosophy & Public Affairs* 33 (2): 181–200. doi:10.1111/j.1088-4963.2005.00029.x.

Sheth, Ujash, Nicole Simunovic, Guy Klein, Freddie Fu, Thomas A. Einhorn, Emil Schemitsch, Olufemi R. Ayeni, and Mohit Bhandari. 2012. Efficacy of autologous platelet-rich plasma use for orthopaedic indications: A meta-analysis. *Journal of Bone & Joint Surgery* 94 (4): 298–307. doi:10.2106/jbjs.k.00154.

Shippee, T. P., K. F. Ferraro, and R. J. Thorpe. 2011. Racial disparity in access to cardiac intensive care over 20 years. *Ethnicity & Health* 16 (2): 145–165. doi:10.1080/13557858.2010.544292.

Silverman, Elaine, and Jonathan Skinner. 2004. Medicare upcoding and hospital ownership. *Journal of Health Economics* 23 (2): 369–389. doi:10.1016/j.jhealeco.2003.09.007.

Siminoff, L. A., C. J. Burant, and S. A. Ibrahim. 2006. Racial disparities in preferences and perceptions regarding organ donation. *Journal of General Internal Medicine* 21 (9): 995–1000.

Siminoff, L. A., C. J. Burant, and S. J. Youngner. 2004. Death and organ procurement: Public beliefs and attitudes. *Kennedy Institute of Ethics Journal* 14 (3): 217–234.

Siminoff, L. A., R. H. Lawrence, and R. M. Arnold. 2003. Comparison of black and white families' experiences and perceptions regarding organ donation requests. *Critical Care Medicine* 31 (1): 146–151.

Siminoff, L. A., M. B. Mercer, G. Graham, and C. Burant. 2007. The reasons families donate organs for transplantation: Implications for policy and practice. *Journal of Trauma* 62 (4): 969–978.

Singh, Tajinder P., Michael M. Givertz, Marc Semigran, David DeNofrio, Fred Costantino, and Kimberlee Gauvreau. 2010. Socioeconomic position, ethnicity, and outcomes in heart transplant recipients. *American Journal of Cardiology* 105 (7): 1024–1029. doi:10.1016/j.amjcard.2009.11.015.

Sinnott-Armstrong, Walter. 1984. "Ought" conversationally implies "can." *Philosophical Review* 93 (2): 249–261. doi:10.2307/2184585.

Sirovich, Brenda, Patricia M. Gallagher, David E. Wennberg, and Elliott S. Fisher. 2008. Discretionary decision making by primary care physicians and the cost of U.S. health care. *Health Affairs* 27 (3): 813–823. doi:10.1377/hlthaff.27.3.813.

Slamon, Dennis J., Brian Leyland-Jones, Steven Shak, Hank Fuchs, Virginia Paton, Alex Bajamonde, Thomas Fleming, et al. 2001. Use of chemotherapy plus a monoclonal antibody against HER2 for metastatic breast cancer that overexpresses HER2. *New England Journal of Medicine* 344 (11): 783–792. doi:10.1056/NEJM200103153441101.

Slaughter, Mark S., Anna L. Meyer, and Emma J. Birks. 2011. Destination therapy with left ventricular assist devices: Patient selection and outcomes. *Current Opinion in Cardiology* 26 (3): 232–236. doi:10.1097/HCO.0b013e328345aff4.

Smally, Alan J., Bob Carroll, Michael Carius, Fred Tilden, and Michael Werdmann. 2011. Treatment of VIPs. *Annals of Emergency Medicine* 58 (4): 397–398. doi:10.1016/j.annemergmed.2011.05.009.

Smith, Adam. [1759] 1969. *The Theory of Moral Sentiments*. New Rochelle, NY: Arlington House.

Smith, Thomas J., and Joann N. Bodurtha. 2013. The "Good Planning Panel." *Hastings Center Report* 43 (4): 30–32. doi:10.1002/hast.192.

Smith, Thomas J., and Bruce E. Hillner. 2010. Explaining marginal benefits to patients, when "marginal" means additional but not necessarily small. *Clinical Cancer Research* 16 (24): 5981–5986. doi:10.1158/1078-0432.ccr-10-1278.

Smits, Jacqueline M., George D. Nossent, Erwin de Vries, Axel Rahmel, Bruno Meiser, Martin Strueber, and Jens Gottlieb. 2011. Evaluation of the lung allocation score in highly urgent and urgent lung transplant candidates in Eurotransplant. *Journal of Heart and Lung Transplantation* 30 (1): 22–28. doi:10.1016/j.healun.2010.08.006.

Sofi, F., B. Giusti, R. Marcucci, A. M. Gori, R. Abbate, and G. F. Gensini. 2011. Cytochrome P450 2C19*2 polymorphism and cardiovascular recurrences in patients taking clopidogrel: A meta-analysis. *Pharmacogenomics Journal* 11 (3): 199–206.

Sondak, Vernon K., Susan M. Swetter, and Marianne A. Berwick. 2012. Gender disparities in patients with melanoma: Breaking the glass ceiling. *Journal of Clinical Oncology* 30 (18): 2177–2178. doi:10.1200/jco.2011.41.3849.

Song, M. K., S. E. Ward, M. B. Happ, B. Piraino, H. S. Donovan, A. M. Shields, and M. C. Connolly. 2009. Randomized controlled trial of SPIRIT: An effective approach to preparing African-American dialysis patients and families for end of life. *Research in Nursing & Health* 32 (3): 260–273. doi:10.1002/nur.20320.

Spiro, Topher, Emily Oshima Lee, and Ezekiel J. Emanuel. 2012. Price and utilization: Why we must target both to curb health care costs. *Annals of Internal Medicine* 157 (8): 586–590. doi:10.7326/0003-4819-157-8-201210160-00014.

Squiers, Linda B., Debra J. Holden, Suzanne E. Dolina, Annice E. Kim, Carla M. Bann, and Jeanette M. Renaud. 2011. The public's response to the U.S. Preventive Services Task Force's 2009 Recommendations on Mammography Screening. *American Journal of Preventive Medicine* 40 (5): 497–504. doi:10.1016/j.amepre.2010.12.027.

Stabile, Mark, Sarah Thomson, Sara Allin, Seán Boyle, Reinhard Busse, Karine Chevreul, Greg Marchildon, and Elias Mossialos. 2013. Health care cost containment strategies used in four other high-income countries hold lessons for the United States. *Health Affairs* 32 (4): 643–652. doi:10.1377/hlthaff.2012.1252.

Stahl, J. E., A. C. Tramontano, J. S. Swan, and B. J. Cohen. 2008. Balancing urgency, age and quality of life in organ allocation decisions—what would you do?: A survey. *Journal of Medical Ethics* 34 (2): 109–115. doi:10.1136/jme.2006.018291.

Starr, P. 1982. *The Social Transformation of American Medicine.* New York: Basic Books.

Stehlik, Josef, Leah B. Edwards, Anna Y. Kucheryavaya, Christian Benden, Jason D. Christie, Fabienne Dobbels, Richard Kirk, Axel O. Rahmel, and Marshall I. Hertz. 2011. The Registry of the International Society for Heart and Lung Transplantation: Twenty-Eighth Adult Heart Transplant Report—2011. *Journal of Heart and Lung Transplantation* 30 (10): 1078–1094. doi:10.1016/j.healun.2011.08.003.

Steinbrook, Robert. 2009. Controlling conflict of interest—Proposals from the Institute of Medicine. *New England Journal of Medicine* 360 (21): 2160–2163. doi:10.1056/NEJMp0810200.

Stone, Deborah. 2011. Moral hazard. *Journal of Health Politics, Policy and Law* 36 (5): 887–896. doi:10.1215/03616878-1407676.

Streiner, David L. 2002. Breaking up is hard to do: The heartbreak of dichotomizing continuous data. *Canadian Journal of Psychiatry* 47 (3): 262.

Sudore, R. L., and T. R. Fried. 2010. Redefining the "planning" in advance care planning: Preparing for end-of-life decision making. *Annals of Internal Medicine* 153 (4): 256–261.

Sullivan, Kip. 2013. How to think clearly about Medicare administrative costs: Data sources and measurement. *Journal of Health Politics, Policy and Law* 38 (3): 479–504. doi:10.1215/03616878-2079523.

Sutherland, Jason M., Elliott S. Fisher, and Jonathan S. Skinner. 2009. Getting past denial—the high cost of health care in the United States. *New England Journal of Medicine* 361 (13): 1227–1230. doi:10.1056/NEJMp0907172.

Sutrop, M. 2011. Viewpoint: How to avoid a dichotomy between autonomy and beneficence: from liberalism to communitarianism and beyond. *Journal of Internal Medicine* no. 269 (4):375-379. doi:10.1111/j.1365-2796.2011.02349_2.x.

Swaminathan, Shailender, Vincent Mor, Rajnish Mehrotra, and Amal Trivedi. 2012. Medicare's payment strategy for end-stage renal disease now embraces bundled payment and pay-for-performance to cut costs. *Health Affairs* 31 (9): 2051–2058. doi:10.1377/hlthaff.2012.0368.

Swan, K. G., and K. G. Swan, Jr. 1996. Triage: The past revisited. *Military Medicine* 161 (8): 448–452.

Tatesihi, John, and William Yoshino. 2000. The Japanese American incarceration: The journey to redress. *Human Rights (Chicago)* 27:10–11.

Tavaglione, Nicolas, and Samia A. Hurst. 2012. Why physicians ought to lie for their patients. *American Journal of Bioethics* 12 (3): 4–12. doi:10.1080/152651 61.2011.652797.

Teno, J. M., P. L. Gozalo, J. W. Bynum, N. E. Leland; S. C. Miller, N. E. Morden, T. Scupp, D. C. Goodman, V. Mor. 2013. Change in end-of-life care for Medicare beneficiaries: Site of death, place of care, and health care transitions in 2000, 2005, and 2009. *Journal of the American Medical Association* 309 (5): 470–477. doi:10.1001/jama.2012.207624.

Thabut, G., J. Munson, K. Haynes, M. O. Harhay, J. D. Christie, and S. D. Halpern. 2012. Geographic disparities in access to lung transplantation before and after implementation of the lung allocation score. *American Journal of Transplantation* 12 (11): 3085–3093. doi:10.1111/j.1600-6143.2012.04202.x.

Thomas, W. John. 1995–1996. The Clinton health care reform plan: A failed dramatic presentation. *Stanford Law & Policy Review* 7:83–105.

Thorpe, K. E., L. L. Ogden, and K. Galactionova. 2010. Chronic conditions account for rise in Medicare spending from 1987 to 2006. *Health Affairs* 29 (4): 718–724. doi:10.1377/hlthaff.2009.0474.

Tilburt J. C., and C. K. Cassel 2013. Why the ethics of parsimonious medicine is not the ethics of rationing. *Journal of the American Medical Association* 309 (8): 773–774. doi:10.1001/jama.2013.368.

Tilburt, J. C., M. K. Wynia, R. D. Sheeler, et al. 2013. Views of US physicians about controlling health care costs. *Journal of the American Medical Association* 310 (4): 380–388. doi:10.1001/jama.2013.8278.

Tinetti, M. E. 2012. The retreat from advanced care planning. *Journal of the American Medical Association* 307 (9): 915–916. doi:10.1001/jama.2012.229.

Tocqueville, Alexis de. 2004. *Democracy in America*. Trans. Arthur Goldhammer. Literary Classics of the United States. New York: Library of America.

Tong, A., K. Howard, S. Jan, A. Cass, J. Rose, S. Chadban, R. D. Allen, and J. C. Craig. 2010. Community preferences for the allocation of solid organs for transplantation: A systematic review. *Transplantation* 89 (7): 796–805. doi:10.1097/TP.0b013e3181cf1ee1.

Tong, Allison, Stephen Jan, Germaine Wong, Jonathan C. Craig, Michelle Irving, Steven Chadban, Alan Cass, and Kirsten Howard. 2013. Rationing scarce organs for transplantation: Healthcare provider perspectives on wait-listing and organ allocation. *Clinical Transplantation* 27 (1): 60–71. doi:10.1111/ctr.12004.

Tonry, Michael. 2009. The mostly unintended effects of mandatory penalties: Two centuries of consistent findings. *Crime and Justice* 38 (1): 65–114.

Treanor, John. 2004. Weathering the influenza vaccine crisis. *New England Journal of Medicine* 351 (20): 2037–2040. doi:10.1056/NEJMp048290.

Trivedi, Amal N., Regina C. Grebla, Steven M. Wright, and Donna L. Washington. 2011. Despite improved quality of care in the Veterans Affairs health system, racial disparity persists for important clinical outcomes. *Health Affairs* 30 (4): 707–715. doi:10.1377/hlthaff.2011.0074.

Truog, Robert D. 2007. Tackling medical futility in Texas. *New England Journal of Medicine* 357 (1): 1–3. doi:10.1056/NEJMp078109.

Truog, Robert D. 2009a. Counterpoint: The Texas Advance Directives Act is ethically flawed. *Chest* 136 (4): 968–971. doi:10.1378/chest.09-1269.

Truog, Robert D. 2009b. Screening mammography and the "R" word. *New England Journal of Medicine* 361 (26): 2501–2503. doi:10.1056/NEJMp0911447.

Tsuchiya, A., L. S. Miguel, R. Edlin, A. Wailoo, and P. Dolan. 2005. Procedural justice in public health care resource allocation. *Applied Health Economics and Health Policy* 4 (2): 119–127.

Tsukimoto, Ichiro, Akio Tawa, Keizo Horibe, Ken Tabuchi, Hisato Kigasawa, Masahiro Tsuchida, Hiromasa Yabe, et al. 2009. Risk-stratified therapy and the intensive use of cytarabine improves the outcome in childhood acute myeloid leukemia: The AML99 trial from the Japanese Childhood AML Cooperative Study Group. *Journal of Clinical Oncology* 27 (24): 4007–4013. doi:10.1200/jco.2008.18.7948.

Tulsky, J. A., G. S. Fischer, M. R. Rose, and R. M. Arnold. 1998. Opening the black box: How do physicians communicate about advance directives? *Annals of Internal Medicine* 129 (6): 441–449.

Tversky, Amos, and Daniel Kahneman. 1973. Availability: A heuristic for judging frequency and probability. *Cognitive Psychology* 5 (2): 207–232. doi:10.1016/0010-0285(73)90033-9.

Tversky, Amos, and Daniel Kahneman. 1981. The framing of decisions and the psychology of choice. *Science* 211 (4481): 453–458.

Ubel, Peter A. 2001. *Pricing Life: Why It's Time for Health Care Rationing*. Cambridge, MA: MIT Press.

Ubel, Peter A., and Susan Dorr Goold. 1998. "Rationing" health care: Not all definitions are created equal. *Archives of Internal Medicine* 158 (3): 209–214. doi:10.1001/archinte.158.3.209.

Ubel, Peter A., and George Loewenstein. 1996. Public perceptions of the importance of prognosis in allocating transplantable livers to children. *Medical Decision Making* 16 (3): 234–241. doi:10.1177/0272989x9601600307.

Unroe, K. T., M. A. Greiner, A. F. Hernandez, et al. 2011. Resource use in the last 6 months of life among Medicare beneficiaries with heart failure, 2000–2007. *Archives of Internal Medicine* 171 (3): 196–203. doi:10.1001/archinternmed.2010.371.

U.S. Preventive Services Task Force. 2009. Screening for Breast Cancer: U.S. Preventive Services Task Force Recommendation Statement. *Annals of Internal Medicine* 151 (10): 716–726. doi:10.7326/0003-4819-151-10-200911170-00008.

U.S. Renal Data System (USRDS). 2011. *US Renal Data System, USRDS 2011 Annual Data Report: Atlas of Chronic Kidney Disease and End-Stage Renal Disease in the United States*. Bethesda, MD: National Institutes of Health, National Institute of Diabetes and Digestive and Kidney Diseases.

Uyeki, Timothy M., and Nancy J. Cox. 2013. Global concerns regarding novel Influenza A (H7N9) virus infections. *New England Journal of Medicine* 368 (20): 1862–1864. doi:10.1056/NEJMp1304661.

Vaughn, Bryan T., Steven R. DeVrieze, Shelby D. Reed, and Kevin A. Schulman. 2010. Can we close the income and wealth gap between specialists and primary care physicians? *Health Affairs* 29 (5): 933–940. doi:10.1377/hlthaff.2009.0675.

Vernale, C., and S. A. Packard. 1990. Organ donation as gift exchange. *Image—the Journal of Nursing Scholarship* 22 (4): 239–242.

Volk, Michael L., Scott W. Biggins, Mary Ann Huang, Curtis K. Argo, Robert J. Fontana, and Renee R. Anspach. 2011. Decision making in liver transplant selection committees: A multicenter study. *Annals of Internal Medicine* 155 (8): 503–508. doi:10.1059/0003-4819-155-8-201110180-00006.

Volk, R. J., and A. D. Wolf. 2011. Grading the new US Preventive Services Task Force prostate cancer screening recommendation. *Journal of the American Medical Association* 306 (24): 2715–2716. doi:10.1001/jama.2011.1893.

Wailoo, K., J. Livingston, and P. Guarnaccia. 2006. *A Death Retold*. Chapel Hill: University of North Carolina Press.

Walker, Rebecca L., and Andrew W. Siegel. 2002. Morality and the limits of societal values in health care allocation. *Health Economics* 11 (3): 265–273.

Wallace, Steven P., Jacqueline M. Torres, Tabashir Z. Nobari, and Naderah Pourat. 2013. Undocumented and Uninsured. Barriers to Affordable Care for Immigrant Populations. Los Angeles: UCLA Center for Health Policy Research. http://www.commonwealthfund.org/~/media/Files/Publications/Fund%20Report/2013/Aug/1699_Wallace_undocumented_uninsured_barriers_immigrants_v2.pdf.

Walter, Stephen D., Xin Sun, Diane Heels-Ansdell, and Gordon Guyatt. 2012. Treatment effects on patient-important outcomes can be small, even with large effects on surrogate markers. *Journal of Clinical Epidemiology* 65 (9): 940–945. doi:10.1016/j.jclinepi.2012.02.012.

Wansink, Brian. 2002. Changing eating habits on the home front: Lost lessons from World War II research. *Journal of Public Policy & Marketing* 21 (1): 90–99. doi:10.2307/30000711.

Weeks, J. C., P. J. Catalano, A. Cronin, M. D. Finkelman, J. W. Mack, N. L. Keating, and D. Schrag. 2012. Patients' expectations about effects of chemotherapy for advanced cancer. *New England Journal of Medicine* 367 (17): 1616–1625. doi:10.1056/NEJMoa1204410.

Weimer, David L. 2010. Stakeholder governance of organ transplantation: A desirable model for inducing evidence-based medicine? *Regulation & Governance* 4 (3): 281–302. doi:10.1111/j.1748-5991.2010.01082.x.

Weinstein, M. C., and W. B. Stason. 1977. Foundations of cost-effectiveness analysis for health and medical practices. *New England Journal of Medicine* 296 (13): 716–721. doi:10.1056/NEJM197703312961304.

Weismüller, Tobias J., Panagiotis Fikatas, Jan Schmidt, Ana P. Barreiros, Gerd Otto, Susanne Beckebaum, Andreas Paul, et al. 2011. Multicentric evaluation of model for end-stage liver disease–based allocation and survival after liver transplantation in Germany—limitations of the "sickest first"-concept. *Transplant International* 24 (1): 91–99. doi:10.1111/j.1432-2277.2010.01161.x.

Wells, Shirley A. 2009. Health disparities in kidney transplantation: An equity analysis. *Journal of Health Disparities Research and Practice* 3 (2).

Werner, Rachel M., G. Caleb Alexander, Angela Fagerlin, and Peter A. Ubel. 2004. Lying to insurance companies: The desire to deceive among physicians and the public. *American Journal of Bioethics* 4 (4): 53–59. doi:10.1080/15265160490518566.

Williams, Alan. 1997. Intergenerational equity: An exploration of the "fair innings" argument. *Health Economics* 6 (2): 117–132. doi:10.1002/(sici)1099-1050(199703)6:2<117:aid-hec256>3.0.co;2-b.

Wilmot, Stephen, and Julie Ratcliffe. 2002. Principles of distributive justice used by members of the general public in the allocation of donor liver grafts for transplantation: A qualitative study. *Health Expectations* 5 (3): 199–209. doi:10.1046/j.1369-6513.2002.00176.x.

Witkowski, Terrence H. 1998. The American consumer home front during World War II. *Advances in Consumer Research (Association for Consumer Research)* 25 (1): 568–573.

Woolf, Steven. H., and Aron Laudan, eds. 2013. *U.S. Health in International Perspective: Shorter Lives, Poorer Health.* Washington, DC: National Academies Press.

Worchel, Stephen, Jerry Lee, and Akanbi Adewole. 1975. Effects of supply and demand on ratings of object value. *Journal of Personality and Social Psychology* 32 (5): 906–914. doi:10.1037/0022-3514.32.5.906.

Wynia, M. K., D. S. Cummins, J. B. VanGeest, and I. B. Wilson. 2000. Physician manipulation of reimbursement rules for patients: Between a rock and a hard place. *Journal of the American Medical Association* 283 (14): 1858–1865. doi:10.1001/jama.283.14.1858.

Yankelovich, D. 1995. The debate that wasn't: The public and the Clinton plan. *Health Affairs* 14 (1): 7–23. doi:10.1377/hlthaff.14.1.7.

Young, E. W. 1994. Rationing—missing ingredient in health care reform. *Western Journal of Medicine* 161 (1): 74–77.

Young, Pierre L., and LeighAnne Olsen. 2010. *The Healthcare Imperative: Lowering Costs and Improving Outcomes: Workshop Series Summary.* Washington, DC: National Academies Press.

Youngclaus, James A., Paul A. Koehler, Laurence J. Kotlikoff, and John M. Wiecha. 2013. Can medical students afford to choose primary care? An economic analysis of physician education debt repayment. *Academic Medicine* 88 (1): 16–25. doi:10.1097/ACM.0b013e318277a7df.

Zhang, B., A. A. Wright, H. A. Huskamp, et al. 2009. Health care costs in the last week of life: Associations with end-of-life conversations. *Archives of Internal Medicine* 169 (5): 480–488. doi:10.1001/archinternmed.2008.587.

Ziogas, Dimosthenis, and Dimitrios H. Roukos. 2009. Genetics and personal genomics for personalized breast cancer surgery: Progress and challenges in research and clinical practice. *Annals of Surgical Oncology* 16 (7): 1771–1782. doi:10.1245/s10434-009-0436-2.

Zweiniger-Bargielowska, Ina. 2000. *Austerity in Britain: Rationing, Controls and Consumption, 1939–1955.* Oxford: Oxford University Press.

Index

Basic Bioethics

Arthur Caplan, editor

Books Acquired under the Editorship of Glenn McGee and Arthur Caplan

Peter A. Ubel, *Pricing Life: Why It's Time for Health Care Rationing*

Mark G. Kuczewski and Ronald Polansky, eds., *Bioethics: Ancient Themes in Contemporary Issues*

Suzanne Holland, Karen Lebacqz, and Laurie Zoloth, eds., *The Human Embryonic Stem Cell Debate: Science, Ethics, and Public Policy*

Gita Sen, Asha George, and Piroska Östlin, eds., *Engendering International Health: The Challenge of Equity*

Carolyn McLeod, *Self-Trust and Reproductive Autonomy*

Lenny Moss, *What Genes Can't Do*

Jonathan D. Moreno, ed., *In the Wake of Terror: Medicine and Morality in a Time of Crisis*

Glenn McGee, ed., *Pragmatic Bioethics, second edition*

Timothy F. Murphy, *Case Studies in Biomedical Research Ethics*

Mark A. Rothstein, ed., *Genetics and Life Insurance: Medical Underwriting and Social Policy*

Kenneth A. Richman, *Ethics and the Metaphysics of Medicine: Reflections on Health and Beneficence*

David Lazer, ed., *DNA and the Criminal Justice System: The Technology of Justice*

Harold W. Baillie and Timothy K. Casey, eds., *Is Human Nature Obsolete? Genetics, Bioengineering, and the Future of the Human Condition*

Robert H. Blank and Janna C. Merrick, eds., *End-of-Life Decision Making: A Cross-National Study*

Norman L. Cantor, *Making Medical Decisions for the Profoundly Mentally Disabled*

Margrit Shildrick and Roxanne Mykitiuk, eds., *Ethics of the Body: Post-Conventional Challenges*

Alfred I. Tauber, *Patient Autonomy and the Ethics of Responsibility*

David H. Brendel, *Healing Psychiatry:Bridging the Science/Humanism Divide*

Jonathan Baron, *Against Bioethics*

Michael L. Gross, *Bioethics and Armed Conflict: Moral Dilemmas of Medicine and War*

Karen F. Greif and Jon F. Merz, *Current Controversies in the Biological Sciences: Case Studies of Policy Challenges from New Technologies*

Deborah Blizzard, *Looking Within: A Sociocultural Examination of Fetoscopy*

Ronald Cole-Turner, ed., *Design and Destiny: Jewish and Christian Perspectives on Human Germline Modification*

Holly Fernandez Lynch, *Conflicts of Conscience in Health Care: An Institutional Compromise*

Mark A. Bedau and Emily C. Parke, eds., *The Ethics of Protocells: Moral and Social Implications of Creating Life in the Laboratory*

Jonathan D. Moreno and Sam Berger, eds., *Progress in Bioethics: Science, Policy, and Politics*

Eric Racine, *Pragmatic Neuroethics: Improving Understanding and Treatment of the Mind-Brain*

Martha J. Farah, ed., *Neuroethics: An Introduction with Readings*

Jeremy R. Garrett, ed., *The Ethics of Animal Research: Exploring the Controversy*

Books Acquired under the Editorship of Arthur Caplan

Sheila Jasanoff, ed., *Reframing Rights: Bioconstitutionalism in the Genetic Age*

Christine Overall, *Why Have Children? The Ethical Debate*

Yechiel Michael Barilan, *Human Dignity, Human Rights, and Responsibility: The New Language of Global Bioethics and Bio-Law*

Tom Koch, *Thieves of Virtue: When Bioethics Stole Medicine*

Timothy F. Murphy, *Ethics, Sexual Orientation, and Choices about Children*

Daniel Callahan, *In Search of the Good: A Life in Bioethics*

Robert Blank, *Intervention in the Brain: Politics, Policy, and Ethics*

Gregory E. Kaebnick and Thomas H. Murray, eds., *Synthetic Biology and Morality: Artificial Life and the Bounds of Nature*

Dominic A. Sisti, Arthur L. Caplan, and Hila Rimon-Greenspan, eds., *Applied Ethics in Mental Healthcare: An Interdisciplinary Reader*

Barbara K. Redman, *Research Misconduct Policy in Biomedicine: Beyond the Bad-Apple Approach*

Russell Blackford, *Humanity Enhanced: Genetic Choice and the Challenge for Liberal Democracies*

Nicholas Agar, *Truly Human Enhancement: A Philosophical Defense of Limits*

Bruno Perreau, *The Politics of Adoption: Gender and the Making of French Citizenship*

I. Glenn Cohen and Holly Fernandez Lynch, eds., *The Future of Human Subjects Research Regulation*

Philip M. Rosoff *Rationing Is Not a Four-Letter Word: Setting Limits on Healthcare*

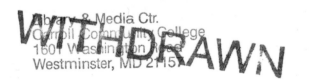